# BREAST INTENTIONS

# BREAST INTENTIONS

How women sabotage breastfeeding
for themselves and others

Allison Dixley

*Breast Intentions:*
*how women sabotage breastfeeding for themselves and others*

First published in the UK by Pinter & Martin Ltd 2014

ISBN 978-1-78066-215-2

Also available as an ebook

Edited by Susannah Marriott
Index by Helen Bilton

British Library Cataloguing-in-Publication Data
A catalogue record for this book is available from the British Library

Printed in Great Britain by TJ International Ltd, Padstow, Cornwall

This book has been printed on paper that is sourced and harvested from sustainable forests and is FSC accredited

Pinter & Martin Ltd
6 Effra Parade
London SW2 1PS

pinterandmartin.com

*To the doubters, the cynics and the apologists,*
*for keeping the fire in my belly to prove them wrong.*

# Contents

# Introduction

'Like tears, milk is functional;
but it also has a lot to say about us'.
Fiona Giles, 2003, *Fresh Milk: The Secret Life of Breasts*[1]

The issue of breastfeeding vs formula feeding is under the media lens now more than ever. The tabloid press prints stories of alpha mums who – shockingly – breastfeed well beyond the eruption of their baby's first tooth. Broadsheets roll out schizophrenic arguments that extol the virtues of breastfeeding one day and diminish them the next morning. Television shows invite 'breastfeeding experts' to lecture the public on the perils of jealous husbands and what to do when your milk 'runs out'. Academic journals pour over the physiological, societal and even philosophical aspects of a mother's infant-feeding choice. Google the phrase 'giving up breastfeeding' and the internet explodes.

Many women having babies today were formula-fed as infants. And the world around them is dominated by perceptions of infant feeding that can only be described as regressive: as a species, we have moved from the uncostly, self-regulating and environmentally friendly breast to the unquenchable industrial teat – a capitalist's dream. In essence, the human race has rejected a wholesome, biologically normal way of nourishing its young and replaced it with an illusion of normalcy built on the consumption of synthetic goods (well, okay, not the entire human race, just the so-called 'developed' sector of the species). In the UK for instance, only 23 percent of six-week-old babies are receiving the optimum nutrition for their species by being exclusively breastfed according to the NHS Infant Feeding Survey (2010). The rest have been removed – quite abruptly in evolutionary terms – from their mothers' breasts and are fed instead via plastic breast replicas containing the milk of an alien species. Consequently, the sight of a mother suckling her offspring – once common in our collective consciousness – is now foreign, and often framed as a vision of repulsion. The bottle has become culturally synonymous with infancy; it symbolises our exchange of natural excellence for man-made mediocrity.

Even if a mother can defy this culture, deciding to breastfeed does not ensure success. At six months of age, just 34 percent of British babies are receiving some breast milk, the same survey tells us; most of them, in conjunction with formula. Why? You might think research instruments like the NHS Infant Feeding Survey could tell us. But their focus is on breastfeeding initiation, and while their research is quantitatively useful, it provides little qualitative understanding of women's unique experiences and conflicts – of why they take up or give up nursing. The truth is that breastfeeding is not, for a woman, simply a means of getting nutrition into a baby; it is part of her psychosocial transition to motherhood.[2] The nebulous nature of breastfeeding makes answers to why it is so difficult elusive and strategies for change evasive.

The contemporary mother-child relationship is characterised by tension from the very start – some studies describe early motherhood as 'a moral minefield'.[3] Why the wartime language? Because infant feeding has become an increasingly probed domain; rightly so, considering its vital importance to the healthy development of babies. Exclusive breastfeeding for six months provides numerous protective factors for both baby and mother. Chief among these is protection against infant gastrointestinal infections, observed not only in developing but also industrialised countries. Adults who were breastfed as babies are slimmer. Children and adolescents who have been breastfed are smarter, even when confounding factors are accounted for.[4] Indeed, most women know breastfeeding is 'better' for baby,[5] and as the saying goes, 'When you *know* better, you *do* better'. So why aren't women translating their knowledge about breastfeeding's supremacy into action?

## SOCIETY VS WOMAN

Since most contemporary women fail at breastfeeding, society readily accepts the idea that mothers are in no way to blame for the failure – if everyone is failing, this must be down to the difficulty of the task. Such reactive explanations convey the idea that breastfeeding is something women have little control over. This idea is now so taken for granted that it pervades mainstream opinion and prevents us from obtaining a deeper and truer understanding of women's breastfeeding experience. Currently, women are expected to fail at breastfeeding; it fits in with our pro-formula society's self-fulfilling raison d'être. The argument that individual women aren't responsible for their failure to breastfeed appears plausible, comprehensible and consistent with the timeless and persistent world-view of women as the weaker sex. Some commentators (ironically defining themselves as feminists) are so bent on over-framing breastfeeding as a sociological issue, that they have taken to describing the biological process of lactation as a 'reproductive ritual' (notice the hyper-cultural word 'ritual', implying that nursing one's baby is some sort of man-made ceremony),[6] while others describe lactation as bordering on a patriarchal conspiracy, a misogynistic net in which to snare women, tethering them to their babies and thus to the often-ridiculed domestic sphere.[7]

Yet this response to a normal bodily function is needlessly reactive and awkwardly paternal. A blame-free breastfeeding culture infantilises women, framing them not as active agents capable of controlling their destiny and achieving their goals, but as passive wallflowers at the mercy of forces they are powerless to defy. I concede that social influences play a role in breastfeeding, but I believe they are merely a small part, not the whole, of a woman's breastfeeding journey. Culture may predict aspects of a woman's breastfeeding performance, but not its totality.

The aforementioned sociological stance on understanding breastfeeding – that the likelihood of success is as fickle as the flip of a coin – is clearly not working. The best conclusion sociological studies have come up with for mothers quitting breastfeeding is that the reasons 'lie buried deep within our culture'.[8] Even the statistics emerging from sociological studies are not clear-cut. In some, older mothers are found to have higher breastfeeding rates;[9] in others, younger women out-breastfeed their elders.[10] In some studies, women with relatively high levels of education have stronger breastfeeding performances;[11] in others, the lower Mum's educational attainment, the likelier she is to breastfeed,[12] while in more studies maternal education has zero bearing.[13] Sociological fetishes like age, education and socio-economic status paint only a cursory picture of what is really going on. To illustrate, consider this universal fact: when mothers are given the exact same opportunities and the exact same constraints, some will succeed while others fail. Why? Previous scholarly discourse hypothesising the 'cause' has tended to look to habits and customs. But one piece of the puzzle has so far evaded the discourse – *personality*.

A mother's personality has a direct effect on how she interprets and transforms her circumstances. Rather than adopt the same old defeatist and paternalistic 'society is to blame' rhetoric, in this book I will argue that a mother's responses to breastfeeding are acutely idiosyncratic. Until now, personality has been neglected and downplayed in the infant-feeding debate. Neglected because its varied nature makes personality difficult to study; downplayed because looking at personality arouses uncomfortable thoughts and emotions that hinge on 'anti-collectivist' notions, such as personal responsibility and individual determinism. Mothers being responsible for their actions? Who'd a thunk it!

## AN INDIVIDUALISTIC APPROACH

I contend that all behaviour begins with a mother's personality and ripples outwards. These ripples often take the form of emotion. Maternal emotion is of pivotal importance to a mother's breastfeeding performance, acting as it does as an intermediary between her personality and the culture surrounding her. Yet the emotional world of women's interactions with regard to infant feeding remains largely unacknowledged – it represents a 'private' sphere, and private experiences are not easy to discern. Nevertheless, an awareness of the emotions that arise during the infant-feeding journey is pivotal if we are to understand mothers' behaviour, and thus make sense of the infant-feeding statistics. Why aren't mothers in contemporary society coping well with breastfeeding? This question has been hypothesised to death. Sociological theories[14] would have us believe the answer lies in factors beyond the mother's control – fetishism of the breast, formula-company advertising, vague notions of 'lack of support' and 'a disabling social environment' – in other words, we are led to believe that individual mothers are not responsible for the outcome of their attempts at breastfeeding. This assumption is defeatist and disempowering.

'Social support' is the buzzword of this apologetic era and dominates breastfeeding discourse. Yet social support is a broad umbrella term that can be conceptualised in so many different ways that it becomes redundant as a definition. Even so the term persists, hanging around like a fart trapped in an elevator. And, like a fart, the 'support' rhetoric functions as a comforting if elusive scapegoat, nifty at deflecting attention from other salient issues – issues I will cover in this book.

On the occasions that attention drifts away from the support rhetoric, it stagnates on the outcomes of breastfeeding failure rather than on how that failure came about. Restricting dialogue to breastfeeding outcomes rather than processes reflects our preoccupation with a medical model of health. The medical model paints women as passive; indeed, the existence of the medical model relies on it. The model assumes that an expert 'professional' (health practitioner or formula company) is serving an inexpert mother, and thus depends on a hierarchical relationship based on often-biased knowledge gained from textbooks. It focuses on atomised mothers and babies, places them in a clinical setting and separates them from their personal 'cognitions': their thoughts, their emotions, their dreams and their nightmares. By religiously adhering to this model, we neglect part of the story – a huge part, an essential part – women's voices.

In defiance, this book adopts a radically different approach, looking at the topic of breastfeeding through the lens of the individual. It aims to unpack the murky depths of a mother's emotional life and to reveal the complex, often conflict-ridden reality it obscures. The ways in which mothers interact with one another are fascinating. As we look at them closely through the chapters of this book, we will see a peculiar mixture of behaviour, involving intersecting agendas and a creative flair for improvisation. Mothers' interactions reveal how clever and discerning they sometimes are, yet how biased and simple-minded they can also be. For too long we have been living in the dark, not understanding the deeper network of a mother's psychosocial life – the way her thought processes interact with her social environment and entwine with those of other mothers. It is imperative that we explore the underbelly of these relationships if we are to fully understand how breastfeeding lives and breathes – or more likely, is choked.

This book is provocative precisely because it focuses on the issues most relevant to the way mothers live and interact with each other. The decision to breastfeed or formula feed – whether from day 1 or day 21 – does not occur in an emotional and cognitive vacuum, and therefore should not be discussed in one either. We experience our choices through our emotions, and it is our emotions that give our choices meaning. In fact, our emotions are inseparable from our engagement with others, which begs the question why the support rhetoric has largely neglected them.

The philosopher Nietzsche warned that we are most clueless about what is closest to us. Our emotions are our most private, most intimate experiences. In this book I move away from the 'cold' analysis of statistics and the medical model and instead examine the effects of a mother's emotions on her judgement, choice and conduct. Emotions drive our behaviour, yet we have a relatively ignorant understanding of them. If we want more women to choose breastfeeding in the 'real world', then we need to understand more about 'real women' – that is, women influenced by emotion. This book explores how mothers relate and respond to each other, how they understand themselves, and how they manipulate both themselves and others. The chapters examine, in turn, the most common emotions emerging from mothers' experience of breastfeeding, from guilt through to sabotage. It reveals how emotions affect a woman's concept of herself as a mother and the substantial impact they have on the dynamics of her interpersonal relationships.

*Breast Intentions* brings together various fields and disciplines, including psychology, biology, philosophy, anthropology, sociology and even economics to produce a new understanding of how women cultivate breastfeeding 'success' or 'failure' in their everyday lives. I have no intention of competing with any text already in print; rather, my goal is to create a dialogue I feel has not been available until now.

A word of warning: the ground covered is largely depressing. It also has the potential to be threatening, striking a chord of recognition in the reader that may trigger feelings of shame, embarrassment or unease. This book is about untruth, about deception and about lies, interior and ulterior. It lifts the veil on the way women pathologise their relationships in the quintessentially strategic arena of motherhood – where self-interest and manipulation reign supreme. As you plough through these chapters, your instinct will be to think, 'How shocking! You'd never catch me behaving like that!' Yet, many of the behaviours explored in this book do not involve conscious awareness or deliberate planning. For this reason, I cite academic studies to support my assertions. Many of these studies are the seedlings of long-established theories, subsequently tried and tested by exhaustive empirical research. In such cases, I aim to cite the founder of the theory. So for instance, when I discuss the psychological concept of 'the ego' I cite its creator, Sigmund Freud. Although some of these references are decades old, they are still valid, and some represent monumental breakthroughs in our understanding of human behaviour.

I'll say it again: in *Breast Intentions* you may read things you would prefer not to. Indeed, there is a darker, more malignant side to the breast vs formula debate, particularly concerning women's relationships with each other. This book exposes the unforgiving and angry constituents of the maternal character, revealing a mother's capacity to deprave as well as to nurture.

In exploring the mechanics involved in deception, guilt, envy, contempt, defensiveness and sabotage, the book penetrates emotions that often feel too ugly or too unacceptable to talk about, particularly in such a feminine domain. Yet this dark and opaque side of motherhood is one we leave untreated at our peril.

In the infant-feeding context, the issue of corruption has typically been regarded by scholars and social commentators as an exclusively commercial phenomenon occurring between big business on the one hand and consumers on the other.[15] This approach is, of course, valid. It holds an important (albeit partial) key to the analysis of widespread breastfeeding failure – but it makes up only one strand of a far more complicated story. Focusing solely on the marketing of breast-milk substitutes – with the well-meaning intention of solving the breastfeeding drought – neglects a fundamental truth: corporate interests don't operate in a vacuum. Until the demand is examined and addressed, there's no point in fighting the supply; it's an inadequate and wasteful endeavour. Our over-occupation (indeed preoccupation) with the macro reality of the infant-feeding debate overlooks the micro reality of what's going on at grass-roots level, between mothers themselves. As my good friend James Akre, founder, chairman and CEO of the International Breastfeeding Support Collective and member of the Scientific Advisory Committee La Leche League France, has justly said:

'A prescription for change in feeding behaviour that focuses primarily on commercial interests and is filtered through a regulatory prism is doomed to failure. The buying public is as responsible for creating, accepting and maintaining an artificial child-feeding status quo as are formula manufacturers themselves'.[16]

Indeed, it is women's behaviour that needs to change rather than the so-called higher political or public-health authorities advising them. Commercial interests have long understood this reality: since women consumers decide, their objective is to convince women consumers. The process of grass-roots change begins with a deep understanding of what is going on in the lives of women and mothers that makes their attitude so incompatible with breastfeeding. In taking an individualistic approach to the infant-feeding debate, this book focuses on empowerment. Rather than being at the mercy of their environment, in this book mothers are shown (through phenomenological insight) engaged in the rational considerations that govern their infant-feeding choices. As such, these choices are open to mothers' control. *Breast Intentions* argues that while 'society' provides the backdrop for mothers' breastfeeding journeys and can structure the range of opportunities available, it is the mothers themselves who exploit or fail to exploit the opportunities available. Some researchers have given, at best, tentative acknowledgment of these murky waters, declaring that, 'The process is much more complex than just women with positive experiences and conditions tend to breastfeed, whereas those less fortunate do not'.[17]

This book shows that mothers are not merely passive passengers on their breastfeeding journey, but quite active in picking out the route. A mother's behaviour is determined by her intentions – her explicit plans or motivation regarding when to quit breastfeeding, and indeed, whether to begin in the first place. As we see in the first chapter, a mother's motivation to breastfeed mostly, if not entirely, reflects her personal attitudes: the extent to which she perceives breastfeeding as desirable or favourable. In fact, intention is such a strong indicator of whether a woman will start to breastfeed and continue to nurse that it *transgresses* sociological factors such as education, age and that elusive holy grail of apologist rhetoric, 'social support'.[18]

## A CAVEAT ABOUT TERMINOLOGY

I use the terms 'breastfeeding success' and 'breastfeeding failure' not to be provocatively dichotomous, but because these are terms commonly used by women – indeed, they overwhelm their discussions of breastfeeding.[19] Yet success and failure are tricky to define. These are dynamic labels, deeply subjective and forever morphing, depending on which theoretical lens is used to view them and the era in which they are used.[20] To one woman, breastfeeding for two months is a noteworthy success, whereas to another it is an embarrassing failure. This subjectivity forms the bare bones of a mother's perception of her reality – from which can spring guilt, pride or apathy. For my purposes, I use 'failure' in a fluid sense, to refer to a performance that falls below a certain standard, resulting in dissatisfaction. Said dissatisfaction and said standard may belong to an internal source (the mother herself), an external source (the media, health professionals, organisations) or indeed both, depending on the context.

## WHO IS THIS BOOK FOR?

Besides the obvious answer – anyone with an interest in breastfeeding – *Breast Intentions* may be of particular use to:

- Mothers, whether exclusive breastfeeders, veteran formula feeders or someone somewhere in between.
- Family members, immediate, extended or estranged.
- All those involved in counselling mothers.
- Psychologists and professionals employed in preserving the mental health of women.
- Policy-makers, particularly those with an interest in health-promotion and maternal and infant welfare.
- Other social architects, including feminists and other activists, commercial regulators, academics and the media.

I recommend that you read the book in chronological order, starting with the first chapter, Deception. This beefy chapter lays the foundations for what follows. Deception begins at the very start of a woman's breastfeeding journey and colours her entire narrative. The subsequent chapters – Guilt, Excuses, Envy, Contempt, Defensiveness and Sabotage – mirror a mother's emotions as they flow in this largely linear fashion. This cycle becomes self-affirming. It begins with, and is facilitated by, the mother herself.

# 1

# DECEPTION

'Choice requires us to think more deeply about who we are, both within ourselves and in the eyes of others'.

Sheena Iyengar, 2010, *The Art of Choosing*[21]

'Choice', the buzzword of our neoliberal era. The rhetoric of choice is becoming increasingly deafening in discussions about parenting – hardly surprising when, at its core, good parenting is framed as making prudent choices. As long as nothing forces us to act in a certain way, our parenting behaviour (and therefore our children) is a manifestation of our choices. Through our choices we construct a parenting legacy for which we are sole author. No pressure then.

Choice means that women, and mothers in particular, have become progressively liberated – at a price. We can choose to work inside the home or outside, vaccinate or not vaccinate, babywear or pram push, spoon wean or go baby-led. However we now have to suffer the backlash of accountability that follows the thrill of an overflowing catalogue of options. The choices a mother makes – for instance whether to breastfeed or formula feed – carry social meanings that affect the impressions others form of her, the way they treat her and the way she views herself. Choice in infant feeding is a paradoxical predicament from which mothers can never escape – it's like being trapped in a car with the uncle you love so much, but who had chicken balti for lunch and just let out a whopper. Choice is simultaneously appealing and burdening in equal measure. Put crudely, a mother has no choice about the fact that she has choice. Since formula milk became mainstream, mothers *have had to* choose, and be held accountable. As the locus of power falls upon the mother, the question of who she is – what her goals and motivations are – moves centre stage. Choosing to breast or formula feed is not only a private activity, it is a social one. It necessitates a level of self-scrutiny that is both confusing and menacing. Mothers have to confront difficult personal questions, requiring them to balance competing interests and construct complex hierarchies of priority. It is chronically overwhelming. I'm tired just telling you about it.

## THE FALLACY OF CHOICE

In the context of infant feeding, the over-esteemed, almost sacred commodity of choice is a tragic fallacy: a big fat fuck-you to mothers. For those in the middle of their breastfeeding journey, the road is rocky. To *choose* to continue breastfeeding or to switch to formula requires mothers to compare options – and in order to do this, they must determine the value of each option. To put it bluntly: the extent to which breastfeeding difficulties influence a mother's decision to switch to formula depends on the focus of her attention. Convenience or consummation? Immediate release or delayed gratification? Maternal well-being or infant welfare? To put it even more bluntly: how 'mum enough' is she? The task is both cognitively and morally challenging. At what point do present suffering and anticipated future suffering appreciate so much that formula seems preferable? Or how much hope – calculated as the probability of overcoming present challenges – must a mother accumulate before deciding to continue breastfeeding? Does a mother factor in emotional stress, financial pressures and the effects on other family members when making her choice, or does she put this child's needs ahead of everything else? Decisions, decisions....

Essentially, choice requires mothers to fix a price on something that's priceless – a bit like Wall Street bankers. And just like those guys, Mum doesn't have a clue what she's doing. What I'm saying is that mothers often pay a mental and emotional tax for their freedom of choice. By virtue of biology, they are forced into stressful judgements – stressful precisely because we tend not to assign comparative values to things we feel emotionally connected to. Know what I mean? Try putting a price on your husband's left testicle. You can't do it. Yet pricing up our valuables is precisely what the infant-feeding decision demands: a mother must assign a measurable, fixed value to her baby. There is so much for her to consider, so much to bear responsibility for, it's no surprise that sometimes mothers long for an easier path. To take another quote from Sheena Iyengar's book *The Art of Choosing*, 'To face our future equipped only with the complicated tool of choice scares us as much as it excites us'. Choice is that dry-clean-only dress that flatters you, but is a bugger to maintain. Choice brings the burden of gathering information; it places the onus on mothers to identify, select and implement the 'correct' choice – and it puts them at risk of feeling guilt and a sense of blame if they make the 'wrong' choice. Even if no one explicitly confronts a mum demanding that she justify her choices, she will continually be asked to do so symbolically. For instance, in the cash she hands over in exchange for the powder and paraphernalia necessitated by her choice to formula feed. Or the breast she exposes in public as she latches on her babe. A mother's everyday behaviour is a re-enactment of her choices. The heat is on.

## CAN WE PREDICT BREASTFEEDING FAILURE?

Here's a common misconception embraced by exponents of the rhetoric of choice.[22] To successfully breastfeed, a mother must:

1. Possess functioning breasts.
2. Have an intention to breastfeed.
3. Exert effort in the direction specified by the intention.

Sounds entirely plausible. How can we argue with such a logical statement? Yet breastfeeding data tell a different story. While NHS figures proudly flaunt that 81 percent of mothers initiate breastfeeding at birth, the tail feathers of the strutting health service peacock wilt remarkably fast. By three months, the number of mothers breastfeeding exclusively is a mere 17 percent, and at four months it's a pitiful 12 percent. Exclusive breastfeeding at six months is a quite frankly shameful one percent.[23] So, while the Breast is Best message is getting through to new mothers,[24] simply knowing the 'best' choice doesn't mean a mother can bring herself to stick with it. While eight out of ten mums intend to breastfeed, their feeding plans are far from static. Their reasons for starting to breastfeed appear to be very different to their subsequent reasons for maintaining it – or not. To help us understand why mothers are not carrying through their original intentions, we must first pinpoint the moment when the proverbial tits go up.

Fortunately, academics have provided the tools to do just that. Psychology boffins created a nifty theoretical device called the Transtheoretical Model of Behaviour Change. The people responsible – researchers Dr James Prochaska and Dr Carlo DiClemente[25] – identified several stages that typically occur when an individual undergoes 'a change in lifestyle', which breastfeeding certainly is. These stages can vary in duration depending on the individual. The model is cyclical, in that someone can start at any point in the circle and also drop out or relapse at any stage. She can also go from one stage to the next and back again without moving to any further stage in the model.

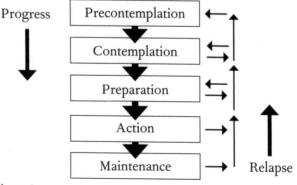

*Figure 1*

To help people understand what they were on about, Prochaska and DiClemente used smoking cessation as the theme when they conceived the model.[26] I'll use breastfeeding to illustrate it:

*Stage 1: Precontemplation* ('I won't')
At this stage, a mother does not intend to breastfeed. She may be unaware of the superiority of breastfeeding, or if she is aware, typically underestimates the pros while overestimating the cons.

*Stage 2: Contemplation* ('I might')
The mother is unsure about whether to breastfeed. Whether conscious of it or not, she makes a 'decisional balance sheet' of comparative potential gains and losses.[27] Though mothers in the contemplation stage are usually now more aware of the pros of breastfeeding, they perceive the cons as about equal to their pros, leading to ambivalence.

*Stage 3: Preparation* ('I will')
Here, the mother has decided to breastfeed and has taken steps towards some kind of action (telling family and friends about her intention, buying nursing bras, attending antenatal breastfeeding classes and so on).

*Stage 4: Action* ('I am')
Woot! The mother has initiated breastfeeding and is attempting to get it established. She needs to work hard to keep moving ahead while fighting urges to quit. The formula industry love to get a handle on mothers in this stage.

*Stage 5a: Maintenance* ('I have')
Now the mother has fully established breastfeeding and has a firm commitment to it. However she may become complacent and may not be aware of situations that may tempt her to quit – particularly stressful situations. Ouch! We'll look at those shortly.

*Stage 5b: Relapse*
Oh dear. The mother has ceased breastfeeding and returned to the Contemplation or Precontemplation stage. This can occur at any stage in the model.[28]

Okay, so providing a mother intends to breastfeed and makes it to the Action stage, why is she then highly likely to jump ship within a few measly weeks? She made it through Stages 1–4 just to walk the plank? The fancy-pants Transtheoretical Model of Behaviour Change doesn't help us figure out why that happens. It would appear that mothers reach a sort of breaking point that no one understands. In 2011, the *British Medical Journal* carried out a series of interviews with women and their families in two health boards in Scotland. The process identified 'pivotal points where families perceive that the only solution that will restore family well-being is to stop breast feeding or introduce solids'.[29] I argue that deciphering this conundrum need not involve copious epidemiological head-scratching. Nope, in fact, it's as simple as A, B, C….

## THE ABC OF BREASTFEEDING FIDELITY

Sorry, here's another theoretical model, but stay with me, because this bad boy is one I have devised myself – and it's a much simpler, three-factor framework.[30] My framework[31] gives a nod to the cultural context of women's lives, but is not engulfed by it. Here's the skinny: a mother's breastfeeding fidelity – and thus outcome – can be determined by looking at just three factors, which we'll investigate in turn through this very long chapter:

A: *Attitude*
Her personal attitude regarding breastfeeding.

B: *Belief*
What she believes her friends and family think about her breastfeeding.

C: *Control*
Her perceived control over breastfeeding.

## ATTITUDE

### 'Inconvenient', 'embarrassing', 'cumbersome', 'restrictive', 'primitive', 'ugly', 'unpleasant'

No, I'm not going off on a rant about my in-laws, rather, these are just some of the words mothers have used to describe breastfeeding.[32] Note that each word shares one salient point – they are focused on the mother. They reflect mother-oriented reasons for not breastfeeding. For 'self-focused' women (those for whom self-gratification is a key behavioral incentive), the mother-orientated benefits of breastfeeding can be turned around. For instance, while breastfeeding is widely recognised as an unparalleled opportunity for bonding, self-focused mums see this as negative, believing that bonding will make it more difficult for them to leave their babies with others, meaning their lives become more difficult.[33] This behavioural approach to breastfeeding is so important that my A B C of Breastfeeding Fidelity begins with A for Attitude.

Attitude refers to a mother's overall evaluation of breastfeeding. It comprises two interacting components: a mother's beliefs about the benefits of breastfeeding – or the consequences of not breastfeeding – and her corresponding positive or negative judgements of those beliefs.

Research has demonstrated that a mother's attitude is a good predictor of breastfeeding behaviour.[34] I know, no shit! Attitude regulates behavior: who knew? Put even more simply: we do things that give us satisfaction and refrain from doing things that make us feel dissatisfied. So we make judgements and decisions by first consulting our attitude. Sometimes mothers delude themselves into thinking that they made a rational decision – weighing all the pros and cons of various alternatives – when in fact their choice was determined by little more than their simple likes or dislikes, in the same way we choose the jobs we 'like' and buy houses we find 'attractive', then justify these choices. In other words, 'intention to perform a behaviour is mainly motivated by the desire to carry out the behavior'.[35] Psychologists call this 'the affect heuristic'.[36] In psychology, 'affect' refers to the experience of *emotion.* Our emotional attitude drives our beliefs about such factors as benefits and risks. If a mother dislikes breastfeeding from the get-go, she will probably believe its risks are high and benefits negligible. So to use a few common examples, she sees the health benefits as outweighed by the 'risk' of not knowing how much milk baby has consumed, the 'risk' of having sore nipples, the 'risk' of having to spend copious amounts of time with baby, and the 'risk' of marital disharmony because one's husband is given carte blanche to shirk his obligations in the feeding department. Mothers' attitudes towards breastfeeding come before – and direct – their judgements about its risks and benefits. The impact of this attitude ebbs and flows according to how far breastfeeding evokes images that mothers tag with positive or negative emotions.

And yes, I'm suggesting what you think I'm suggesting: some women (perhaps more than we care to imagine) don't quit breastfeeding as reluctantly as they would have you believe; rather, they have an implicit desire – an attitude – to quit. They then go through a process of mental gymnastics, applying all kinds of strategies to manipulate events to this end. That way, they can quit, but at the same time keep up the appearance – to themselves and others – that they were victims of circumstance.[37] Over the following pages, I will discuss the deceptive mechanisms at play.

### Personality

First up: personality. Most often, a mother's social environment is dubbed the architect of her breastfeeding outcome. Yet a handful of studies have looked at how a mother's personality rather than social environment impacts upon whether she breastfeeds or not. Many of the results of these studies are self-explanatory, for instance mothers with more anxious personalities are less likely to breastfeed[38] and high anxiety is associated with shorter breastfeeding duration than low levels of anxiety.[39]

However one rogue study has gone above and beyond the call of duty in deciphering the link between parental attitude and parental behaviour. Dr Belsky[40] designed an influential model to predict and explain individual differences in parenting. This model is one of the few to recognise maternal character traits as an implicit determiner of parenting style. Indeed, of the three 'determinants' of parenting recognised by the model – caregiver characteristics, child characteristics and contextual factors – the personality of the parent was deemed the most crucial component. So, if one of the three components remains healthy while the others fail, breastfeeding is more likely to be successful if that component is the personality of the parent. As an example, mothers who struggle to regulate their emotions have a harder time breastfeeding, due in part to the frequent intimate contact required in nursing an infant. Many of these mums respond to infant crying with an over-reaction of self-focused anxiety and irritation or inappropriate laxness.[41] Such responses are incompatible with the dyadic (the term means two people as one) harmony required for successful breastfeeding. Successful breastfeeding asks a mother to perform a purposeful and non-impulsive behavior – breastfeeding – often in the face of negative emotions, such as stress, pain or exhaustion.[42] Herein lies an uncomfortable fact: mothers cannot respond appropriately to their infants if they are unable to respond appropriately to their own emotions.[43]

To see another fascinating facet of parental personality illustrated, feast your eyes on the following pair of contrasting quotes:

'The big contradiction is that breastfeeding is so natural, and yet so completely unintuitive. What's really natural is for women to have a love-hate relationship with it'.

Florence Williams, 2012,
*Breasts: A Natural and Unnatural History*[44]

'Disadvantages to breastfeeding are those factors perceived by the mother as an inconvenience to her because there are no disadvantages for the normal infant'.

Ruth Lawrence, 2009,
*Breastfeeding: A Guide for the Medical Professional*[45]

Notice the dichotomy? One is parent-orientated and the other is infant-orientated. The degree to which a parent is self-orientated or infant-orientated is an important facet of personality. Yup, I'm talking about the elephant in the Mommy Wars arena: selfishness. Egocentrism, narcissism, self-absorption – call it what you like. A mother's emotional responses to her baby, for instance to him crying, can range from empathy (an infant-orientated reaction) to irritation (a self-focused indulgence).[46] Empathy focuses on and prioritises infant well-being, while irritation focuses on and prioritises adult sentiment. Mothers with a more empathic response to their babies will be more willing to breastfeed when their baby is crying, fuelled by a desire to help the baby, which they prioritise above perceived personal inconvenience.[47] They may also be better able to discern their baby's hunger cues.[48] Another infant-orientated virtue is patience: patience to help baby latch properly, patience while baby finishes his often-long feeds, patience to 'get your body back' (presumably from the baby who has stolen it).

### Learning to Choose, Choosing to Learn

With her personality as her flashlight, a mother sets off on an epic journey. The mission normally begins in pregnancy, when the issue of infant feeding is considered in earnest for the first time. Mothers have a choice in the infant-feeding dilemma: breast milk (home-grown or donated), formula milk (homemade or purchased) or a combination. Remember, mothers have no choice about having a choice – they must make a decision. In the hope of reducing the risk of making an erroneous decision, a mother will typically go through three key processes:[49]

1. She acquires information.
2. She searches through the information.
3. She combines the information to make a judgement.

The whole three-stage process is uniquely personal to her and specific to the context of her life.

Let's begin with the first process, acquiring the information about infant feeding: where does the mother look? Her strategy of what information to seek (and how much) ultimately depends on the relative weight she places on the goal – making an accurate infant-feeding decision – versus saving effort. With finite time and resources, most mothers have to select a handful of avenues of enquiry. Popular go-to sources of infant-feeding info for the time-strapped woman include books (okay), magazines (uh-oh), television documentaries (oh my), the internet (oh dear), friends (oh no), family (God no) and health professionals (God help us).[50]

Once mum has ascertained her sources, how does she choose what areas of infant feeding to research, and in what order? Social scientists have studied exposure to information prior to making a choice and have found evidence of – gasp – selective exposure to information. So, for instance, a mother who likes the idea of rapid infant weight gain might choose to focus on this when comparing breast milk or formula, whereas a mother fixated on sleep might choose to look at that area. Often the process is a conscious trade-off between the *accuracy* of the information and the *effort* involved in acquiring it.[51] 'Experts', such as midwives and GPs, are a common source of information, but studies show that decision-makers typically consult experts only after completing more than 75 percent of their own information search.[52] This is problematic – because the mother is not unbiased in her research efforts. She has a propensity to steer away from topics she is ignorant about,[53] while seeking out information that confirms her existing beliefs. If a mother has come to the conclusion that formula is just as good as breast milk, her belief is likely to be reinforced by a bias in the information she pays attention to. She will be less interested in information favouring breastfeeding than mothers uncertain about which method to choose.[54] She may, for instance, be drawn to formula-company literature or consult formula-feeding parents rather than a pro-breastfeeding pal.

We all have a tendency to give more weight to evidence that confirms our beliefs than to evidence challenging them; it's a quirk of human cognition known as 'confirmation bias'.[55] Often, it's a passive act, a form of wilful negligence: a mother simply fails to look for any information that could contradict her beliefs. But in order to do this, the mother must know enough to avoid it. For instance, a mum wanting to protect herself from information that highlights the risks of formula feeding knows to discard the midwife's pro-breastfeeding pamphlet and not ask too many questions. In a sense, she is both the giver and receiver of deception. Such inaction has obvious self-serving advantages: if a mother can manage to remain largely ignorant about the consequences of her choices, she can evade the pain that often accompanies being informed. As the prolific psychologist Abraham Maslow succinctly put it:

'Often it is better not to know, because if you *did* know, then you would have to act and stick your neck out'.[56]

So once Mum has acquired information (albeit through dodgy research methodology), how does she search through and process it? Step up Parent-Offspring Conflict Theory. I hope you have your hard-hat at the ready; it's about to get nasty.

### Parent-offspring Conflict Theory – aka Maternal Selfishness

A common argument from the pro-breastfeeding camp is that formula feeding does not make evolutionary sense. After all, breasts evolved to lactate and providing milk is their primary purpose. Sincere apologies to any 'lactivists' reading, but this argument is not entirely foolproof.

To explain this, we need to look at the cognitive process of decision-making more closely. Central to a mother's decision of whether to breast or formula feed are her expectations of what outcomes each choice would produce. Whether conscious of it or not, mothers decide to initiate, reject or terminate breastfeeding based on expected pay-offs.[57] They make tenuous mental lists of gains and losses for each feeding option.[58] However, the mother's personal attitude makes a big difference to how she sees and responds to various infant-feeding factors when she evaluates them, for instance, whether she labels some things as pros and others as cons. This seems fairly straightforward: if the mother wants and expects to get more sleep by formula feeding, she will focus on this perceived advantage when choosing to formula feed.

From an evolutionary perspective, a cost/benefit risk analysis seems reasonable. We can't fault women for doing it. Breastfeeding is intensive. It draws on finite pools of maternal time and energy. Think about the mum you know (and we all know at least one) who slathers herself in bio oil as soon as blue lines appear on that stick she just peed on. The mum who schedules her C-section around manicures, for whom the thought of a sleepless night triggers a rash. You know that mum? Well, you can't be that mum when you breastfeed. Frequent breastfeeding is the biological norm for babies thanks to their tiny stomachs and the ease with which breast milk is digested.[59] Breastfeeding takes up a lot of a mum's day (and night). Both the NHS and La Leche League – the go-to global organisation for breastfeeding – have instructed mothers to feed their babies 'at least 10–12 times in 24 hours', waking them if necessary.[60] Because it is all babies want to do in their early days, feeding dominates mother-baby interaction.[61] A new mother can expect to be feeding her baby every other hour around the clock, with feeds lasting up to an hour in length. And, after baby's seventeenth trip to the Milk Bar, not only are there no compliments for the chef, but he fails to clean up after himself and leaves no tip. This pattern of regular refuelling results in fragmented maternal sleep,[62] which, surprise, surprise, is a pet hate of many mothers.[63] The pleasure the mother anticipates deriving from breastfeeding's 'benefits' to her baby is overshadowed by the displeasure of the 'loss' to her, namely her bodily autonomy, sleep and the rest of it.

It gets worse. Research has consistently demonstrated that losses loom far larger in our minds than gains.[64] We are compelled to do whatever we can to avoid losing the things that are important to us. The mother attempting to breastfeed typically has several established 'valuables' that are important to her and which she would be loath to loose – her bodily autonomy, her belief in marital equity through shared division of chores, her consumer choices, her social life. The snag is that these values can, at times, be in conflict with the mechanics of breastfeeding. And when this happens, something has to give.

Either the mother reframes her values or does away with the conflicting agent – breastfeeding.[65]

So far, the list of losses related to breastfeeding is really stacking up – autonomy, sleep and sanity all get a bashing when one has to produce food for an infant who seems to eat more than a teenage boy with a weed habit. But what about the gains? The 'gains' of breastfeeding revolve around enabling the breastfed child to reach his or her genetic potential in terms of mental and physical health. However, typically in our culture, our dialogue frames these factors as 'benefits' rather than what they really are: the natural sequence of human biology. In a sense, there are no 'benefits' to breastfeeding; rather, breastfeeding is the biological norm for our species. Breastfed babies are – from a biological perspective – our species' neutral reference point, and formula-fed babies are deviations. This is important in decision-making terms because we humans tend to perceive gains or losses as relative to a neutral reference point.[66]

Now, here's where it *really* gets problematic for breastfeeding. Our culture takes evolution and shows it the finger: formula feeding is erroneously viewed as the neutral reference point and breastfeeding as a deviation. Breast milk is placed on a pedestal; it is seen as 'liquid gold'. Rather than appreciate the risks of formula, mothers consider the benefits of breast milk. When formula is framed in a neutral position like this, mothers do not acknowledge the risks involved in using it, and they do not comprehend a 'loss' to the baby. This is particularly troublesome in light of the fact that people are more averse to losses than they are attracted by corresponding gains. The true attractiveness of breastfeeding is diluted by the way we frame breastfeeding as a deviation. We are inclined to take whatever option requires least effort, or the path of least resistance. For most mothers, this is formula feeding. Richard Thaler and Cass Sustein explain the consequences of this inclination in their book, *Nudge: Improving Decisions About Health, Wealth and Happiness*:

'If, for a given choice, there is a default option – an option that one will obtain if the chooser does nothing – then we can expect a large number of people to end up with that option, whether or not it is good for them... These behavioural tendencies toward doing nothing will be reinforced if the default option comes with some implicit or explicit suggestion that it represents the normal course of action. Defaults are ubiquitous and powerful'.[67]

In our society, formula feeding is the default. Almost everyone does it. This leads decision-making women to think, 'If formula is the norm then that means if I formula-feed I will not fall outside the boundaries of normality and acceptability, then my fate will be like the fate of the majority'. Comforted by herd mentality, some mothers choose the bottle from birth. This choice is particularly self-protective in the breastfeeding context because those who want to breastfeed and try to breastfeed, but fail, paradoxically feel *more regret* than those who want to breastfeed but do not try. Rolf Dobelli described this irrational fallacy as, quite unremarkably, 'the fear of regret'.[68]

Alongside breastfeeding's cultural characterisation as 'deviant', the abstract invisibility of many of its benefits further fuels its downfall. Many of breastfeeding's pro-points are in the future, and their remoteness varies enormously (allergy protection and IQ actualisation for example), whereas almost all of formula's pro-points are immediate (ability to measure baby's intake and redistribution of feeding duties, for example). Unfortunately for breastfeeding, our judgement is clouded when choices and their consequences are separated in time. When the benefits seem so vivid but their tangibility so questionable, they are easy for mothers to cognitively minimise.[69] Is a mother consciously aware that her baby doesn't have a chronic disease? How readily does she visualise her baby without asthma, without diabetes? Indeed, one seldom thinks how one's life could suck more. The threat of breast cancer several decades from now or the obese teen seem so far removed from today's priorities as to be irrelevant. In other words, it is hard for mums to envisage a profit to offset the maternal cost. For the breastfeeding mother, the pleasure to be derived from seeing her child reach his or her potential in intelligence and health is at least a decade off, whereas the disruption to her bodily autonomy is immediate.

The behavior of the formula-feeding mother has rewarding effects immediately, but longer term – and thus more remote – harmful effects on health and wealth.[70]

So where does this leave our decision-making mum? In evolutionary terms, she is wise to commit to the burden of breastfeeding 'only when prospects for success are reasonable and only to a degree that optimizes lifetime reproductive success'.[71] According to Darwin and friends, parents strive to raise healthy offspring who survive to reproduce at a minimal cost.[72] The alternative to breastfeeding – formula – fits this bill. It enables a baby to 'survive' and the cost (in energy, if not economics) is minimal. Formula frees mothers to spread their energies across a spectrum of family members, rather than localising it upon one tiny, loud, projectile-pooping machine.[73] Succumbing to the allure of formula feeding is therefore – contrary to popular belief – evolutionarily sound. Mothers and babies are, after all, participants in a broader family unit.[74] The infant-feeding decision is a choice between prospects and gambles.

Numerous studies have validated the theory that the decision to quit breastfeeding hinges on a mother's subjective cost/benefit calculation. Anthropologists Dr Kristen Tully, and my very own PhD supervisor Professor Helen Ball[75] explored the mindset of breastfeeding quitters. First, they ascertained a theoretical time of maximum 'profit' – when the difference between the baby's benefit and the maternal cost is greatest and most favourable. In other words, when Mum is able to provide the greatest benefit to her baby at the lowest cost to herself. For many mothers, this happens at around the one-week mark, when Mum's milk has come in and settled down and her baby is typically piling on the pounds.[75b] At this point, she is feeling relatively calm and pleased with herself. Consequently, it's easiest to maintain breastfeeding during this window, which normally lasts but a few short weeks. Later on, breastfeeding challenges pop up.[76] Infant weight gain may stall, Mum may be venturing outside the home more and feeling embarrassed nursing in public, a growth spurt will kick in leading to marathon cluster feeds, and exhaustion hits a new level. At this point, when Mum perceives the cost/

benefit analysis to be turning against her, she is vulnerable to relapse. Suddenly, formula is looking like her Diet Coke bloke. Her immediate desires and priorities (the wish for more sleep and more bodily liberty, for instance) seem so different from – and more compelling than – her baby's theoretical long-term health outcomes. In the words of Professors Tully and Ball, at this point, she 'subconsciously resists investment' because she deems the additional time and effort is not worth what she sees as a modest additional benefit to her baby. Many things contribute to this steep curve in mothers' perceptions of the losses of breastfeeding. Let's take a brief gander at these factors:

### The Burden of Breastfeeding

'For a piece of finely tuned evolutionary machinery, mine often malfunctioned. They became objects of betrayal, frustration, self-doubt, and excruciating pain'.

Florence Williams, 2012,
*Breasts: A Natural and Unnatural History*[77]

The new or expectant mother does not have to look hard to discover that most people find breastfeeding difficult. The evidence is all around her. Indeed, breastfeeding – even in circumstances when it turns out to be relatively-speaking 'easy' – is labour-intensive and time-consuming. The majority of mothers, even the most crunchy and committed, concede that breastfeeding entails a loss of independence, of difficulty going anywhere *sans* babe because only mum has the requisite equipment. Studies speak in weighty terms of 'The isolation and confinement that result from having sole responsibility for nourishing a child while not feeling confident doing so publicly'[78] and of 'solitary confinement in the home'.[79]

Then there's the perceived indignity. In a culture where women are expected to look and feel as fresh as a daisy, the messy and often animalistic nature of breastfeeding can be hard to handle. Breasts swell and then have the nerve to leak without written warning; milk patches appear on clothing at inopportune moments; the cry of random infants triggers the milk-ejection reflex; and at the end of a long day, a pool of sweat and milk is one's bedfellow. When lost adrift a sea of breast pads, soggy bras and plastic pump parts, that 'livestock feeling' is hard to evade, even for the staunchest lactivist.

But is all this strife really breastfeeding's fault? Or is it simply part of navigating the unfamiliar terrain of being responsible for another human? Getting to grips with motherhood takes time, but many women seem to have very unrealistic expectations of what motherhood entails. This is, in part, because we live in a society that romanticises infancy and parenthood on one hand, while bowing to egotism on the other.[80] Many health professionals and parenting books exacerbate this widespread misunderstanding by maintaining that babies should feed only four hourly or be sleeping through the night by X weeks. Consequently, normal breastfeeding behaviour isn't explained to women and their expectations are skewed by generations of formula feeding.

Regretfully, as a result of this knowledge deficit, at the first sign of inconvenience or a potential problem, many mothers are apt to rashly and imprudently blame breastfeeding, rather than simply having a baby. Often, new mothers' feelings of being 'suffocated by breastfeeding'[81] is actually an indirect expression of shock aroused by new motherhood itself. The loss of freedom that accompanies having a baby is magnified by breastfeeding, and breastfeeding often takes the blame for a lot of things that aren't necessarily to do with feeding. No matter how a woman decides to feed her baby, the first few weeks require a monumental adjustment. Many expectant mothers cannot comprehend quite how much their baby will require of them around the clock, and how urgent the baby's needs will be.

And that's just the bog-standard everyday stuff. When serious challenges arrive, as they inevitably do for most mothers – mega-engorgement, blanched nipples, latching mishaps, the threat of low milk supply (real or imagined) – the charm of those lovely mummy-baby bonding moments promised by La Leche League pamphlets evaporates faster than steam off a chapped nipple. Suddenly, mothers describe wanting to regain a 'normal' body and a 'normal' routine, especially in relation to sleep.[82] They swiftly develop a drive to re-establish their identities as 'more than a mother'. Others feel that being a mother 'was never a major part of their identity'.[83] Funny that.

### *'I Had No Choice' – Feigned Reluctance to Quit*

A mother's breastfeeding outcome hinges on whether she can bear frustration and whether, indeed, she wants to. If she doesn't want to carry on, she faces a sticky situation: by holding the power to give immeasurable vitality to her baby, Mum is bound by immeasurable moral obligation. Therefore, to quit breastfeeding is to put oneself in moral danger. Quitting intentionally is viewed by others far more negatively than unintended quitting.[84] Mums who are less convinced about their desire to breastfeed are going to require some trickery, some invention, some deception if they are to convince *others* of their commitment, much less themselves. Deception is the cloak mothers don to mask weak resolve.

Such mothers presume a sense of omniscience – the capacity to know everything there is to know – about what they are fleeing from, partly powered by an inability to comprehend and endure delayed gratification. They believe – or at least want to believe – that breastfeeding will always be an unpleasant experience and so they had better quit now. These mothers make systematic errors by assuming that what they are feeling now will extend into the future.[85] They seek to evade frustration rather than working out ways to cope with it. Let's contrast this viewpoint with the view of satisfaction held by determined breastfeeding mothers, a feeling encompassing the sensations of pride and pleasure that reward those who persevere. Each mother, whether irresolute or determined, conjures up her own mental images of satisfaction to make her choices bearable, plausible and attractive. Each mother takes these predicted outcomes for granted. They are presumed just.

Mothers secretly intent on quitting give the illusion that they accept and support the Breast is Best message; however, subtle tweaks in their language and behaviour reveal their true ambivalence. Women may, for example, use 'disowning words' when they refer to breastfeeding's benefits by saying 'They say breast is best' rather than 'I believe…'.[86] These women may not see possible strategies to combat breastfeeding challenges because their perceptions are constrained by the determination to quit.[87] A pertinent example is advice-seeking: when facing difficulties, it is human nature to consult other people for advice, and more often than not people relish the opportunity to oblige. It is not uncommon for struggling breastfeeding mothers to have advice flung at them from every Tom, Dick and Harry. Now, let's say numerous people respond to the mother's plight by encouraging her to keep on breastfeeding. Then, eventually, the mother runs into someone who suggests she should quit. Logic would suggest heeding the advice of the majority rather than the single minority voice. However, for many mothers in the throes of quitting, the rogue suggestion to quit – the lifebuoy flung to them – is too tantalising an escape route and they abandon logic. The first suggestion to quit is taken as permission to quit, and Mum gladly, willingly buckles. The process of consulting various sources until one gives the desired advice allows a mother to justify the choice she really wanted to make – by tracing the roots of the decision to someone else. Slick.

If this someone else happens to be a health professional, even better! Many health professionals pick up on mothers' desperate desire to quit, and respond by indulging them. Otherwise sincere, they are forced to forsake their patients' – the babies' – well-being because their patients' parents are showing such a pitiful demand for it. Take midwives, for example. Many confess to functioning in a reactive way, prioritising the needs of the mother often at the expense of the child. They speak of picking up on a mother's 'signals',[88] and then concentrating on resolving concerns based on the mother's wishes, aiming to accommodate her without attempting to influence her with new knowledge.[89] In one study, midwives confessed to adjusting their breastfeeding support so that their primary source of information was the woman, rather than the baby.[90]

In a culture that prizes work, struggle and earnestness, all mothers need to do to alleviate the impact of their impending throwing in of the towel is to make it clear that they exerted great effort in their attempt to breastfeed. Citing numerous visits to health professionals is a great way to do this. Mothers can lament over their turmoil at 'having' to quit, listing assorted hurdles that have impeded them and the lengths they went in their attempt to resolve the issues. This process feeds into our cultural preoccupation with means to the exclusion of concern with ends. Picture the father turning to his son after his team loses a football match, 'At least you tried your best son; it's the taking part that counts'. In other words, as long as a mother is seen to have conscientiously tried breastfeeding, it matters less if she was successful or not. Success, when it matters, only has importance in terms of successful deception.

To be successful at deception, a mother's actions must not contradict and undermine her words. For instance, if she reluctantly switches to formula claiming 'insufficient milk' as her motive, whether or not she continues to breastfeed with the milk she has left, is a telling sign. Women with agenesis of mammary tissue (a *very rare* condition in which the breasts don't develop normally) are still able to breastfeed, with supplementation, for a year or longer – because some breast milk is far better than none at all.[91] So, when a mother cites insufficient milk yet doesn't attempt to mix feed, she holds up a red flag revealing her true desires: to be done with breastfeeding in the first place. Thus, a mother's desires and her commitment are irrevocably interwoven. For breastfeeding, this marriage begins even before a mother conceives her baby....

### 'I'll Try' – Famous Last Words

A woman's pre-birth commitment to breastfeeding is widely recognised as playing a central role not only in starting to breastfeed, but in how long she keeps it up. Mothers who are committed to breastfeeding before they are pregnant are more likely to breastfeed for longer than those who make the commitment during pregnancy.[92] Still, women who commit to breastfeed in pregnancy are more likely to continue breastfeeding at three months, compared with undecided mothers.[93] If Mum can pin a date on how long she will breastfeed for, all the better! In one study[94] the most important of all variables associated with longer breastfeeding duration was the mothers' anticipated length of breastfeeding – mothers who planned to breastfeed longer actually did so. It seems that when mothers achieve a level of 'confident commitment' before the birth of their baby, they are able to withstand lack of support and common challenges. However, without this element of 'confident commitment', a decision to breastfeed is likely to fall apart once it is challenged.[95]

Commitment is not a fate-massaging golden ticket, however. It can act simultaneously as a help and a hindrance. As a help, commitment leads towards success, channelling a mother's thought processes and actions in productive pro-breastfeeding directions. 'The more a mother commits herself 'to' breastfeed (as opposed to "try"), the more she is able to do so'.[96] Philosopher Bob Mandel[97] explains it with this eloquent analogy:

> 'It's like a tree. You plant it and nourish it. Over time its roots take hold. Storms and droughts test the will and purpose of the tree. Each time a test is passed, a sense of deepening conviction and greater permanence emerges'.

Commitment also defines a person, and in this case it can become a hindrance. The pledge to breastfeed hangs around a mother's neck, and it hangs heavy. No one else can own it in the same way. Subsequent success or failure is her burden to bear.

*True* commitment rests upon a mother's attitude. I say 'true' in italics, because in this context, truth is seldom disclosed. A mother keeps her true commitments locked in an internal dialogue with herself, and in that sense, the process is highly deceptive. When the topic of breastfeeding arises antenatally, rather than disclosing their true commitments and thus intentions, many mothers strategically opt for the purposively tentative one-liner 'I'll try'.

'I'll try' is an example of how the way in which we frame our intentions can create a self-fulfilling prophecy. As one of

America's most quoted writers, William Arthur Ward, said, 'If you can't imagine it you can't do it'. The first step towards being a successful breastfeeding mother is the ability to imagine – to see yourself as a successful breastfeeding mother. It sounds so simple, doesn't it? Yet so many mothers topple at this first hurdle.

Often, pregnant women fear (rightly so if their cultural role models are anything to go by) that their forthcoming breastfeeding actions could be construed as a poor performance. To dilute this fear, they attempt to lower both the internal (their own) and external (everyone else's) expectations of their forthcoming performance. A common caveat from the lips of the expectant mother is, 'I'll give breastfeeding a try'. By taking such a cautiously innocuous stance, the mother bags herself a double-whammy of social advantage: first, she gives the impression of being broad-minded, moderate and rational, and second, she retains maximal flexibility for later. The word 'try' is ambiguous. It props the door open for future reinterpretation and even abandonment. 'Try' is a self-deprecating, middle-of-the-road stance that mothers use to evade accountability.[98] It's safe territory, a proactive and strategic manipulation of the context so that others can only infer desired things about her personal qualities. By appearing to have no attitude, mothers who say 'try' evade the possibility of having what turns out to be the wrong attitude. They reset expectations so that later, when faced with the genuine act of breastfeeding, they can shift to either side of the fence and defend each side with some credibility, concomitantly avoiding any threat of appearing hypocritical. Indeed, it is difficult to suffer embarrassing failure when one is defending a moderate stance. Saying 'I'll try' thus limits a mother's personal risk and responsibility to manageable proportions. It's a win-win scenario for her. If the expected failure results, it can be discounted, with the difficulty of the task taking the responsibility. If a more positive result occurs and the mother succeeds at breastfeeding, she can claim she triumphed despite the difficulty of the task.

'I'll try' is so vague as to feasibly encompass a broad spectrum of behaviour, from steel-willed determination to half-arsed puffery. A telling indication of where a mother falls on this spectrum is whether she supplements her 'I'll try' speech with a few finely sculpted excuses for why breastfeeding might go wrong. This pregnant lady, for example, is so far at the latter end of the spectrum as to be hanging off the edge:

'I'm just dying to get my own body back and know that I can eat that and not worry about it or drink that and not worry about it.... It's always been at the back of my mind that I'll probably switch to bottle feeding'.[99]

Other common examples include, 'I might end up having a c-section', 'I might not produce any milk' and 'the baby might not 'take' to breastfeeding'. These 'anticipatory excuses' (as social psychology terms them) are a treasure trove for the non-committed mother to dip in and out of. If she can generate a plausible excuse in anticipation of her failure, this disclaimer or 'defence in hand' allows her to impart less effort than she would have without such prepared excuses. Sneaky. So sneaky in fact, that Professor Elizabeth Murphy of the University of Nottingham decided to get to the bottom of it.[100] She carried out longitudinal qualitative interviews examining how mothers account, in advance, for the possibility of breastfeeding failure. Her findings were astonishing: anticipatory excuses are so common in breastfeeding discourse that almost all the mothers in her study dabbled in it, regardless of socioeconomic background. But wait, there is more! Mothers who had offered anticipatory excuses for abandoning breastfeeding were much more likely to go on to abandon breastfeeding than those who did not. In fact, of the woman who had offered anticipatory excuses, one hundred percent – ONE HUNDRED PERCENT – had quit breastfeeding by 16 weeks.[101] Wow.

So, after a mother makes the decision to breastfeed, anticipatory excuses give her an escape route to countermand that decision. She fantasises, in advance, acceptable motives for quitting. And here we see the strange thing about quitting: its anticipation precedes its realisation. The mere acceptability of anticipatory excuses for quitting increases the probability of quitting.[102] Excuses that precede quitting make quitting possible, and even encourage quitting by making it more palatable – not only to a mother's external audience but also to her internal self, as Professor Murphy concluded at the end of her study:

'The anticipatory accounts which many of the women produced, represent a powerful means of "speaking back", not only to actual others who may question their behaviour, but also to the generalised other of their community and, hence, to self. In doing so, they may, literally, be making such untoward behaviour "thinkable" and, as a result, "do-able"'.[103]

A mother's reluctance to breastfeed lowers her motivational standard,[104] and poor motivation is a precursor of breastfeeding failure. The amazing ability of antenatal maternal dialogue to predict breastfeeding outcome supports the politically unpalatable truth that ATTITUDE determines breastfeeding success MUCH MORE THAN FATE.

Then, there's another deceptive game. Some pregnant ladies favour a slightly less moderate approach to anticipatory excuses, and soften the road to their anticipated poor breastfeeding performance by derogating breastfeeding itself. 'It's not that important' and 'I'll try but if I fail, it's not the end of the world, formula is just as good' are common assertions. The rationale is that if they can convince their audience that breastfeeding is not valuable, their level of performance becomes less important.

And mothers are not only seeking to convince an audience. Although the 'try' rhetorical safety net is cast publicly, it is even more often reassuringly affirmed in the privacy of a mother's own mind. And herein resides a not-too-subtle secret: she has 'weak self-efficiency beliefs' – she does not believe that she can actually breastfeed. This affects a mother's breastfeeding goals and aspirations. The weaker a mum perceives her 'self-efficiency', the lower the goals she sets for herself and the weaker her commitment to them.[105] A mother with low efficiency expects not to be able to breastfeed successfully, and her verbal warning paves the way for it. Later, when the time comes to breastfeed, mothers with 'low efficiency' are easily convinced of the futility of effort in the face of challenges and quickly give up trying.[106] A mum could soak up the Breast is Best message with the efficiency of an industrial-strength breast pad, but this will never trump a crippling void of self-efficiency.[107]

So where does low self-efficiency come from? To understand this, we need to look at two powerful human emotions: fear and hope.

## FEAR OF FAILURE VS HOPE OF SUCCESS

Here's a self-affirming fact: how a woman chooses to channel her emotional energy significantly predicts her breastfeeding outcome; specifically, whether she channels it into fearing breastfeeding failure, or whether she channels it into hoping for breastfeeding success. And before you poo-poo this as mere motivational rhetoric – like the cheesy quotes you find on mugs in gift shops – it's not. The distinction is genuine and hinges on our old friend: personality.

Psychoanalytical research has consistently shown that people with personalities that channel emotional energy into hoping for success prefer situations in which their own actions, rather than external factors, heavily influence the outcome. In other words, people who hope for success prefer situations in which they are in the driving seat. Great, because that's exactly where breastfeeding puts you.

People with a high fear of failure, on the other hand, do not have this preference, and indeed, may even show a reverse tendency, preferring situations where external dynamics are the deciding factor.[108] Arguably, those whose hope for success is stronger than their fear of failure are better equipped for breastfeeding. Studies reveal that women planning to breastfeed are more likely than women planning to formula feed to identify themselves as having an 'internal locus of control', that is, to perceive themselves as having control over the health of their baby.[109] Which is great, because by its very nature, breastfeeding is an internalised act. While external support – qualified health professionals, doting family members, decent maternity leave – is helpful, breastfeeding success ultimately hinges upon the mother's own behaviour.

Sadly, most women are destined to set up shop in the 'fear of failure' camp. There are two reasons for this: firstly, breastfeeding is an irrevocably feminine act, and fear of failure is characteristically more common in women than in men.[110] Secondly, contemporary mothers, particularly first-timers, do not carry with them a stable sense of their own breastfeeding abilities.[111] Even La Leche League concede in their breastfeeding bible *The Womanly Art of Breastfeeding* that, 'Mothers have become bogged down in scales and charts and schedules and have lost confidence in their own abilities'.[112]

Thus, for the majority of women, the negative consequences of failure outweigh the positive incentives of success. Breastfeeding, with its innately individualised nature, creates tension, ironically exacerbating the fear of failure, growing it further. Many women on the cusp of attempting breastfeeding even experience what psychologists call 'anticipatory grief', a type of unduly pessimistic emotional preparation for expected failure designed to reduce grief after it occurs. This mindset has the self-sabotaging effect of weakening a mother's attachment to breastfeeding, even before she has attempted to breastfeed.

Women plagued with a fear of failure – and thus an expectation of failure – are drawn to focus on the relative hardships involved in breastfeeding. They resent the inability to share the feeding 'chore' with others; they fret over the uncertainty of their baby's exact intake; they are offended by the prospect of having to feed in public. Some of these women even avoid breastfeeding altogether, opting to head straight to formula feeding, because for them, the net effect of doing nothing outweighs the perceived consequences of trying. We commonly speak of breastfeeding as a choice, but ironically, for these mothers, breastfeeding becomes the ultimate 'unchoice'.

Many of those with the balls to initiate breastfeeding regard the outcome of their journey as so predetermined that they fail to seek relevant education or support. Philosophers call this the Idle Argument – if something is fated, then it would be pointless or futile to fight against it, and effort decreases in anticipation of failure. By dwelling on possible uncontrollable outcomes (the unlikely threat of anatomical failure, for instance), a mother can protect herself against disappointment – at a cost. In doing so, she must relinquish her sense of control. She must become passive rather than engaging. This attitude of passive resignation, this fatalism, produces a paradox. Rather than triggering the mother's anxiety, it can generate comfort. People thrive from predictability. Predictability is a psychological comfort blanket. Certainty of failure is much easier to bear than uncertainty of success. As a bonus, a belief in fatalism can provide a ready excuse for poor decision-making: 'I had no choice'. Formula feeding is framed as an imperative.

What about those women, on the other hand, who hope for success? These women focus on the consolations of breastfeeding: the health rewards, the convenience of having a portable food source, the freedom from having to sterilise utensils. Whether fearful or hopeful, each mother chooses to focus on the various facets of breastfeeding that relate to how she sees her journey turning out. Pessimistic mothers focus on the negatives; optimistic mothers focus on the positives. Motivational speaker Harvey Mackay understood this process when he said, 'Optimists are right. So are pessimists. It's up to you to choose which you will be'.

### Self-Deception – Denial Turned Inwards

So far, we have established that mothers like to dabble in the deception of their nearest and dearest. However, can you guess what is even better for the mother than deceiving others? Why, deceiving herself of course! As options go, self-deception is more attractive than Colin Firth, and its practice is more prevalent than most of us are prepared to concede. In fact, we all have a proclivity for self-deception because we are all drawn to believe privately in things that reflect favourably on us.[113] For mothers who have quit breastfeeding, or who are on the verge of doing so, self-deception is the BFF that keeps on giving.

Firstly, the main advantage, indeed the main function, of self-deception is that you fail to give off cues that go with conscious deception – no poker face necessary – thus boosting your chances of successfully deceiving others. As they say, 'Fooling yourself, the better to fool others'. A sense of self-esteem is achieved when a mother's breastfeeding outcomes match or exceed her 'perceived reality constraints'.[114] 'Perceived' is the key word here. If a mother can convince herself that the constraints on her breastfeeding success were tighter than they were in reality, she is more readily able to soak up her own deception that she 'tried hard enough'. In this way, self-deception serves as a shield to protect a mother from feelings of humiliation and guilt.

Secondly, the actual process of deceiving others is rendered easier (or to use psychobabble, 'cognitively less expensive') by keeping part of the truth in the unconscious store cupboard. You see, our brains act more efficiently when they do not have to deal with ongoing contradiction. When we dabble in a spot of self-deception, the cognitive consequences don't feel as severe as they do with a full-blown lie.

Thirdly, self-deception acts as a type of emotional defence mechanism. Morally threatening emotions can be buried in the subconscious. At this junction you may be noticing that there's a lot of talk about the subconscious behaviour buried deep beyond layers of awareness, but it is important to recognise that self-deception is *not* a wholly passive exercise. We suppress information by storing certain emotionally satisfying truths in the conscious mind, and other less palatable but equally valid truths in the subconscious. This is why philosophers refer to self-deception as motivated lying to oneself.[115]

An excellent example of self-deception – and one prolific in discussions of breastfeeding – is the sacrosanct notion of 'luck'. For instance, in the popular parenting book *A Rough Guide to Babies and Toddlers*, the author presents a wish list of prerequisites for successful breastfeeding, which includes, 'Luck: you need to be one of the people who can breastfeed'.[116]

Collectivist political movements such as socialism are big believers in luck – and formula-feeding apologists mirror their rhetoric. Hardship is inflicted upon the individual rather than being brought about by the individual. Yet resigning successful breastfeeding to the trashcan of luck is harmful to women's pursuit of breastfeeding. As we will see later in this chapter, the vagueness of luck generates in women an anxious uncertainty that can lead to self-handicapping strategies, propelling women to create impediments that make breastfeeding success less likely. Irrevocably linking successful breastfeeding to luck encourages mothers to reserve their energy and emotional investment for other situations. In other words, the effort they expend in breastfeeding is dramatically reduced. This reduction in effort is rationalised if a mother tells herself that 'luck' rather than effort is the deciding factor. To illustrate the mother's 'disengaged' mindset, I am going to apply a tennis analogy used by Ed Smith (2012) in his aptly titled book, *Luck: What It Means and Why It Matters*:[117]

> Do you have free will when a ball is thrown at you? In fact, your response is conditioned, like a tennis return. There's almost no decision-making involved. You do not think through how you are going to react to the ball. However, when you serve a ball you have more choice. Which provokes the question, is the nature of life like serving, or like returning (which flows along more preordained tracks)?

Mothers who believe breastfeeding success is marred with luck approach breastfeeding problems with a return serve – they see problems as not requiring conscious consideration. They are passive rather than dynamic. Whereas positive, more determined mothers approach problems with a serve. In essence, it boils down to how much control mothers believe they have over their success in breastfeeding. So subjective reality largely determines how successfully breastfeeding goes, rather than objective reality.

The physiological reality for the vast, vast, VAST majority of women is that breastfeeding success does *not* boil down to luck. It is high time we supplanted luck with a more scientific understanding of how the lactating body really works. The human species didn't get this far by relying on 'luck'. If we were to banish the notion of luck from discussions of breastfeeding and replace it with a renewed faith in self-determinism, mothers would truly feel that success was within their grasp. Abandoning the discourse of luck would smooth the transition from fate to free will, and therefore to empowerment. I suggest ways health professionals and breastfeeding advocates can do this – by directing a mother's awareness to positive feedback signs, such as wet and dirty nappies, baby sedation and so on – on page 67.

## BELIEF

The B in the A B C of Breastfeeding Fidelity stands for Belief. This is where I grudgingly tip my hat to 'cultural conditioning' – but be forewarned, this is a short section. In accordance with the book's aim towards empowering women, I will not dwell on external constraints beyond a mother's control. In any event, as I argue in the introduction, the power of such constraints pales in comparison to the power of a mother's internal will.[118]

It is a prevalent, if somewhat lazy, argument that a woman's behaviour is brought about by external constraints, as if society (whatever that is) 'plays' a mother like a puppet. The argument maintains that society prescribes what acceptable motherhood is, and mothers are acutely faithful to whatever 'society' tells them they must be. So if society tells mothers that motherhood is a sacred role that demands selfless dedication and commitment, this ideology 'makes' mothers submit to being primarily responsible for shaping the destiny of their child. Dominant ideology 'forces' them to be martyrs. This role becomes internalised as part of mothers' self-image, providing them with 'self-constructs' – a baseline for how they should be acting – and expectations related to the role. Or so the theory goes.

However, this Cultural Martyrdom of Motherhood is not the all-powerful bully lamented over by communitarian commentators, the same folk who believe the individual is helplessly directed, like Lemmings in the video game, by the mouse cursor of 'society'.[119] If we were to stop and actually look at the lived reality of mothers, we would see that they weigh society's external standards for how they 'ought' to act against their own personal attitudes and the social messages emitted from friends and family. The result is that mothers hear the Breast is Best/Martyr message as nothing more than static noise. Moral relativism (the subjectivism of what is deemed right and wrong) makes it impossible for such dogma to influence norms or behaviour when the martyr stratagem is perceived by individual mothers as an inaccurate, and thus sanctimonious, reflection of their everyday reality. Rather than soaking up such messages, mothers feel they are intended for other reasons, such as an insidious and unexplainable government agenda to make them 'feel bad'.

To truly appreciate and understand mothers' lived experiences, we need to radically tighten the scope of power we attribute to 'cultural influence'. Culture has noteworthy impact upon the success of breastfeeding only in as far as 'culture' includes a mother's family and close friends – those people important to her. Everyone else – media, society, government et al – can claim mere marginal impact at best.[120] A mother's family and friends – her 'homies' as I call them – are where the real influence stems. The importance of these people to the mother affects the extent to which their approval will shape her breastfeeding intentions. You'll be learning a lot about the behaviour of family and friends in the Sabotage chapter, but for now, we are going to focus on what the *mother* believes her homies think about her breastfeeding. These beliefs are entirely subjective estimates of the kinship pressure to breastfeed (or not breastfeed, as the case may be). Belief, in this sense, is summed up by the following internal dialogue: 'How would my family and friends react to my breastfeeding?'

The *Guinness Book of Records* slot for most unremarkably obvious research outcome must have gone to the following finding: 'Women whose family and friends share their pro-breastfeeding stance tend to breastfeed longer'.[121] Woah, someone call Sherlock; his job is on the line. The revelation that familial environment is a pivotal player in breastfeeding outcome is hardly ground-breaking. Many, if not most, mothers are dependent on immediate and/or extended family members for support;[122] consequently the expectations and beliefs of these family members are a salient voice in mothers' lives. There's a reason why successful breastfeeding mothers tend to have been breastfed themselves, and that formula feeders tend to have been formula-fed themselves.[123] Having a supportive band of merry men (or even better, women) is an undeniable asset to the breastfeeding mother, as one mum gushed in an interview:

'I really needed somebody to tell me "Keep going. It's going to be okay", especially for the three-week period where I was by myself and I had this one nipple that was really, really sore. I needed somebody almost every two days to tell me, "Keep going, it's going to be all right". So there were people that, you know, if you really didn't want to quit you could call them and they would really give you a pep talk. That would get me going again'.[124]

Both pessimism and optimism are viral. A mother's confidence in her ability to breastfeed increases around people who radiate assurance. Likewise, her doubts flare up around the cynical.[125]

But not all women have such fortunate taste in family. Many women deliberating over breastfeeding find themselves dissuaded by the negative experiences of friends or relatives.[126] One major reason why a mother's homies wield such a powerful influence is their omnipresence. A mother sees her friends and family frequently, if not constantly. The more available certain information is, the more a mother will perceive it to be frequent, probable and causally important.[127]

If a woman's family and friends never breastfed, she misses out on the experience of observing breastfeeding behaviour, a process that results in what sociologists call 'embodied knowledge' – the kind of knowledge associated with confidence in breastfeeding. This knowledge is way more important than soaking up the Breast is Best message.[128] Indeed, while women are generally aware that breast is best, many express distrust in this message if they have not been breastfed themselves. These women prefer their infant-feeding choice to be guided by the perceived norm among family and friends.[129]

It is hard for a new mum to make a good decision when she has trouble translating the choices she faces into the experiences she will have. So she looks to her nearest and dearest for hints of what she should be doing. In doing this, she is driven by the assumption that the people around her possess more knowledge of the situation than she does. Even though she has created a brand new family herself, she will intuitively rely on her old family for support and guidance. Such sheep-like imitative conformity is not passive and senseless. Rather, it has a curious internal logic. If lots of people are doing something, there must be a good reason why. Psychologists call this powerful cognitive drive 'social proof'. The fallacy of this human tendency – and we all do it to a certain extent – can be summed up by my own mother's favourite catchphrase (the soundtrack to my childhood), 'If all your friends jumped off the Tyne Bridge, would you jump too?' Large groups can easily conform to choices, even if they are disadvantageous.

Although social proof reflects a rational motive to take into account the information possessed by one's kin, it can also cause a mother to converge too quickly on a single choice, with the result that her decision is grounded in very little information. Social proof is a particularly powerful – indeed incomparable – influence in the infant-feeding domain, firstly because culture places importance on the accuracy of the decision (infant feeding has been granted 'big issue' status) and secondly, because one's family, particularly elders with more experience of childrearing, are perceived by novice mothers as especially knowledgeable. It's easy to see how a particular method of infant feeding can easily become entrenched in a family group over time.[130] Of course, the group may change its behaviour if it can be shown that the practice is causing serious problems. However, if there is uncertainty on that question, the group will often continue doing what they have always done.[131] This 'pluralistic ignorance' is a common human fallacy. We may follow a practice not because we like it, or even think it is the best choice, but merely because we think our peers like it. Shall we take a closer look at the peers of a typical mother? (You: bring it on mofo).

### The Influential Klout of Peers

Women thrive on solidarity, and for mothers, there is a no greater, more mutual peer than a fellow mum. Psychology professor Daniel Stern has spoken of the maternal craving for a mutual network. His studies revealed that right after their babies were born, mothers had a 'huge' amount of daily contact with other mothers.[132] A prime meeting place for these 'mummy peers' is the culturally standard 'baby group'. In a

UK study of 2,000 new mothers[133] nearly half the women said they made friends at baby groups, while a fifth said they kept in touch with mothers they met at antenatal classes.

It is not unusual for a new mother's peer group to be populated at some point by a number of breastfeeding mothers. At present, 81 percent of women begin motherhood by breastfeeding.[134] However, the number of breastfeeding mothers drops dramatically in relatively quick succession. Every year, more than 200,000 British mothers stop breastfeeding in the first few days and weeks – 90 percent of these mothers would have liked to continue.[135] This means the make-up of the baby-group environment takes a dramatic shift in a very short space of time, from a group of novice but enthusiastic breastfeeders to a group of disillusioned and regretful formula feeders. For the few breastfeeding mothers who survive the initial struggles that often colour the first few months of breastfeeding, the baby-group environment does not adapt in line with their experience. As their peers switch to formula, the resulting atmosphere is one of tense social awkwardness. We'll have fun exploring this awkwardness in dramatic depth later in the Envy chapter, but for now let's focus on how a mother's perception of her peers influences her own behaviour.

In a landmark series of studies, psychologist Solomon Asch[136] highlighted the sheer strength wielded by an individual's perception of their peer-group, and specifically, the desire of individuals not to face the disapproval of their peers. Asch found that people often go along with the rest of the group even when they think – or know – that everyone else has blundered. When the vast majority of a peer group choose an incorrect course of action, their influence in numbers drives the minority members to also take the incorrect cause of action, even if the action is clearly and obviously wrong!

In a group scenario with only two non-conformists, Asch found that the removal of one of them halfway through the experiment influenced the other's level of conformity, namely their level of conformity increased once the ally had been removed. The methodology developed by Asch has been utilised by many researchers and the paradigm is now firmly established in social psychology. We see the phenomenon too often played out in the baby-group environment: as numbers of breastfeeding mothers dwindle, the ethos of the group shifts from a pro-breastfeeding mentality to a pro-formula-feeding one. This leads to increased pressure to formula feed. The new group average exerts significant influence. Conformity tends to increase as the size of the group increases. The few remaining breastfeeding mothers become effectively 'non-conformists', and as their numbers dwindle it becomes increasingly socially hostile for anyone to continue breastfeeding. The pressure of conformity increases the more difficult a task is perceived to be. When individuals are uncertain, they look to others for confirmation. The issue of conformity is central to infant feeding. People tend to conform more when asked to behave publicly, and infant feeding is an unavoidably public act.

## CONTROL

Control, a priceless commodity. Who doesn't want control? The C in the A B C of Breastfeeding Fidelity is Control. It is human nature to gravitate towards control. When we speak of choice, what we really mean is the ability to exercise control over our lives. Thus in order to choose to breastfeed, a mother must first believe that she has control. There are two aspects to control: first, how confident Mum feels about her ability to breastfeed in the first place, and second, how much control she feels she has over the breastfeeding process. Thus, control in the world of breastfeeding is interwoven with perceptions of ability and mastery – of both internal factors and 'situational' ones (responses to one's situation and challenges that arise).[137] Let's look at ability and mastery in turn.

### Ability to breastfeed

Albert Bandura, a renowned psychologist who's been in the business for almost six decades, has explained the importance of control, and described it thus:

'Unless people believe they can produce desired effects by their actions, they have little incentive to act or to persevere in the face of difficulties. Whatever other factors may serve as guides and motivators, they are rooted in the core belief that one has the power to produce desired changes by one's actions'.[138]

Bandura could well be describing the typical new mum – the breastfeeding novice. This mother is fuelled by a fear of the unknown and a belief that she has no control should challenges arise.[139] She feels stranded in an endless limbo that is too open, too ill-defined, too uncomfortable. The level of apparent uncertainty inherent in the nature of breastfeeding leaves many mothers feeling ill at ease, unable to relax or feel secure.[140] Concerns about milk supply are the most common reported.[141] Breastfeeding's inability to tell a mother precisely how much her baby is consuming makes it appear infinitely more 'risky' than using bottles. Formula feeding carries with it a level of almost clinical certainty that breastfeeding simply cannot match.[142] The new breastfeeding mum feels as though she is floating in a dangerous area between being in control and being utterly helpless. She understands the basic mechanics of breastfeeding, but this limited knowledge doesn't provide the guarantees that would make her feel comfortable. She imagines her baby starving or becoming malnourished or her milk suddenly drying up (that's if she's confident she even has any milk to start with). Such fears are a striking example of how perceived control is not always an accurate indication of actual control.[143] The resulting feeling of helplessness is stressful. If it persists, a mother becomes passive, feels incompetent and may even sink into depression.[144]

Most mothers make their decision to quit while undergoing breastfeeding difficulties. How a mother reacts to breastfeeding difficulties depends on whether she sees the ability to breastfeed as entrenched – unchanging, unquestionable, a fixed state – or as flexible and likely to change. Those who believe the ability to breastfeed is entrenched often 'hit a wall', experiencing high degrees of helplessness and hopelessness – both enhanced by the environment and by the intrinsic features of lactation – which ultimately leads to them stopping.

In contrast, those who view the ability to breastfeed as flexible tend to respond to difficulties with a problem-solving focus, remaining motivated to overcome any obstacles, exerting greater effort and being willing to experiment with different strategies.[145] Interestingly, these mothers – who take personal responsibility for their breastfeeding success – are more resistant to depression.[146] They develop not only confidence in their own breastfeeding ability, but also a sense of mastery of the breastfeeding process. Let's take a closer look at the concept of breastfeeding mastery and why it is so important.

### Mastering Breastfeeding

Commentators have observed that, more often than not, mothers 'lack the confidence and skills needed to take control over their own breastfeeding practice'.[147] At the beginning of their breastfeeding journey, women report feeling uncertain and vulnerable.[148] Control is a central theme in their dialogue. Talk of feeling 'overwhelmed and out of control' is common.[149]

Unsurprisingly, mothers with lower feelings of control over the breastfeeding process are more likely to turn to formula.[150] Furthermore, mothers who are uncomfortable with their body shape or their capacity to control their body – such as women with eating disorders and other kinds of dysmorphia and obsessive-compulsive disorder – are substantially less likely to attempt breastfeeding in the first place.[151] These facts demonstrate that rather than being a subtle factor, a mother's thoughts and feelings are in fact a vital determinant of her breastfeeding performance, by far outweighing environmental influences.

One of these maternal feelings is prominent yet deadly silent, particularly in the early days of motherhood: resentment. Mothers resent their babies having control over them. The once autonomous adult woman finds herself yielding to the unforgiving and relentless shrieking demands of an infant barely days old. For many mothers, this dyadic set-up – in which two beings are meshed as one by virtue of their interdependency – symbolises a major loss of independence.[152]

In one study, formula-feeding mothers described formula as a partial antidote to this tug of war 'because feeding routines could be controlled by the mother rather than by the infant'.[153]

Those attempting to breastfeed, on the other hand, also comprehend the centrality of maternal control. They understand that having control over the breastfeeding process means having control over the baby, because the baby is integral to the process. Some try to do this by installing strict feeding and sleeping routines or with the aptly named 'controlled crying' technique.[154] These mothers believe their babies should conform to parental wishes. Yet far from helping a mother to gain mastery over breastfeeding, such widespread techniques have been proven to decrease breastfeeding success.[155]

Embarrassment about breastfeeding in public is another often-cited barrier to feelings of control,[156] with many women describing a self-imposed dichotomous choice between feeling isolated at home or formula feeding.[157] Is it any wonder then, that for the vast majority of mothers quitting is the answer and formula feeding the destination? But is formula *really* the easy way out?

## FORMULA FEEDING – THE CONTROL PARADOX

Is formula feeding the easy option? I'm going to give an evasive answer, just to irritate you: yes and no. The 'yes' camp is arguably populated by the majority of breastfeeding quitters, because as a counterpoint to the 'difficulty' of breastfeeding, formula tends to come up trumps in the maternal mindset. Even one of the most vocal of formula apologists, Dr Ellie Lee, a reader in Social Policy at Kent University, has admitted that, 'Formula feeding is predominantly experienced by mothers as "easy", enabling them to address a wide range of demands and difficulties that mothering a small baby poses for them'.[158] The majority of women in one of Dr Lee's studies experienced formula feeding as 'a pragmatically advantageous option for feeding babies'.[159]

To the anxious mother, formula feeding offers an opportunity to circumvent uncertainty and gain a sense of control. The promise of being in control that formula feeding provides is pleasurable. Using bottles gives mothers the comforting illusion that the feeding process is stable and knowable. Even if a mother is aware of the risks of formula feeding, those risks seem pretty abstract when compared with the immediate practical and emotional utility of bottle feeding. The bottle is celebrated as an almost sacrosanct utensil which, relative to its competitor – breastfeeding – is 'convenient', 'easy', 'provides freedom from the baby', 'provides a means of getting back to normal'... the list is endless. Indeed, so amazing is the bottle that some even claim it enables mothers 'to re-establish an identity as non-mothers'[160] – a ship that in all logic has surely sailed?

Yet formula feeding is far from the easy option – if done properly. Besides sterilising all the equipment, measuring the formula correctly and ensuring precise water temperature, safety guidelines direct parents to, 'Make up feeds, one at a time, as your baby needs them'[161] in order to protect babies from pathogenic bacterial nasties. Yet many mothers, after shunning breastfeeding guidelines, go on to shun formula-feeding guidelines too, all in the name of 'ease'. In one study, a mother was interviewed boasting that formula feeding was 'just easier... like you can make up the bottles for the whole day, either last thing at night, first thing in a morning, and you're done'.[162] For those mothers who, unlike this one, quit breastfeeding and actually adhere to formula-preparation guidelines, the exhaustion of cluster nursing is replaced with the exhaustion of a never-ending bottle preparation conveyor belt. Easy it is not.

Besides the burden of utensil management, another even crueller irony comes to light when mothers switch to formula. Women make the switch in order to capture a sense of control, a reasoning that's understandable yet fatally flawed. Let me explain why. Formula feeding routinises a baby's care. Mothers are told how to prepare a feed, how often to feed and how much to feed. In such a predictable feeding environment, there is little for mothers to think about. Reliance on formula actually exacerbates the uncertainty mums feel about their own mothering abilities. They are robbed of the mindful state needed to perceive control. Instead, they are being told what to do by a relatively disinterested third party: a formula company.

Those few mothers who don't succumb to the bottle and instead persist with breastfeeding find themselves dropping their time-honoured hobbies: a gym class here, polo-neck fashion there, booze-guzzling nights out, coffee-fuelled mornings in, sexy MILF bras. In their place, breastfeeding mothers take up a new pastime – self-talk. To be successful, they must engage in this hobby frequently in order to prod themselves through the challenges, strains and encumbrances of breastfeeding. When the going gets tough and the bed gets soggy, when baby won't latch or latches like a barracuda, mothers find themselves playing pretend friend with an internal dialogue in which difficulties and doubts battle against a drive to continue and stand firm. It is on bad days – typically characterised by exhaustion, emotional stress and the pain of peeing with fanjo stitches – when such internal prep-talks are most needed.

What happens in a mother's mind during those bad days is so central, so imperative, to breastfeeding success or failure that it deserves more in-depth analysis. And I'm not one to disappoint. But a word of warning before we continue: the workings of the human mind are unavoidably complex, so this chapter is about to get a tad technical. I suspect the complexity of psychology is one of the reasons why books about breastfeeding seldom explore mothers' idiosyncratic experience with much penetration. Yet explore we must if we are ever truly to understand and appreciate the lived reality behind infant-feeding statistics.

### Breaking Point – Visceral Influences

The bleak days of new motherhood are when most women take the mortal leap from breast to formula. Such days are characterised by pain, discomfort and tiredness.[163] These unyielding and unforgiving sensations find a mother longing for her previous life: a life in which her body was not expected to produce meals every couple of hours, when she could take day-long shopping trips, and when she could get a solid night's kip.

Back in 1996, psychologist Dr George Loewenstein[164]

identified what he called 'visceral' influences – which, he ascertained, have a disproportionate effect on our behaviour. These rewarding or punishing sensations – for example the urgent desire to escape pain – tend to alter the attractiveness of certain activities. When you're pounding the treadmill at the gym and lactic acid begins to course through your appendages, suddenly having Beyonce's butt no longer seems as attractive as having a sit down on your own butt. At their most fundamental, visceral influences slot into the well-established paradigm of hedonism: people seek pleasure and avoid pain. Visceral influences affect the relative desirability of goods and actions. Discomfort or shock, for example, increase the desirability of withdrawal behaviours. One only has to take a shower at the same time as another member of the household decides to do a spot of dish washing to understand this.

The granddaddy of psychoanalysis, Sigmund Freud[165] recognised these impulsive surges, but used a different name for them – 'the id'. This part of our personality, he explained, embodies our primitive and instinctual natures. The id is biological; it knows no values and no morality. Its goal is the instant elimination of all tension and the instant gratification of all needs – in complete disregard of outside forces. Let me put it in parenting terms: the id is the boisterous toddler of the psyche, unable to comprehend constraint, practise delayed gratification or act logically. Were the id left to run free, we would all be feral. However, this toddler has a parent, what Freud called 'the ego'. While the id is the biological component of our personality, the ego is the psychological component. The ego serves as a mediator between the id and the outside world. In this sense, human beings are not really rational beings; we are quasi-rational. The id and the ego are in periodic conflict, with – thankfully – the rational ego usually prevailing.

How does this relate to the breastfeeding scenario? When struggling with breastfeeding difficulties, a mother is subject to conflicting forces, with some influences promoting continued breastfeeding and some inhibiting it. Take formula milk, for example. Giving formula seldom improves breastfeeding, yet its use is regularly recommended to struggling mothers by family, friends and even health professionals. It's not difficult to see why. Formula provides instant relief for both mother and baby. It appeals to the id. Anyone can stick the bottle in the baby's mouth. The baby will then devour the contents and may even fall asleep. The environment then becomes, at least for now, serene. To the struggling mother-baby unit, the allure of formula goes without saying. For baby, literally, because he can't talk. And for Mum, figuratively, because her mouth is otherwise occupied by teeth gritting. Indeed, formula is firmly framed in the collective consciousness as a magic bullet in times of breastfeeding crisis. It also promises the illusion of control, and with it unrealistic expectations of being able to influence future events – for instance, getting more sleep and more convenience.

I say an 'illusion' of control because as we discussed earlier, the popular equating of formula feeding with control is a misguided paradox (see page 54). Nonetheless, the misconception continues to thrive, partly facilitated by the promises of formula companies and health professionals. Under pressure, struggling mothers can let their best intentions (breast intentions?) slip and, when their attention is diverted, succumb to the misplaced allure of formula. In Freudian terms, the id overwhelms the ego. The mother finds herself dominated by her biological needs; all other needs are pushed into the background or temporarily forgotten. Pain or exhaustion can have a disproportionate effect on a mother's behaviour – with the result of 'crowding out' virtually all goals. In the dead of night, with George Foreman infomercials and a suckling piranha as your only companions, visions of throwing a tin of formula and a bottle at your husband (preferably at his balls) don't seem so dramatic. Unsurprisingly, formula's ability to calm immediate visceral forces like tiredness and pain has been shown to lead to changed maternal assessments of what is 'best'.[166]

To make matters worse, visceral influences, although extremely powerful 'in the moment', are often profoundly underweighted or even denied by mothers first before they arise and then after they have gone.[167] This inadvertently increases their power. To prepare for a fully rational infant-feeding choice, mothers should anticipate visceral factors and plan for when they kick in. Strategies for pain-relief, for example, are routinely deliberated over and prepared for in relation to childbirth, but much less so for breastfeeding. Consequently, when visceral factors are triggered during breastfeeding, a mum finds herself, in a moment of weakness, embracing the misguided reassurance of a family member or health professional that, 'Just one bottle of formula won't hurt'. Like Esau in the Book of Genesis, who sold his birthright for a mess of 'pottage', the mother sacrifices her breastfeeding goals for more sleep or less pain.

In normal circumstances, the ego would take control. The mother would give her full attention to a whole range of features and weigh them up in the course of making the decision to reach for and prepare the bottle: the current context, her mood and motivational state, the dietary impact on her baby, the impact of reducing her supply of breast milk, the risk of nipple confusion and so on. But when a mother's 'attentional resources' are diverted (by tiredness or pain perhaps), her focus of attention narrows and things drop away so that only the most salient and immediate features remain for her to consider when making a choice. If those salient features (sedating the baby, for instance) happen to be strongly tied to the visceral attractiveness of the formula (formula marketing aims to ensure this is the case), then the bottle is more likely to be given.

Another unfortunate feature of visceral factors is their uncanny time-narrowing effect. Pain or exhaustion lead to a collapsing of our time-perspective towards the present. When a mum looks down at her misshapen breasts, which now represent a sock full of stones, and then looks up at her future in its bawling red face, her breastfeeding goals begin to fade into the horizon. She is likely to make short-sighted trade-offs between immediate and delayed satisfaction. Many mothers understand that, logically, using formula is a detrimental to their long-term breastfeeding goals, but are unable to translate this belief into action. The process is not unconscious; as Dr Loewenstein noted, 'Visceral factors cause people to behave contrary to their own long-term self-interest, often with full awareness that they are doing so'.[168]

A fun way to conceptualise visceral factors was proposed by American economists, Richard Thaler and Cass Sunstein. They used the metaphor of temperature and described visceral influences as a continuum ranging from cold to hot. Let's take hunger as an example: when an individual is very hungry and appetising aromas are wafting from the kitchen, we can say she is in a hot state. Conversely, when someone is thinking in an abstract way about what to have for dinner the following day, she is in a cold state. 'We call something "tempting" if we consume more of it when hot than when cold'.[169] Formula is tempting to a mother when she is in a 'hot' state —when she's under emotional or physical pressure. This is why keeping a container of formula in the house 'just in case' is such an effective tool of self-sabotage.

Various dimensions of proximity – temporal, physical and sensory – can intensify visceral drives and thus change our behaviour. The vividness of that packet of formula intensifies the immediate emotions that arise when a stressed new mother thinks about the anticipated relief formula can bring. The scenario is worsened by a hard-wired psychological mechanism persistent in all of us: 'hyperbolic discounting'. Put bluntly, the closer a reward is – in this case, access to formula and thus baby sedation – the higher our 'emotional interest rate' rises and the more we are willing to give up in exchange for it. In this instance, mothers often are willing to put their breastfeeding relationship on the line for a few hours of sleep or relief from discomfort. Such immediacy magnetises us. A breastfeeding mother's decision to use formula is seldom the result of rational, objective planning. Formula companies are, of course, aware of this. They orchestrate timed mail-outs of marketing materials and free samples to arrive on mothers' doorsteps during their babies's early infancy, when breastfeeding difficulties are likely to peak.[170] Formula marketing is the ideal masquerading as real. Its use promises autonomy, sanity and sleep.

Another noteworthy feature of visceral factors is their attention-narrowing bias towards the self. If, whenever her baby latches onto her breast, a mother experiences searing pain, that pain will narrow her focus inward, undermining her altruism. To put it crudely, people who are in pain or exhausted tend to act selfishly.

A humbling, if sadly pessimistic, reality is that most women abandon breastfeeding as a result of visceral influences. The driving force of these instinctive states is too primitive and too urgently felt for most women to suppress. The fact that breastfeeding is no longer a matter of life or death for babies and that a substitute is readily available means that women heed their own visceral factors more now than ever before in human history. The widespread availability of formula for non-emergency use has relegated breastfeeding in the public consciousness to little more than an act of 'self-actualisation': something worthwhile to do, but not essential. Consequently, the desire to breastfeed no longer dominates the visceral response system like it did for our ancestors. At one point in history, a mother's goal was to breastfeed in order to prevent her baby from starving to death. Today, mothers' breastfeeding goals reflect the less pressing need for achievement, mastery, satisfaction, social recognition, dignity, competence and reputation.

The often-visceral reality of breastfeeding is in conflict with women's contemporary breastfeeding goals. Visceral factors operate in the here and now. The visceral need to alleviate her exhaustion is more immediately compelling to a mother than the need to bolster her maternal kudos by becoming a competent breastfeeder. In fact, the less imperative a need is for sheer survival, the easier it is for that need to disappear. Take the universal example of the new mother. Most women in the initial stages of motherhood feel exhausted. Their need to alleviate this exhaustion, bolstered by its visceral nature, becomes of great concern to them. The more exhausted the mother becomes, the louder her need for rest bellows. Being visceral, if this need were audible, it would have the decibel level of a jackhammer. Meanwhile, the secondary need to enhance her self-confidence by reaching self-imposed breastfeeding goals is drowned out.

For most mothers, only when their visceral needs – to rest, to be free from pain – have been satisfied can their long-term breastfeeding goals regain their position as a primary concern.

This is an intrinsically human trait. When opportunities for analytic deliberation are reduced by visceral factors, we are more likely to rely on our biological drive. Then, when the visceral need is satisfied, another lesser need can emerge and take centre stage.[171] When a mother's need for rest is tended to, its volume is turned down and the need to tend to her breastfeeding goals can be heard again, first subtly and then more clearly as the need for rest becomes more sated and thus quieter. We can explain this process through percentages. If by switching to formula a mother feels more able to rest, after formula feeding for one day her physiological need for rest would be partially satisfied, say by 10 percent. At this point, her need to fulfil her breastfeeding goals may not be audible at all. However, as her need for rest becomes satisfied by 25 percent, her need to establish breastfeeding competency may emerge by 5 percent. As her need for rest becomes satisfied by 75 percent, her need to fulfil her breastfeeding goals may emerge by 50 percent, and so on. However – and here's the snag – by the time her breastfeeding goals become sufficiently audible again, there is a possibility her milk will have dried up.[172]

The visceral nature of many breastfeeding challenges reflects the importance of thorough antenatal planning and timely postnatal support. When a mother's breastfeeding relationship – not to mention her nipple – is hanging by a thread, time is, quite literally, of the essence. Even if Mum later swears blind that she made a fully informed, deliberate decision to quit, one would be forgiven for raising an eyebrow if visceral factors were involved. Most people believe their actions result from deliberate decisions.[1173] However, it is questionable whether these claims reflect the results of fully conscious, reality-based decision-making processes or are simply a result of the retrospective rationalisation and esteem-massaging behaviour to which we are all susceptible.[174]

Then there are the emotions of the struggling mother – another undervalued force driving the switch from breast to bottle, and a sibling of visceral factors. Emotional reactions such as fear, confusion and resentment work in concert with cognitive thought processes – attention, judgement and evaluation – to guide a mother's reasoning and decision-making.[175] Her cognitions and emotions diverge during this dynamically volatile time and lead to her behaving quite differently than she would if she considered things in a purely cognitive way. For instance, a mother may overweigh small and extreme possibilities – such as the risk that she is one of the five percent of women who physically can't breastfeed. Even if she were aware that almost all women can produce enough breast milk (for at least two babies at a time – fact!), during the storm of her angst, this knowledge would recede out of her awareness. In such emotional times, an irrational hypothesis can seem rational. A mother becomes hyper-sensitive to departures from certainty, so for instance in her mind the five percent risk that she won't be able to breastfeed represents the crossing of a threshold from a consequence of no concern (zero percent risk) to one that becomes a source of worry. The weight she assigns to the two percent probability is great in part because the consequences of being in that two percent are great: baby's failure to thrive.

The cultural acceptability of formula exploits a mother's visceral and emotional weaknesses. During breastfeeding difficulties, the most powerful and attractive features of formula tend to become 'cognitively salient', that is, more accessible to her awareness. However if, in contrast, the salience of the *risks* of formula are enhanced, the greater weighting of those features will incline a mother to avoid formula. So if we frame the infant-feeding choice in terms of the risks of formula feeding, fewer mothers will make the switch from breast to formula in times of weakness.

It sounds logical and straightforward, and indeed there is a scientific basis to bolster this somewhat radical approach. As the descendants of quick decision-makers, we rely on mental shortcuts called 'heuristics'. One of the mechanisms that I mentioned earlier (the 'affect heuristic', see page 25) is designed to help us make decisions and solve problems quickly and efficiently. So if a mother is given information about the benefits of formula, her affective evaluation of formula will rise and she infers – via a mental shortcut – that the risks associated with formula are low. In future chapters we'll see how this inference is often reflected in mothers' public defence of formula, 'If formula was so bad, they wouldn't be allowed to sell it' being a common chant of justification.[176] Similarly, if a mother is told that the risks of formula are high, her affective evaluation is lowered and she infers that formula is low in benefits. In other words, providing information about one attribute (a risk) has a carryover effect on the attribute about which no information has been provided and nothing has been learned directly (the benefit).

The risks associated with formula use are indeed numerous. Some are relatively common, such as gut problems; some are much more remote, such as SIDS (sudden infant death syndrome). There is still value in emphasising remote risks to mothers. Studies have shown that even when the chance of an event occurring is low, people are less willing to engage in the behaviour the more negative the event.[177]

## EMPOWERING MOTHERS

This chapter has, thus far, been pretty depressing, hasn't it? Chin up! Research has clarified that maternal feelings of control can be improved by breastfeeding education, particularly focusing on self-care programmes and particularly when this education is given early in the postnatal period.[178] Aside from showcasing the risks of formula-use, there are numerous important ways that breastfeeding advocates can empower a mother to adhere to her breastfeeding goals. Each hinges on giving the mother an invaluable gift – a sense of control. Here are just several of my suggestions for breastfeeding advocates:

1. Shift a mother's state of mindfulness from passive to active. One way of doing this is to encourage women to seek out new information, weigh up alternatives, plan, strategise, and so on. The iPad is your friend.
2. Enhance a mother's feelings of control by altering her interpretation of breastfeeding. Essentially, someone is deemed to be in control when a desired outcome is dependent on her responses. I'm talking about self-determination here; success is dependent upon a mother's

actions, and being passive won't cut it.[179] Breastfeeding fits this bill in the vast majority of cases. Establish a correct latch and your baby will be able to feed effectively. Feed more often and you will provide more milk. Feed less often and you will produce less. Mothers need to see breastfeeding for what it really is – a time-honoured and predictable biological to-and-fro process.[180]

3.   During the antenatal period, empower mothers by supplying them with appropriate breastfeeding information containing accurate warnings about what to expect, together with pertinent reassurances. This 'emotional inoculation' to challenges reduces feelings of helplessness if those challenges subsequently materialise. Evidence from a number of laboratory experiments indicates that preparatory information, when accompanied by reassurance, can reduce the emotional impact of subsequent stressful or painful stimuli.[181] Interestingly, when this kind of information is given without reassurance, stress and pain tolerance decreases.[182] This explains why novice mothers told 'horror stories' by failed breastfeeders are at a distinct disadvantage. Indeed, it is seldom the process of breastfeeding itself that causes stress, but rather the view people take of it and the attention mothers give to those views.

4.   Encourage a mother to attribute her successes to herself – and indeed to reframe what she considers a success (perhaps each day of breastfeeding rather than a distant goal in the future). With a feeling of success comes a sense of control.

5.   Increase the predictability of a mother's personal, social and physical environment – yet another way to foster a maternal sense of control. Examples include encouraging safe co-sleeping, giving a mother access to telephone helplines, ensuring other family members support her desire to breastfeed, linking the mother to regular breastfeeding workshops, teaching techniques for discreet public breastfeeding if this is an issue for her, to name but a few.

6.   If you like a more systematic approach, focus a mother's efforts on three areas of control: behavioural, cognitive

and decisional.[183] *Behavioural control* involves 'directing action to the environment' to minimise a threatening event. For example, you could pacify potential milk supply fears by teaching mothers new skills (such as hand expression) and remind them of skills they already have (recognising infant hunger cues). *Cognitive control* means changing how a mother interprets threatening events, for instance, reinterpreting cluster feeding as an aid that boosts milk supply rather than an inconvenience or a sign of low milk supply. *Decisional control* is the ability to choose between various courses of action, like between positional holds such as cross-cradle vs football.

7. Talk up the efficiency and reliability of human lactation, encouraging women to trust their body's ability, even if this means encouraging them to fake confidence long enough for it to be established naturally. Supplement this approach by exposing mothers to breastfeeding success stories, countering the culture of failure in which many women find themselves immersed.[184] Increased maternal confidence means fewer maternal perceptions of breast milk insufficiency – and that's a fact![185]

8. Last, but absolutely not least, help mothers cultivate a sense of 'learned optimism', encouraging them to adjust their vision to see that they really do have control. In her landmark book *The Psychology of Control*, Ellen Langer described the reality of control as a linear process: 'People experience control as they master their internal (mental) or external environments – as they make the unfamiliar familiar'.[186] In a culture where successful breastfeeding is an alien concept, a mother cannot feel much control because it is unfamiliar. It is the job of breastfeeding advocates to help mothers exercise control by making the unfamiliar familiar. For instance, a mother's thoughts can be directed to appreciate the consistent pattern of outcomes she has already experienced – the regular sensation of let-down, the passage of meconium, wet and dirty nappies, infant alertness, achieving developmental milestones and so on. 'Ways of making the invisible visible have potential to increase women's confidence'.[187]

Since people tend to be motivated to see themselves as causal agents responsible for their own success, mothers are particularly receptive to the notion that sequential outcomes represent proof of their personal success – a cue signalling that breastfeeding is going well. Then a mother can appreciate that success and failure stem from purposeful rather than arbitrary acts. It is this very process of making the unfamiliar familiar that gives rise to the perception of control and the feeling of mastery.

## SELF-HANDICAPPING – TRYING NOT TO TRY

We humans not only instinctively seek to control processes like breastfeeding, we also seek to control the conduct of other human beings, especially how they respond to us. New mothers feel a heightened version of this drive – a sense of impending scrutiny, fuelled by responsibility. When one is responsible for an event, one is answerable for it. Gulp! Few variables are as important in our lives as our perceived moral status. Responsibility has a social function; it serves to channel admiration and criticism to appropriate destinations. It is therefore in the interest of mothers to pave the way for evading responsibility when failure seems likely. Some mothers do this by attempting to set the stage for failure before they even embark on their breastfeeding journey. Their goal is to fog the path of blame, so that possible causes of events (such as the mother's characteristics and capacities) become lost in the mist. In essence, a mother mitigates against uncomfortable feelings of scrutiny by influencing the way in which people come to assess her breastfeeding journey. This shady behaviour is commonly known as 'self-handicapping'. There are two methods of self-handicapping: 'behavioural' and 'claimed'.

### Behavioural Self-handicapping

Here, a mother actually makes breastfeeding harder for herself, fearing her ability to master it successfully. Then, when she does in fact fail, she can simply place the blame on the obstacles rather than placing it on herself. When applying this strategy, a mother actively searches for opportunities to latch onto an escape route. Strategies include preparing for breastfeeding to an inadequate degree; not putting in enough effort; constraining circumstances, such as putting baby to sleep in a different room or leaving him for prolonged periods; using inhibitory devices like dummies; seeking advice from people with a poor breastfeeding reputation, and so on. By focusing on failure, mothers disengage from the breastfeeding process – and therefore from success. It is as though there is something about success they would rather not know about (or do): the effort required, the authorities shunned, the body-image reframed, the culture ignored, the peer pressure defied.

A good example is the mother who shuns 99 percent of good advice that comes her way in favour of the 1 percent of bad advice. By following the health professional's recommendation to top-up with formula, for example, the mother decreases her chances of breastfeeding success. Then, if failure results, it is not necessarily because of poor ability or lack of commitment – the health professional can be faulted. Consider the doctor who suggests formula as the medically superior option; this scenario makes the mother feel better about her decision to formula-feed. Irresolute mothers prefer less breastfeeding-friendly health professionals to those who adhere to their professional remit by merely presenting the options without voicing a preference.[188] Mothers look to sources of authority and expertise to alleviate the burden of their difficult decision. They relinquish their difficult choices to others, thus neatly avoiding having to face the distress, harm and loss of face that would result from choosing wrongly.

Indeed, advice and information are threatening to the uncommitted breastfeeding mother. Having a wealth of information available implies that she should be able to make best use of it. Then she cannot use the excuse of ignorance. The availability of information and advice makes demands on her to be better, to do better. Consequently, self-handicapping mums actively avoid situations where information and advice will be given – a breastfeeding support group for example. This wilful ignorance is reflected in the often unconscious thought, 'I can't act on what I don't know'. And when advice is given, this mother makes herself aware of the general tenor of the information but avoids its details.

Another common example of behavioural self-handicapping in the breastfeeding context is the pregnant mother who purchases formula 'just in case'. Rather than a sensible precaution, this is a tell-tale sign of weak intentions. The reality is that there's really very little a mother needs for breastfeeding – Mother Nature has supplied her with the essentials. A tin of formula is nothing but superfluous. Yet, if an item is more readily available, you are more readily going to use it. For example, if you were in the middle of nowhere and had a splitting headache but no painkillers, you would have to develop strategies to help yourself deal with the pain. If you were at home and there were painkillers in the cupboard you'd be more likely to use them. Likewise, if you were about to go on a diet, it would be akin to self-sabotage to buy chocolate and fill your cupboard with it. Science explains why. The proximity to objects of desire can lead people to be disproportionately influenced by the anticipated rewards of immediate gratification rather than the risks of 'consummatory behavior': the unnecessary consumption of products. In one lab study, participants were given the choice of playing a game in which they risked time in the lab to win chocolate chip cookies. Participants who could see and smell the cookies while they made their decision were less sensitive to risk information than participants for whom the cookies were merely described.[189]

To illustrate behavioural self-handicapping in more depth, it helps to look at an inverse scenario. This tale involves another foodie lab experiment, this time involving cutesy preschoolers. In the infamous Stanford marshmallow experiment,[190] a series of studies were conducted in which a preschool child was offered the following choice: he could have a marshmallow immediately, or two marshmallows if he waited until the experimenter returned (after an absence of approximately 15 minutes). A tray of marshmallows was then placed on a table in front of the child and the experimenter left the room while video cameras recorded the child's reaction.

Many of the preschoolers failed the experiment, opting to eat a single marshmallow before the experimenter returned. But some were able to resist temptation, and the secret to their remarkable restraint was their ability to devise strategies. Some put their hands over their faces so they couldn't see the tray of delights in front of them. Others imagined playing with toys to avoid thinking of the food. Using such tricks, the children physically or mentally hid the treat, thus removing the option of eating it. Bless their socks.

Mothers attempting to breastfeed are faced with a similar temptation to these children – the temptation of formula. The ingrained nature of formula marketing and paraphernalia provides a cultural backdrop in which temptation is not only strong, but omnipresent. Unlike the resourceful preschoolers, the uncommitted mother does not actively seek to avoid temptation – and in the case of behavioural self-handicapping, may even court it. She may seek contact with pro-formula media rather than pro-breastfeeding influences, for instance by signing up to 'baby clubs' facilitated by formula companies in order to receive token free gifts. She may also seek counsel from friends and relatives with little or no breastfeeding experience. In this latter example, the mother passes off the decision of whether to breastfeed or not as an opportunity for other people to express an opinion. This way, she doesn't have to take responsibility for her decision, and the people she asks often enjoy giving advice.

### Claimed Self-handicapping – aka Malingering on the Road to Breastfeeding Cessation

The second way that mothers self-handicap is by coming up with justifications for their potential failure, so that if they do not succeed in breastfeeding, they can point to their excuses as the reasons for their failure. This is known as 'claimed self-handicapping',[191] or our friend the anticipatory excuse. For a mother attempting to breastfeed, an example would be the declaration that she is depressed or experiencing various physical and psychological symptoms. The mother seeks to escape from the pressure, expectation and responsibility of breastfeeding by hinting that she is no longer capable of success.

Other mothers develop an almost obsessive preoccupation with training their babies to feed from a bottle at a young age to ensure babe will be friendly with bottles in the future.[192] Some may jump at the chance to draw attention to their baby's fussiness and showcase it as proof that formula is necessary. No matter the scenario, they can frame it to this end: if baby is gaining weight slowly, then Mum's milk is insufficient. If baby is gaining weight fast, then Mum's milk will be insufficient to 'keep up'.[193]

Another common example of claimed self-handicapping is the scapegoat. Scapegoating is a form of 'victimage' – transferring the burden of blame to a 'vessel' other than the mother, thus declaring the mother herself as under attack. In other words, the mother alleges her behaviour was a response to the behaviour or attitudes of someone else. She relinquishes control to a scapegoat, and so shifts the locus of power – and the spotlight – away from herself and onto another source. The chosen scapegoat must not only be dissociated from the mother, but also plausibly responsible for the actions that led to the breastfeeding failure. An incompetent health professional or unsupportive relative is normally framed,[194] making the scapegoat the straw man of breastfeeding blame. The problem with scapegoating, of course, is that there's a high probability the mother will be labelled as 'easily led' or 'weak willed'. Many mothers are prepared to accept this as the 'least of evils' consequence. Which is less aversive to the mother – being seen as weak-willed or confronting unambiguous information that might confirm her own worst fears of maternal incompetence?

Then there is the heavyweight champion of claimed handicaps – the strategic presentation of medical symptoms indicating incapacity, otherwise known as 'I've got broken breasts'.[195] An impressive array of medical-sounding labels exists to enable a woman to describe herself as having an inability to breastfeed: insufficient glandular tissue, insufficient milk syndrome, lactation failure, failed lactogenesis, suckling failure, hypoplasia. Do we really need all these words to describe a largely fictional phenomenon? They don't even sound like words. Hypoplasia sounds like the noise a baby makes when it farts in the bath.

By claiming an inability to breastfeed, Mum increases the likelihood that when the self-detonated bomb of failure explodes, she can emerge from the debris integrity intact, safe in the knowledge that others will attribute her failure not to her own shortcomings, but to the debilitating impediment. Many sources have referred to not having enough milk as 'a Western problem'.[196] In sling-using communities where it's usual for babies to have unrestrained access to their mother's breasts all day, a physical inability to breastfeed is virtually unheard of. Nonetheless, once a mother has latched onto this desired escape route, the search is on for evidence to confirm it. Studies reveal that those intent on malingering will seek out evidence that supports the desired medical label while evidence that disconfirms it is ignored or given less weight.[197] Ironically, such malingering is unwittingly encouraged by health professionals. There exists an unyielding medical bias towards finding an ailment where there is reason to suspect that one may be present. So if, for whatever reason, baby is unsettled or weight gain has stalled, the apparent existence of a serious problem is taken for granted, rather than the usual culprits: a cold virus, a normal plateau, incorrectly calibrated weighing scales. It is, after all, far more culpable from a legal perspective to dismiss an ill patient than to mislabel a well one, particularly where children are involved.

Once a medical label has been successfully attached, mothers are rewarded for conforming to the role prescribed by their label. Some are given free prescription formula milk or the NHS's unfortunately named 'healthy start vouchers' so they can obtain a formula of their choosing free of charge. For some women, reward is simply the explicit reassurance given by a practitioner that the mother is doing well by switching to formula. Pity and attention are other noteworthy advantages. However, perhaps more importantly, the 'faulty' label reduces any (real or perceived) external pressure to breastfeed. Health professionals, friends and family ask fewer questions, offer less advice and may even avoid the topic of breastfeeding altogether. The consequence is a reduction in the mother's breastfeeding support network. This reduction has the added 'benefit' of arming the mother with a common retort to use at a later date: 'I wasn't given enough support'.

Here we see the mother as opportunist. Notice that her choice of impediment is strategic. For instance, if she wishes to sustain the impression that she can, at some future time, successfully breastfeed a subsequent child – and thus preserve a favourable future competency image – her handicap must be *time limited*, for example, pain. Of all medical complaints, pain is arguably the most subjective and therefore the easiest to feign.

Self-handicapping is particularly prevalent in breastfeeding because of mothers' heightened sensitivity to the shame and embarrassment of being seen to fail their children voluntarily. The more uncertain the mother is of her competence – and paradoxically, the more she *wants* to succeed at breastfeeding – the more likely she is to use self-handicapping. Mothers who self-handicap create an identity for themselves in their own mind. They reach out for impediments and create ceilings over their ability and potential to breastfeed. If a mother thinks it will only be possible for her to breastfeed for a few days, then that's exactly how long she's going to programme herself for. Self-handicapping mothers focus on their inadequacies and weaknesses as a covert way of lowering their own and their audience's expectations.[198] Of course, by indulging in this behaviour, they are ironically increasing the probability of failure. Indeed, this is sometimes the intention. Such mothers may complain dramatically about their impediment but – and here's the important part – they will show little interest in problem-solving. On the contrary, solutions become part of the problem. Helplessness is the desired image.[199] Once a mother has made the decision to quit, she will seek out information consonant with this future and avoid information that is dissonant with it. This results in what psychologist Kurt Lewin – often recognised as the 'founder of social psychology' – has called 'freezing of decisions'.[200] The mother's change of information-seeking behaviour means she finds it difficult to reverse her preference to quit once she has made the mental commitment.

Locked into her decision with a strategy in place, this mother will be eager to call attention to her breastfeeding struggles, and may even deliberately attract the attention of a breastfeeding specialist. However, much to the latter's frustration, a self-handicapping mother has no intention of seeking advice, let alone following it. Rather, she is looking for professional 'permission' to quit. If the specialist senses the mother's vibes and colludes – and many do – this adds credence to the decision the mother had made all along. But there's a dilemma for the mother: the more passionate and committed breastfeeding specialists have an annoying habit of trying to find and address breastfeeding problems. This aggravation leads to the mother adopting passive-receptive mannerisms. Examples include listening half-heartedly, shunning suggestions, neglecting to mention pertinent factors such as dummy use, agreeing to advice but not following it, and so on.

The aforementioned malingering behaviour of mothers is so omnipresent that it can be observed at baby groups and almost all maternal gatherings. The deceptive transaction between the mother and those present takes the guise of a psychological game. The mother begins by initiating what at first appears to be a civil adult conversation, 'I'm going to have to give up breastfeeding because I've got mastitis'. The other 'players' in the game (her peers) adopt a paternalistic attempted-rescue stance, offering solutions to the problem: 'Why don't you increase feeds?', 'Why not see a breastfeeding counsellor?', 'What about expressing?' At this point in the conversation, the deceptive mother can't help but regress into child-mode. Her replies begin with, 'Yes but...'. She asserts that she hasn't got the time to increase feeds, or to express, or to see a counsellor. Even if she has tried some of the solutions presented, she will object to them. The purpose of the game is not to get suggestions, but to reject them. The deceptive mother's behavioural switch from adult to child is a pivotal point in the game. If she is committed to the game, she can stand off her peers indefinitely, until they give up. The advantage of this game is that it massages the mother's ego by providing a form of reassurance. Naomi Stadlen alludes to this behaviour in her bestselling book, *What Mothers Do*:[201]

> 'Most of the time, what mothers seem to want from each other is compassion – without any advice. That's why their stories can sound harrowing. The harrowing quality is to elicit pity. A mother may often give a more one-sided picture than is truly the case. This is because the mother longs to be bathed in her listener's compassion. She has probably spent all morning being patient and compassionate towards her child, and craves some attention for herself. However, her harrowing story may make her listener feel so sorry for her that the listener feels pressured into helping her by giving her practical advice. This makes the first mother try harder to reassert her need for compassion by sounding even more harrowing, but that in turn pressures the listener harder to come up with some acceptable advice. Neither mother can understand why her efforts aren't working'.

### 'Oops, I Did It Again' – the Drawbacks of Self-handicapping

Not only does handicapping provide a self-protective function, it is also has self-promoting qualities. It allows a mother to preserve a sense of maternal esteem and competence in what is essentially a threatening situation in which she is being evaluated. If the mother *does* succeed at breastfeeding in spite of her handicap, she will be deemed all the more entitled to the accolades that success would ordinarily bring. Self-handicapping guarantees no blame for breastfeeding failure and enhanced credit, should a mother in fact succeed at nursing her baby. For 'I'll try' mothers with a shaky commitment to breastfeeding, self-handicapping creates a win-win scenario.

Or so one would think. But social psychology throws a spanner in the works, and that spanner is 'foreseeability'. Human nature means we hold people more responsible for unintended negative actions that were foreseeable compared to those that were unforeseeable.[202] If a mother has numerous children who she also failed to breastfeed, the issue of foreseeability is a blinding beacon shining a spotlight on her grimy facade. Even a faint whiff of self-handicapping can lead people to question her character.[203] Other people's knowledge of the mother's prior breastfeeding failure drains self-handicapping of much of its usefulness as a means of self-promotion. Consequently, first-time mothers (those with a 'blank slate') are more likely to apply self-handicapping than those with a 'lesser' reputation to protect.[204] Mothers who failed at breastfeeding in the past are significantly less likely to even bother pursuing it again. They make the past their default setting. In fact, previous breastfeeding experience is not just a minor influence over a mother's decision to breastfeed her current child, it has actually been found to be THE strongest predictive factor.[205]

### The Culture of Failure

Does self-handicapping lead to pessimism, or does pessimism lead to self-handicapping? The answer to this chicken and egg conundrum is that pessimism appears to be the starting point from which self-handicapping becomes a coping mechanism. Let me explain by referring to what I call the Culture of Failure.

First-time mothers, by their novice nature, are uncertain as to their personal capacity for breastfeeding success.[206] When this self-doubt is combined with an omnipresent cultural pessimism, the motivation for self-handicapping is amplified two-fold.

A widespread lack of confidence in breastfeeding is a contemporary endemic, creating pessimism, both collectively and individually. Once internalised, this collective belief tends to affect the individual.[207] Women live in a culture of failure in which the norm is to try and fail at breastfeeding. All females born into this culture are primed for failure. Because examples of breastfeeding failure are plentiful and readily available – indeed, omnipresent – women develop a 'social schema', an abstract and implicit set of hypotheses about how they think breastfeeding will turn out. Often, this is a distortion and over-simplification tenaciously held onto and resistant to change. Then, when women become mothers and encounter breastfeeding challenges of their own, their existing knowledge structures (that failure is common and unpreventable) help them to fill the gaps in their own pending experience and to make certain bridging assumptions (that their own failure is imminent).

You see, as social creatures, we largely repeat, reapply and reaffirm patterns that are already available to us. The constant presence and the ubiquity of breastfeeding failure makes it more difficult for women to conceive of anything else. When imagining what it will be like to breastfeed, a woman can only conjure up what she has seen in her modest experience – failure upon failure. She can easily visualise specific threats that can lead to her failure because she has heard these specifics from other women. In contrast, the alternative of success is diffuse and hard for her to visualise.

The powerful impact of our culture of failure on mothers' self-appraisals and expectations of themselves exerts a seductive influence on our decisions and actions. Often it creates a self-fulfilling prophecy in which a mother attaches a *false* definition to breastfeeding (failure is the default norm) from the very beginning of her motherhood journey. In turn, this sets up new patterns of behaviour that make the original false conception come *true*. Such a defeatist mindset has a marked effect on a woman's sense of mastery, which subsequently mediates how effectively she is able to deal with breastfeeding challenges. Once we expect to fail, we are likely to continue expecting to fail because we have a bias toward 'perceptual confirmation': we interpret behaviour that is actually ambiguous as consistent with our expectations. We misinterpret cues in our environment, assimilating the information in such a way as to comply with our expectation of failure. For example, we interpret the relative scarcity of stools from our growing breastfeeding baby as proof that she's starving (she's not); we see our deflated breasts as a sign of reduced milk production (they're not); we interpret the thimble-full of breast milk we managed to extract with a pump as evidence that our breasts have dried up (they haven't). Such subjective reality is of far more consequence in determining breastfeeding success than most people imagine. As psychologist Robert Merton observed back in 1948, the self-fulfilling prophecy perpetuates 'a reign of error'.[208] When a mum expects breastfeeding to fail, often she diverts energy into worrying and defensive strategies. Examples include introducing a bottle early on so that baby won't refuse one when breastfeeding inevitably fails, administering formula top-ups to guard against inadequate milk intake, using a nipple shield to prevent sore nipples, attempting to measure her supply with a breast pump and then getting stressed at the results, interpreting baby's fussiness as 'evidence' of poor breast milk supply without considering other causes, and so on. Ironically, these actions unwittingly sabotage a mother's supply of breast milk.

The mother's perceived likelihood of failure creates, for her, a public dilemma. Her decision to self-handicap reflects her attempt to avoid imminent unflattering evaluations of herself by others. Then the deception of self-handicapping feeds the culture of failure, and the cycle continues. The culture of failure is a culture of fatalism. As behavioural psychologist Mark Snyder put it, 'Social beliefs can and do create their own social reality'.[209] When you watch your husband building a flatpack bookcase, you know it will eventually fall apart. Likewise, when a mother attempts to breastfeed, most people – herself included – will invariably expect everything to collapse sooner or later. Whether the notion of impending failure is logically valid or statistically likely is of no concern. Rather, most people determine what is probable based on their prior experience of the world – the kinds of things they have (or haven't) observed before. While some mothers may be aware that their fear of failure is not necessarily accurate, they believe it is probabilistically accurate. This intrinsically human behavioural trait is called 'inductive reasoning' and has been famously explained by philosopher David Hume[210] using a much-quoted and fun analogy – how can you be sure that all swans are white if you have seen only a tiny fraction of all the swans that have ever existed? If we apply this analogy to breastfeeding, successful nursing mothers are black swans and failed nursing mothers are white swans. The black swans are lost in a sea of white swans to the degree that they are virtually invisible. Those pessimistic mothers about to embark on breastfeeding will find plenty of observational data to support their belief in their impending failure, and precious little to contradict it.

The culture of failure twinned with formula's 'paradox of control' (see page 57) has created a widespread perceived absence of control over breastfeeding. The effect on mothers is debilitating. Some find themselves so overwhelmed that they choose the course of action that seems most predictable – they opt out altogether. After all, individuals typically engage in tasks when they expect to be successful. You would not begin a marathon if you anticipated not being able to finish it. By turning straight to formula, women avoid the performance arena, and in doing so also avoid the harsh lights of the critics (both internal and external).[211]

### The Positive Deviant

'Women are like tea bags. You never know how strong
they are until you put them in hot water'.
Attributed to Eleanor Roosevelt

So far I've painted a pretty bleak picture – a set-up in which women's innate behavioural quirks work against breastfeeding. When we combine these psychological flaws with our culture of failure, you might be forgiven for thinking that breastfeeding had better just shut up shop. There's a black swan recession going on, and the future of lactation is surely doomed.

But wait. What about those black swans? Those mothers who, despite sharing the exact same gender, resources, education, marital status, age bracket, income, social structure and so on, defy their statistical destiny and instead go on to successfully breastfeed? How do these mothers manage to overcome the hardship barriers that other mothers cannot? This is where I introduce to you an amazing person: the Positive Deviant. The term 'positive deviant' first appeared in nutrition research in the 1970s and refers to the behaviour of individuals who triumph over scenarios of adversity in which most others fail:

'Positive Deviance is based on the observation that in every community there are certain individuals or groups whose uncommon behaviors and strategies enable them to find better solutions to problems than their peers, while having access to the same resources and facing similar or worse challenges'.[212]

In the breastfeeding domain, this interesting minority of mothers is able to override even visceral factors (see page 59). In an interview, one such deviant was quoted saying, 'If I had listened to myself, just from a physical standpoint, I would have breastfed for one week'.[213] Positive deviants recognise potential breastfeeding challenges but do not present them as legitimate reasons for quitting. Instead, they identify strategies that they would use to overcome them.[214] They seem to recognise, but not reject, the shackles of breastfeeding. They view their ability to overcome challenges as having self-esteem-boosting value in itself.

Yes, that's great, but *how* do these women do it? How do they reach levels of success that most women cannot? My view is radical: I argue that personality is key. Hold your fire. You see, we humans perceive, think and decide in a modular way. We are 'consequentialists', which means we anticipate and evaluate the consequences of available options, and then choose the one most likely to satisfy our true desires. This politically unpalatable statement is supported by a theory called 'goal framing'.[215] This says that individuals tend to pursue one of three sets of goals:

1. Hedonic goals – intended to enhance immediate pleasure.
2. Gain goals – pursued in order to accumulate resources.
3. Norms goals – designed to follow the social norms or conventions of the community.

When a mother frames her breastfeeding goals through the third set of goals, the 'normative view', she thinks of her family and friends first and her deliberations turn to what is better for the group.[216] Alternatively, the urge to pursue hedonic goals – where the focus is on the 'now'[217] – is most attractive when a mother is most concerned with her current situation. Conversely, the gain goals have appeal when a mother tries to improve her future resources, for instance in looking to increase her feeling of achievement or state of health.

Prioritisation is central to this thinking process. We cannot attend to all the 'goal dimensions' of a situation all at once – our attention is selective. A mother's internal values determine which particular goal comes into focus, since these values influence the extent to which each goal is 'cognitively accessible'. What is more important to her – being happy in the short-term present, being happy in the long-term future, or making others happy? I believe that successful breastfeeding mothers – positive deviants – share a common 'thinking strategy': they choose to pursue 'gain goals' and prioritise these over immediate gratification or social conformity. The prioritised goal then becomes the filter through which the mum views any breastfeeding challenges that arise. The mum sees an increase in her baby's and her own lifelong health resources as the option that provides greatest gain and so places it at the top of her preferences.

We might understand this as exercising delayed gratification. Her future health and the future health of her baby are at the foreground of the mother's attention, while immediate gratification and social influences serve as background influences, to which she is only secondarily attentive. Psychologists Edward McCaffery and Jonathan Baron have explained this thinking as 'a kind of tunnel vision in approaching problems and choices'.[218] Daniel Goleman, author of the best-selling book *Emotional Intelligence*,[219] called it 'the master aptitude' – an ability to marshal enthusiasm and confidence. I call it 'discriminative determination'. Mothers discriminate in favour of the goal that is most important to them and situate this goal in the foreground of their attention. Their determination and perseverance acts as a motivational force, helping to counteract negative health issues and tiredness. Studies have found that, for breastfeeding quitters 'Immediate family well-being is the overriding goal rather than theoretical longer term health benefits'.[220] In contrast, our positive deviant mum has framed breastfeeding in terms of future benefit. With her sights set on the future, she has greater motivation to overcome any difficulties and reach her goal. In one study, a positive deviant summed it up with this sentiment:

> 'No, I wanted it so much (laugh). Everything that looked like an obstacle, I got rid of it. For me, breastfeeding came first and everything else was secondary, so, I don't know what else could have stopped me from breastfeeding'.[221]

In fact, persistence is so much a part of the breastfeeding experience that some positive deviants have described persistence as 'a way of life'.[222] Accompanying persistence is another integral strand of positive deviant reasoning: focus on the baby. Positive deviant mums are infant-orientated. Take this explanation:

> 'There were so many times I thought of giving up. But I kept talking to myself, saying, "Well, you have to do this. It's going to get better. Think of him. It's good for him"'.[223]

While quitters focus on what quitting would do for them, positive deviants focus on what quitting would do for their baby. The acknowledgement that quitting seldom enriches infants may explain the powerful 'tunnel vision' of positive-deviant mothers. One study noted that 'the strength of the mother's conviction often was reflected in the guilt they experienced when they thought about stopping'.[224] Again in the words of a positive deviant:

> 'When he breastfeeds good, he looks like he's in heaven. He's just enjoying it so much. This is the ultimate. I don't know if you could get this feeling from a bottle. So all you have to do is look at this little face and think, "Don't be such a loser. Keep going"'.[225]

Psychology professor Daniel Stern, whose work I mentioned above (see page 52), has described a unique 'self-system' – what he calls 'the motherhood constellation'. This collection of self-perceptions emerges in positive deviants during pregnancy and may last for many months or even years. During it, 'The mother's self-sense becomes largely organised around the presence of her baby, its well-being, and their mutual connection'.[226] Stern refers to the attunement of the caregiver: the responsiveness of the mother to the child communicating his needs.

Do you recall earlier that I mentioned how mothers with a low sense of self-efficiency jump ship when the going gets tough (see page 59)? Well, positive deviants approach tough times in a reverse fashion. They trust in the power and process of nature. Because they regard breastfeeding as innate and normal, they tend to have a high sense of 'self-efficacy': a strong belief in their ability to succeed. They are more likely to feel that breastfeeding helps them establish their identity as a mother rather than it inhibiting other aspects of their identity.[227] They view impediments as surmountable – driving them to improve their skills and persevere. They stay the course in the face of challenges.

All sounds stellar, right? But one needs to note a very important fact: even if a mum enjoys strong self-efficiency, she will *always* flounder if she lacks intent. Intention and commitment are absolute prerequisites for breastfeeding success (I didn't just title this book *Breast Intentions* because it sounded snazzy you know!). As one study declared, 'Whilst there is a significant, direct relationship between self-efficacy and breastfeeding behaviour, it is not as strong as the mediated path through intentions'.[228]

So how do positive deviants keep their intentions on the straight and narrow? One way is to combine their belief in efficacy with an appreciation that the advantages of breastfeeding outweigh any temporary lifestyle encumbrances. This way of thinking takes a lot of determination and a lot of foresight – particularly because the future benefits are much less visually and mentally arresting than immediate benefits and social pressure. The costs of breastfeeding – in terms of autonomy, energy and time – are immediate and certain, whereas the rewards are delayed and uncertain. Yet positive deviants are able to subordinate both the immediate benefit of attending to visceral cues – like pain and tiredness – and also the disapproval of a social network. In short, the positive deviant mum is one tough cookie.

### Deception: a Tentative Conclusion

Kudos! That's a lot of information you've just processed. Let's seize this moment to recap on the A B C of Breastfeeding Fidelity:

A: *Attitude*
A mother's personal attitude to breastfeeding.

B: *Belief*
What she believes her friends and family think about her breastfeeding.

C: *Control*
Her perceived control over breastfeeding.

I hope by now you have more understanding of how a woman's breastfeeding success can be predicted simply by looking at these three factors.

But what if the factors contradict one another? A common example is the mother with the Attitude that breastfeeding is worthwhile but who simultaneously holds the Belief that her family and friends do not support her. This is a tricky one. She knows breastfeeding is what she wants to do, but part of her feels uneasy. She is in unexplored, unknown and perhaps even hostile territory. What's more, just as she is facing the challenge of learning motherhood, she comes across many different ideas about the qualities of a 'good mother' from within her social networks. These ideas may suggest that breastfeeding does not necessarily equate to being a 'good mother', particularly if, for example, the baby is unsettled and feeding frequently.[229] In this scenario, it is still possible to predict the odds of this mum's success by ascertaining the most salient factor – the mother's Attitude or the importance to her of her Belief that others do not concur. Her personality determines the winner.

## THREE TYPES OF SELF

Before we finish this chapter, I would like to share another – very simple – three-factor framework to help you understand the processes of the maternal mind in the context of infant feeding: I call it the Three Types of Self. You see, the most important and intimate relationship a mother will ever have is not with her baby, nor with her partner; it is with herself. A mother's relationship with herself involves feelings that fluctuate depending on her recent and past actions. Essentially, every one of us divides ourselves between three views of our self:

1. Our Desired Self.
2. Our Ought-to-be Self.
3. Our Actual Self.

Our Desired Self is the self that could conceivably be realistically attained. It is the self we long for. Abraham Maslow, the Godfather of social psychology, called this goal 'Self-Actualisation'.[230] It embodies a person's desire for self-fulfilment: namely, to become 'actualised' in what one potentially is, or to develop oneself as fully as possible – 'the desire to become more and more what one idiosyncratically is, to become everything that one is capable of becoming'.[222] When driven by her Desired Self, a mother seeks admiration only from her *internal* audience. We saw examples of how mothers attempt to stay true to their Desired Self when we explored their Attitude.

The Ought-to-be Self 'is the self full of our learned "shoulds" and "oughts". This self differs from our Desired Self in the sense that many of the "oughts" are not ours – they are the oughts of our culture, our community, our society – but deep down they are not ours'.[232] When driven by the Ought-to-be Self, a mother seeks admiration from an *external* audience. Pride follows when she feels she has lived up to some aspect of her Ought-to-be Self; guilt and shame if she fails. We saw examples of mothers' awareness of their Ought-to-be-Self when we explored their Beliefs about what others think. If a mother's attitude doesn't match the requirements of her Ought-to-be-Self, any attempts to enact the role will be ineffective and unconvincing. Such failure further reinforces her belief that she can't play that role. Resentment looms.

Finally, the Actual Self is how we perceive ourselves to be. Proverbial warts and all. It 'is the self that has failed in ways we often will not share with others. This is the private self. It holds the thoughts we wish we did not have, the acts we wish we had not done, our beliefs about our worth, our attractiveness, and so forth. It is the self of our secrets and our ambitions. It is the self that most try to change in some way or another at some point in their life – perhaps even perpetually'.[233] We saw mothers battling with their Actual Self when we read about their quest for Control. Self-handicapping behaviour, for instance, is a mother's form of internal control designed to sustain her Actual Self.

We will return to this framework throughout the book. It's important to note that the boundaries between the Three Types of Self are dynamic. So, when a mother internalises the standards of external audiences, the Ought-to-be Self spills over into the Desired Self. Indeed, we are rarely totally unconcerned with how others would judge us. Consequently, it is normal for a mum to be simultaneously concerned with external and internal audiences, as will later be painfully illustrated in the Excuses chapter. But first, let's explore a mother's vain quest to evade the ball and chain of her Ought-to-be Self as we explore that dark, bottomless pit – maternal guilt.

# 2

# GUILT

'Catholics have guilt and Jews have guilt, fine.
But mothers can trump them all'.

Attributed to Diane Lane

Guilt is the soundtrack to motherhood. Behind every baby, there's a mother plagued with the nagging suspicion that she is doing it all wrong. However, while some forms of guilt are actively encouraged in mothers, others are curiously off limits. Paediatrician Nancy Wright explains:

'As paediatricians, we do not hesitate to make our patient's parents feel guilty about having their children wear bicycle helmets, using car seats and seatbelts, and fencing in pools. We use guilt to help adult patients lose weight, exercise more, stop smoking, drinking alcohol and taking drugs, what is it about breastfeeding that makes guilt suddenly off limits?'

In this chapter I will attempt to answer this slippery question. In order to do so, I will have to dig to the core of maternal guilt to find out how it arises, why it arises and why we, as a culture, are so obsessed with it.

## RELIEF – THE SILENT EMOTION

Before we take a trip down the bottomless black hole of maternal guilt, it is important to recognise that not all women feel pure guilt immediately after quitting breastfeeding. Relief is a common consolation. In one survey, for instance, a massive majority (76 percent) of the mothers interviewed reported that upon abandoning breast in favour of formula, they felt relief and were 'pleased to find a solution that made things easier'.[234]

Anonymous surveys aside, every culture has 'feeling rules' which inform people that certain feelings in certain situations are inappropriate. In our culture, feelings of relief and even elation upon ending breastfeeding fall into this forbidden realm. While these feelings may indeed be natural and understandable – particularly if a mother was ambivalent about breastfeeding in the first place – they are deemed offensive. Instead, mothers are expected to display sorrow and painful regret upon the breakdown of their breastfeeding relationship. Our culture effectively encourages maternal deceit by raising the stakes. Failing to show the proper emotion in a given situation is to be accounted morally deficient, or even bordering on mentally ill.[235] When mothers experience joy at breaking up with breastfeeding, they are displaying what sociologists refer to as 'emotional deviance'.[236] They are not expressing the culturally prescribed emotional response. These mothers can end up feeling that they have fallen further from social grace than is actually the case. This leads, ironically, to a great sense of guilt and shame.

For most mothers, then, by 'solving' their breastfeeding problems via quitting, they create a longer standing and much more volatile problem: crippling guilt. After the mist of temporary relief has evaporated, mothers suffer the shockwaves that accompany an awakening to the permanent reality of their choice. Post-breastfeeding guilt is an intense mourning of maternal identity. For many mothers, the experience is unbearable. They are left in the ruins of an emotional bombsite, having to navigate a gaping quarry between intention and outcome. These sensations lead some mothers into a trap of chronic 'victimage'. Through their unsuccessful breastfeeding experience, they learn that the journey through motherhood is uncontrollable, that attempting to influence its path is futile, and hence they become passive recipients, dependent, at best, upon other people's advice.

At this point, it seems only fitting to hand over the mic to a mother who has been there – five times. Doris O'Connor is a mother of nine (Yup, you read correctly, NINE). Five of her children were formula-fed, the rest were breastfed. Here, she describes the bellowing narrative of guilt in her life:

'As a breastfeeding mum it can be easy to feel just like a milk machine and that is all baby wants you for. Everyone else can get a cuddle and the minute baby gets close to you, all baby wants is milk and will not settle until you feed him. You may be sore, you are probably leaking milk everywhere and well, it can all be rather undignified to start with. A far cry from the rose-tinted pictures of mum breastfeeding baby happily that you imagined! Rather than looking adoringly down on your newborn, you are probably busting for the loo, as you haven't managed to get off the settee for the last few hours!

I am deliberately painting a negative picture, because breastfeeding can be blooming hard work to start with, and that's when all is going well. Throw in a baby who is not latching well, thus causing mum to be in pain, mastitis, thrush, cracked nipples, etc. and it can be a relief to go over to the bottle. You often hear it don't you, I only started bonding with my baby once we had switched to formula and the pain stopped. I was dreading feeding him as it hurt so much....

I can relate to that, because I have been there, done that. It was a relief at the time; the regrets come later. When you raise your head out of its sleep-deprived state, when you "have your body back", when your baby is not in your arms constantly anymore, when those chubby hands are caressing a plastic bottle instead of your breast. When baby gets excited at the sound of the bottle lid coming off, rather then you lifting your top. When your baby simply doesn't smell like your baby anymore!

When you stand with your seriously ill baby on your shoulder and you look at a breastfeeding display in the children's ward, citing all the things that breastfeeding protects against, all the things that are making your baby so ill, and you know that you have failed that baby.

If only you had tried harder, the pain wasn't really that bad if only, if only, if only....'

## THE GUILT-TRIGGERING PROCESS

Here's a question to ponder: does guilt distort a mother's judgements of her failure or does it give them a purpose or value? Like most issues in psychology, the answer is complex. Once a mother's wish to end breastfeeding is gratified – and it does indeed come in gratifying form ('I now know exactly how much my baby is consuming; this gives me satisfaction and confidence') – she begins to take reality into account ('But now my baby is regurgitating more, so now can I cannot, in fact, know exactly how much she is consuming'). The mother experiences an emerging – sometimes subtle, often not-so-subtle – disillusionment with her choice. Undeniably, the story of breastfeeding cessation is a story of tragedy – forget Hamlet; in the climax of this story, the protagonist discovers, to her despair, that she had been chasing the wrong carrot of satisfaction. She believed that formula feeding would satisfy her – in the most fundamental sense she wanted, or believed she wanted – and in pursuit of it she denied her physiological birthright and that of her baby.

Guilt, by its very nature, is both an inward-directed and internally generated emotion. Contrary to popular perception, no one can 'make' someone else feel guilty. Guilt comes from within. It is a self-conscious and evaluative emotion. Charles Darwin used the phrase 'thinking of others, thinking about us' to make the point that guilt – and its cousins shame and embarrassment – are reliant on a person's sensitivity to the social drama of failure.[237]

So in the infant-feeding arena, how exactly does maternal guilt materialise? The existence and quality of a mother's guilt depends on how she frames her breastfeeding failure – or whether she can place a frame around it at all. When mothers fail at breastfeeding, they experience a range of emotions. These feelings can be split into two neat groups that I am going to call 'outcome dependent' and 'explanation dependent'. Outcome-dependent emotions refer to those primitive feelings and urges a mother experiences following breastfeeding failure: frustration and sadness, for example. In contrast, explanation-dependent emotions are influenced by a mother's specific explanations for breastfeeding failure.[238] So first, a mother may feel sad that she has failed (an outcome-dependent emotion), and then when she tries to make sense of how her failure occurred, she may feel guilt because she knows she was the prime causal agent in her failure (an explanation-dependent emotion). Thus, a mother's emotional response to failure is in fact *created* by her own explanation of it.[239]

Another way of explaining the internalised root of guilt is to revisit our friends from the previous chapter: the Three Types of Self (see page 88). Guilt wracks mothers because they feel accountable to their Desired Self. Remember the Desired Self? It's the self we long for; the type of person we want to be. The first step towards guilt is the mother's acceptance of a set of standards as part of the Desired Self; for our purposes, we'll call these 'breastfeeding goals'. In order for guilt to be triggered, the 'parent' part of her psyche (remember that guy, 'the ego'?) must internalise these goals, latching onto them as a benchmark to aim for: 'I really want to be successful at breastfeeding'. Then, when she fails at breastfeeding, the mother (or more specifically, the ego part of her personality) evaluates her performance and either holds herself responsible for it, or holds herself not responsible. If she concludes that she is not responsible, her evaluation of her performance ceases. However, if she evaluates herself as responsible, she can then evaluate her performance as successful or unsuccessful in relation to her breastfeeding goals. If she deems herself responsible for failing to meet her goals, guilt materialises.

Guilt is responsibility with a magnifying glass. A mother's internal monitoring process, governed by the ego, reflects and is guided by her personal and moral values. By failing to breastfeed, a mother has not violated normative standards (indeed, in our society, failure is expected). Rather, guilt occurs because she has violated personal standards.[240] She feels guilty precisely because she has internalised the standard of Breast is Best. She has accepted the validity of breastfeeding and conceptualised it as the preferred method of infant nourishment. In other words, what a mother defines as breastfeeding 'success' or 'failure' resides within her. It is based on her own subjectively fashioned breastfeeding goals.

Guilt – and indeed pride – are emotional states evoked by the ego's internal monitoring process. The paradox of mothers' guilt is that its intensity directly correlates with the degree of positive concern the mother has for breastfeeding; on her attachment to it. By 'attachment', I mean her binding emotional investment in breastfeeding. This includes the extent to which she projected attributes from breastfeeding to her Desired Self. For many mothers, breastfeeding failure means loss of a way of life, loss of shared understanding with others, and loss of a valued sense of self. In a way, it heralds an identity crisis because attachments that make up the self have been broken. By failing to reach her breastfeeding goals, a mother loses more than her relationship with nursing; she also loses the part of her identity reflected by this relationship. She's lost her mutuality with other breastfeeders, she's lost her private and public role as a nursing mother, she's lost breastfeeding as a source of affirmation, and she's lost the projected future she had envisioned for herself. It's not surprising, then, that breastfeeding failure shakes or shatters a mother's sense of self as well as the structure of her everyday life.

Mothers who do not meet their breastfeeding goals describe feelings of failure and a morphing from 'good mother' to 'bad mother'.[241] This guilt is particularly disturbing to mothers in part because it calls into question not only their confidence in their bodies, but how confident they feel about mothering in its entirety. Breastfeeding failure gives mothers a stark glimpse into the persistent possibility of them failing at other maternal acts, too.

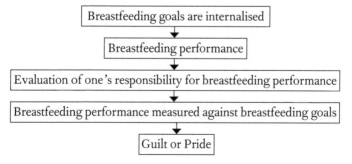

*Figure 2: Breastfeeding Goals and Performance*

A mother's internalised breastfeeding goals are the initial source – the seedling – of her guilt. To use another metaphor, maternal guilt is the phoenix that emerges from the ashes of unmet personal goals. As philosopher Robert Solomon explained in his book *True to Our Feelings: What Our Emotions Are Really Telling Us*, guilt:

> 'Because it is self-imposed, it is by its very nature taken to heart. One can to a considerable extent shrug off other people's criticism and even their contempt, but one cannot shrug off one's own'.[242]

Guilt is a true sentiment of a mother's moral compass enlightened by reason, the natural outcome of regret. In other words: guilt proves that mothers conduct their mothering through a moral lens. Guilt signals to mothers not only that they have failed to complete their optimum reproductive cycle but also – and perhaps crucially – that they recognise that breast really is best.[243] Emma Kwasnica, founder of the Human Milk 4 Human Babies Global Network, concurs:

> 'Guilt is a very good thing! It causes us to re-evaluate our position – lets us know when we are no longer in line with our own principles, our core values. It tells us that something is off, and motivates us to change whatever it is we're doing. In other words, guilt makes us uncomfortable for very good reason!
>
> Rather than blaming others for making us 'feel guilty', we really need to look within ourselves for answers, and stop deflecting our own issues away from ourselves – stop projecting our issues onto others. We must be 100 percent accountable for our own feelings. We need to OWN them. Because they are no one else's but our own.'

For failed breastfeeding mothers, guilt is tied to feelings of disappointment, failure, defeat and helplessness. It triggers and unsettles. In a sense, guilt is aggression turned against the self. Our friend Freud called this self-harming behaviour 'moral masochism'.[244] It is perhaps unsurprising that stopping breastfeeding increases a mother's risk of developing anxiety and depression.[245] Breastfeeding is a relationship that is biologically expected. When a woman does not experience that relationship, or when the relationship is cut short prematurely, she experiences a loss. Like at the end of any relationship, she will grieve for it. Interestingly, grief is a highly gendered emotion. Women tend to experience significantly higher levels of anxiety, sadness and anger upon experiencing a loss.[246] Dr Carlos González, a Spanish paediatrician, has witnessed his fair share of post-breastfeeding maternal turmoil, which he has described as:

> '...a sort of mourning process, similar (though less intense of course) to when a loved one dies.... Unfortunately, our society doesn't seem to understand this sort of suffering. Well-meaning people insist on denying it, eliminating it, blanking it out'.[247]

When you think about it, it's hardly surprising that 'society' (I use the term to mean our social consciousness as projected via media and culture) should downplay maternal guilt. Guilt is a narcissistic emotion. It's impossible to feel the sort of overwhelming, gnawing, tormenting displeasure that some formula-feeding mothers experience without having a self-indulgent interest in oneself. So preoccupied is this mother with what others think that she is almost living life as if she were a celebrity, feeling forever watched by others. By dwelling on guilt – sometimes even marinating in it – a mother can easily lock herself into a limited, self-centred mindset. Such a mindset – a preoccupied concern for oneself – is not a value proudly developed in girls and women, and it is particularly frowned upon in mothers.

Consequently, common stratagems of the guilt-stricken mother range from camouflage to hermit-like isolation. She may avoid public baby groups, feed in out-of-view locations, order formula online or send someone else to the store. To conceal her failure from the public eye, special timing is required. She 'lives on a bungee cord', staying close to places where she can discreetly feed. Travel is restricted to the distance that can be safely traversed in the interval between feeds. This mother's 'bungee cord' is only as long as that interval. When feeding time draws near once again, she springs back to the safety of her HQ.[248] In one study, a formula-feeding mum admitted:

> 'When I went to the clinic to get him weighed I used to hide the bottle in my bag and if there was no-one there then I'd give him a quick sip before and then if someone came, if I could hear them coming up the stairs, I'd put the bottle away. I think now why didn't I just say "I'm bottle-feeding and I'm proud", but no'.[249]

Some mothers even resort to leaving their baby home with someone else so as to appear childless.[250]

But why do women hide if their guilt is not triggered by external sources, but by internal ones? Who is the mother hiding from? The answer to this question reveals another idiosyncratic complexity of maternal guilt: its dual nature. Maternal guilt often features elements of both self-control and social-control. Recall the Ought-to-be Self (see page 88)? That's the part of our personality that reflects our conscious awareness of other people's standards. When the Ought-to-be-Self is absorbed by the Desired Self, Mum becomes concerned with both internal and external judgements of her failure.[251] Rather than seeking approval, mothers in this position – particularly those in the early throws of formula feeding – seek merely to avoid disproval. They spend significant chunks of their time hiding away like social lepers.

So although the Desired Self is the root cause of guilt, its power can be supplemented by the Ought-to-be Self, providing both are in sync, sharing the same standards. In other words, the self-consciousness of a mother's guilt is self-imposed. Back in 1902, American sociologist Charles Cooley[252] identified that a person's 'self-idea' develops through an inherently social lens, the driving force being a preoccupation with how others see us. The process has three major elements: imagining how we appear to our peers; imagining our peer's judgement of that appearance; and the resulting 'self-feeling', such as pride or mortification. In essence, we develop our self through the *imagined* judgements of others. When a mother feels self-conscious guilt about her failure to breastfed, the feeling is not generated merely by the mechanical reflection of herself, but by an 'imputed sentiment' – the imagined effect of this reflection on someone else's mind.

## ADDICTED TO GUILT

By now, you'll have gathered that guilt comes from within a mother herself and that her fear of social evaluation is largely projected from within her own mind. The phrase attributed to Eleanor Roosevelt, 'No one can make you feel inferior without your consent', is particularly apt in this context. But why is guilt – this uncomfortable, often painful emotion – self-generated? Remember, we humans live by the principle of hedonism: we seek pleasure and avoid pain. So why do mothers wallow in a painful emotion? The answer is fascinating: they create and cling to guilty feelings because guilt is useful. I would even go as far as to say that guilt is *rewarding*.

Recall the previous chapter? We found that a 'fashioned impediment' (such as the claim to have faulty breasts, depression or a sick baby) can be used to obtain advantages from the external world (see page 74). These include evoking pity, sympathy, amnesty, attention and privileges. The invention and reward process is called 'secondary gain'[253] and plays an integral role in mothers' addiction to guilt. After failing to breastfeed, a mother is cast into a grieving role, and her friends, family and even health professionals assume roles that complement this script. Facts and home truths are curtailed and sharply controlled.

Indeed, according to what social psychology scholars call 'constructivist theory',[254] emotions should be interpreted in terms of the social functions they serve. Feeling guilty actually serves a purpose for a failed breastfeeding mother. She may even feel unconsciously pleased with herself for feeling guilty. It means she can talk about herself and how she feels for hours. Because that's what guilt is about: her. It's a way of focusing on herself that doesn't feel self-indulgent because she's shining a light on the shameful and disparaging parts of her psyche. It's sort of a back-handed compliment because the fact she feel guilty means she cares, so she can lay claim to being a decent person.[255] The gratification she gains from occupying a morally elevated state makes guilty feelings rewarding, keeping them at the forefront of her mind. 'He who despises himself...' wrote the philosopher Nietzsche, '...thereby esteems himself as the despiser'.[256] Guilt permits – nigh encourages – a mother to wallow in self-pity. It sanctions a preoccupation with the self that in any other context would be deemed egocentric. Some mothers get caught up in this largely unconscious pride in feeling guilty, thus prolonging their guilt rather than discharging it.[257]

## A WORD ABOUT SHAME

Those rare evolutionary anomalies – women unable to breastfeed due to genuine anatomical issues – often cite guilt as a consequence of their predicament. However it is more likely that what they are actually feeling is 'shame'. It's easy to see why guilt and shame often get mixed up; they share many characteristics. But their defining factors are distinctive, and this distinction is particularly important when it comes to breastfeeding failure. Shame results when failure is involuntary. Guilt results when failure is voluntary – an act of choice. Guilt is triggered when our failure is attributed to internal controllable causes, for instance lack of effort. Thus, for true guilt to occur, Mum must have had a genuine feeling of choice. Guilt is associated with lack of effort; shame with lack of aptitude. Guilt springs from controllable causes; shame from uncontrollable ones.

In the context of breastfeeding failure, guilt springs from a mother's painful awareness of betraying her baby's trust and even more so from the self-betrayal of giving up on her own desire. Essentially, guilt is provoked by an internalised awareness of one's unfulfilled potential. The self turns towards the self, evaluating and passing judgement. Shame, on the other hand, is linked to a feeling of inferiority. Experiences of shame 'are experiences of exposure, exposure of peculiarly sensitive, intimate, vulnerable aspects of the self'.[258] Breastfeeding failure cannot be kept private. It places a very intimate part of a mother's physical character on the public stage. It is exposure to oneself that lies at the heart of shame. Shame is 'essentially rage turned against the self'.[259]

## REGRET – THE PERPETUAL CAROUSEL

'The problem with learning from living is that living is like riding a train while facing backward. That is, we see reality only after it has passed us by'.

Friedrich Nietzsche

I like to picture regret as a close cousin of guilt and shame. It involves tension and a sense of remorse, and is the feeling that overshadows lost attachments. A formula-feeding mother experiences regret when she realises her infant-feeding experience could have been more positive had better choices been made. For her, breastfeeding failure becomes part of her past, a past that intrudes into the future. Regretful guilt is a haunting cloud that hovers over a mother for months, even years, whispering the words 'if only'.

Remember the 'visceral factors' we discussed in the previous chapter? This theory explains why physiological feelings such as pain and exhaustion can literally warp a mother's mind, turning her from a logical shrew into a morally inept weakling obsessed with instant gratification (see page 59). Well, those visceral factors have one last masochistic blow to deal. As time passes, people forget the degree of influence visceral factors had on their past behaviour. Then, as a result, the mother who jumped ship and embraced formula in her darkest hour will feel quite perplexed and confused over her 'decision'.[260] Her failure to recall the sources of her compulsion intensify the disabling effects of the guilt. Regret provokes repetitive mental hypotheses about how different the outcome would have been if only she had made different choices. If only she had phoned a lactation consultant, if only she had pumped more often, if only she had slept with the baby.

In this sense, regret is a plague of modern civilisation. You see, as a society we are only just beginning to understand the astonishing interconnectiveness of breastfeeding with the physiological, psychological, economic and environmental well-being of the human race.[261] We are on the threshold of understanding that the choices we make today can have startling effects years from now. By giving up breastfeeding, the quitting mother gives up the positive benefits associated with that choice and accepts the negative features associated with formula. For instance, biochemistry studies have strongly suggested that just one bottle of formula is enough to cause irreversible damage to the lining of a baby's gut. This damage has implications for the health and longevity of a baby's immune system.[262] Even mothers ignorant of such research have an enduring, albeit vague, understanding of the harm caused by formula use: health promotion materials speak of allergies, ear infections and predisposition to obesity. The notion of irreparable injury gives chronic maternal guilt an energy source.

This is where we begin to understand why guilt – and its close cousin regret – are the lifeblood of the post-breastfeeding maternal psyche. Firstly, Mum is helpless to reverse the damage done; atonement is impossible. Her baby has been deprived of breast milk. Job done. Psychologists call this particular brand of guilt 'maladaptive guilt'.[263] Secondly, women are predisposed to spend more time brooding about negative feelings than men.[264] This is what I mean by regret as the 'perpetual carousel'. Mothers caught up in it report a nagging focus on or preoccupation with their breastfeeding failure. They relive the experience that led to their failure over and over in their thoughts, wishing they could somehow undo the damage (perceived or actual). They lose themselves in counterfactual thinking, imagining how events might have unfolded if some aspects of the situation or their actions had been different.

Another reason why guilt and regret encapsulate mothers' post-breastfeeding emotional experience is, quite frankly, because mothers are predisposed to them. Guilt and regret are feminine vulnerabilities. Women feel a moral imperative to care for others, and so are inclined to rely more heavily than men on an ethic of care when they reason about moral dilemmas.[265] Not surprisingly then, compared to males, females of all ages report a greater propensity to feelings of 'dysphoric' self-consciousness, such as shame, embarrassment and guilt.[266] Furthermore, because the marriage between breastfeeding and femininity is undeniable, these mothers feel inadequate as women, too. Failure to breastfeed arouses in women deep feelings of failed attachment and failed responsibility. Feminist scholars Susie Orbach and Luise Eichenbaum have examined how women's sense of self is dependent on their connections with others – in other words, how a woman's subjectivity is *relational*:

> 'She has known herself in connection to, in the service of and for, others. She has no experience of an identity apart from this. Her connection to her child, like any other intimate connection, contains a crucial piece of her psychological selfhood'.[267]

Mothers know themselves as mothers through their attachments to their babies. A mother's breastfeeding failure is marked not only by failure to meet her baby's physiological and psychological need for connection, but also by her failure to meet *her own* physiological and psychological need for connection. She has failed her baby and she has failed herself.

A mother's post-breastfeeding regret varies in length, frequency and intensity. Its ending is often unpredictable and may never occur. Although the regret tends not to be transitory, transitory feelings are part of it. A mother's experience of regret is interwoven with an eclectic range of emotions: sadness, grief, numbness, sorrow, anxiety, fear, anger and depression. From time to time it is punctuated with moments of envy, self-pity, relief and shame. It is a journey that is seldom linear; it ebbs and flows, re-emerging and flooding the mother again and again. Typically, sorrow, sadness and depression are most intense in the weeks and months after cessation of nursing, with feelings of anxiety and sorrow diluting over time. After a while, what were once long periods of painful dwelling and pining become momentary pangs of grief.

What about those mothers who publicise formula feeding as a liberated choice? The mother who openly chants about how 'easy' and 'convenient' it is? Perhaps she is one of the mothers who even decided to formula feed from the very start – and there are plenty: 25 percent of mothers never attempt to initiate breastfeeding.[268] Well, these mothers are digging themselves a grave of isolation. They quite often experience what is known in the psychoanalytic business as 'disenfranchised grief'.[269] This is the black sheep of maternal emotional experience. It is grief that cannot be publicly expressed but is nonetheless privately experienced. Because she is seen to have made the decision to formula feed by choice – and is seen to be content with it – a mother is deemed to have no moral or social 'right' to feel grief. Her grief remains silent, obscure and unsupported. It is, in a word, disenfranchised. This breed of sorrow is particularly unforgiving in that it limits the possibilities a mother has for obtaining support. As her grief is seen to lack legitimacy, it goes unrecognised and unsanctioned by others.

## A MOTHER'S ANTIDOTE TO GUILT – REALITY NEGOTIATION

Our self-identities are anchored in what we do. Our understanding of who we are rests on the existence of integrity and coherence between our actions on the one hand, and our belief system on the other. Through successful breastfeeding, a woman grows more confident in her ability to be a mother. Failure, unsurprisingly, has the reverse effect. Because most of us have a positive self-image, the blow is hard to stomach when we behave in a way we deem to be incompetent, immoral or irrational. Thus, failure to breastfeed creates inconsistency between a mother's positive concept of herself ('I'm a good mum') and her behaviour ('but I didn't breastfeed'). She starts thinking of the negative aspects of formula feeding and the positive aspects of breastfeeding. This triggers major butt hurt because they are dissonant with her decision. The mother's actions produced adverse consequences. That wasn't part of the plan when she set out to be a good mother.

Feeling personally responsible for producing foreseeable aversive consequences has been referred to as the *New Look*[270] version of 'cognitive dissonance'.[271] Cognitive dissonance is a fancy term psychologists use to describe the painful feeling of having to accept responsibility incompatible with your idea of who you are. It is characterised by unbearable inner conflict. On account of being a major pain in the psyche, guilt-induced cognitive dissonance is something mothers crave false solutions to; it lures them into radical inward and outward deceptions. We'll investigate some of the moves in this mental gymnasium in the next chapter: Excuses. But for now, let's focus on one particular cognitive strategy specifically triggered by guilt, a technique called 'Reality Negotiation'.[272] Mothers hold a PhD in it.

So what is reality negotiation, and how does the process work? To understand, we need to look again at 'maternal self-concept'. Most women have an idea of themselves as competent, or at least loving, mothers. The failure to breastfeed seemingly contradicts this important self-image. To stop their self-esteem from being eroded, mothers must sustain the positive image upon which they have built their personal theory of themselves. They must find a way to assimilate their breastfeeding failure into a positive view of themselves.[273] Yet, short of re-lactation, a mother can't rewind time and recapture the breastfeeding relationship she has thrown away. So in an attempt to reassure herself that she is 'still a good mum', she needs to engage in some mental trickery. There are several ways she can do this.

Some mothers remind themselves of other ways in which they have met the 'good mum' standard – be it cooking skills, co-sleeping, staying at home or whatever. A prominent example is the formula-feeding mother who appeals to one particular cultural value that just happens to be compatible with her feeding choice.[274] It's the tantalisingly feminist notion of 'shared parenting':[275] 'I'm a good mum because, through bottle-feeding, I encourage my partner to bond with the baby'.

By diverting attention to her positive attributes, the reality-negotiation process slows down the rate at which a mother has to adapt to her breastfeeding failure, and in doing so, softens the blow.[276] However, because attributes such as cooking, co-sleeping et al are irrelevant to her failure, they serve merely as temporary distractions. Indeed, a focus on these perceived positive aspects of her mothering ironically frames her failure to breastfeed as a discrepancy. This in turn *exacerbates* her guilt. The guilt returns with a magnitude even greater than before.[277]

Another way mothers try (often in vain) to re-conceptualise their reality in order to offset guilt is to re-frame breastfeeding success as something above the normal standard of childcare – on a par with serving organic food or providing a private education. Formula feeding is then awarded the 'default' position. In doing so, mothers direct their attention to outcomes: the decision was good if it produced good outcomes; it was bad if it produced bad outcomes. Mum views the *visible* outcomes of formula feeding to be an unambiguous way of determining the quality of the decision to formula feed. If she sees no visible harm to her child, she concludes that formula feeding was a good choice. Alternatively, if some evidence of harm is present (allergies for example), she will solve this cognitive dissonance by either ignoring symptoms or by attributing them to other causes. The logical flaw in this reasoning is obvious: when a formula-fed baby grows into a toddler with no obvious health issues, is his mother's decision to formula feed now a 'good' one because the resulting outcome appears to be neutral? Clearly not – because of the probabilities involved, the decision to take the gamble was foolish regardless of the outcome. Yet the process of reality negotiation pushes logic to its limits.

Another place we see widespread 'reality negotiation' is in the evolving semantics mothers adopt in their everyday speech. To explain, let me introduce you to a linguistic process that has aptly been called 'the euphemism treadmill'.[278] A euphemism is a bland, inoffensive and often misleading term for things the user wishes to dissimulate or downplay. Examples of euphemisms in contemporary language include 'big-boned' instead of 'fat', 'sanitation engineer' instead of 'garbage man' and 'sleep together' instead of 'have sex'. Each new euphemism soon becomes tainted by what it refers to, so a new euphemism must be invented to take its place. The infant-feeding dilemma is a textbook case: 'artificial feeding' (feeding a feigned substance) has become 'formula feeding' (feeding a synthetic substance), which has morphed into 'bottle feeding' (feeding via a bottle, the contents of which could be formula or breast milk). It seems that mothers are running from the negative connotations of words just to re-establish the association and then have to keep on running. The latest 'bottle-feeding' euphemism seeks to remove stigma altogether by lumping formula feeders and pumping breastfeeders together under the same umbrella, presupposing a faux moral solidarity.

The reframing process reminds me of Aesop's fable 'The Fox and the Grapes'; perhaps you read it at school. After trying in vain to reach some grapes hanging from a tall vine, the fox gives up and wanders away muttering, 'They were probably sour anyway'. Like the bitter fox, mothers lessen the negativity of their breastfeeding failure by asserting that breastfeeding is not important after all. In essence, breastfeeding is analogous with sour grapes. Nifty, huh? In other words, a mother may not have wanted to quit – it wasn't her plan – but now she has, breastfeeding wasn't that special anyway. The author of one study called the reality-negotiation game of guilt-stricken failed breastfeeders 'deconstructing best'. The study concluded that many women renegotiate their initial attitude that, 'It's really best to breastfeed', replacing it with the purposively evasive, 'Everybody's best is different'.[279] It is as if mothers engage in post-hoc re-evaluations of their breastfeeding failure along the lines of, 'Well it didn't work out too bad in the end', adding a rose-tinted gloss to their predicament. This bias has implications for any improvement in future breastfeeding experience. If mothers persuade themselves to be more or less content with the way formula feeding has turned out, they will be less likely to breastfeed future offspring.[280]

In this way, the reality-negotiation process represents a type of psychological Lego play-set. Mum dismantles the self that dissatisfies her and rebuilds a new, more palatable self. She may try different combinations until she finds the easiest 'model' to assimilate into her personality and circumstances. The revised self-image that results from this process is a 'negotiated reality'.

The beating heart of reality negotiation is denial. For the

strategy to succeed, the mother, quite literally, has to deny reality. Then denial creates a hole that needs to be filled. For example, when a mother denies her personal mis-judgement ('I decided not to nurse my baby on demand despite knowing it was preferable') she necessitates a projection onto someone else – a midwife or health visitor, for example ('I was following their advice'). Denial and projection go hand in hand – the negation of reality and the creation of a new reality. The process of denial makes guilty feelings even more complex. Mum's denial works as a defence mechanism, attempting to 'bypass' feelings of guilt. It does not obliterate the mother's recognition of her failure, but appears to prevent the development of full-blown guilt.[281]

We see even more denial when mothers attempt to protect their newly negotiated reality. Many avoid contact with pro-breastfeeding people and literature wherever possible, adopting a fingers-in-the-ears 'la-la-la, I'm not listening' stance. To such a mother, the enemy is anything that arouses her guilt-stricken anguish. So she associates only with fellow formula feeders and those sympathetic to her cause, acquiring psychological reinforcement in numbers. She seeks the affirmation of like-minded others in order to make the fragile morality of her choice seem more robust. The unfortunate knock-on effect of this social engineering is that she becomes willfully ignorant of breastfeeding facts. This in turn sabotages her chances of successfully breastfeeding in the future.

## THE INCONVENIENCE OF REALITY

You may be thinking that this reality-negotiation lark sounds useful, in a self-pacifying sense – a formula feeder's Get Out of Jail Free card. Alas, every rose has its thorn. When dabbling in reality negotiation, a mother must also keep in touch with external reality. She has to take into account just how far she can be economical with the truth before being labelled 'deluded'. A mother's negotiated reality must reflect a biased compromise between fantasy and reality.

Alongside a mother's subjectivism sits an objective response to the question of what constitutes breastfeeding success and failure: cultural expectations. These expectations are informed, for instance, by government guidelines. In the UK, the National Health Service recommends exclusive breastfeeding for six months,[282] and then is largely mute on the issue of so-called extended breastfeeding. In the US, the Department of Health and Human Services recommends that mothers breastfeed for at least 12 months,[283] with exclusive breastfeeding for the first six months. Meanwhile, the World Health Organization encourages both developing and developed nations to breastfeed for at least 24 months.

Such clear guidelines are bad news for the failed breastfeeder. Her reality-negotiation process must operate within the constraints of external reality (defined by such sources).[284] The clearer the standard to which a mother is expected to perform, and the more influential the source, the more she will feel that others perceive her failure as unacceptable.[285] In the aftermath of breastfeeding failure, the best a mother can hope for is a compromise between how she wants to view herself and what other people will believe. Negotiating reality enables her to pull her self-image closer to her Desired Self (an identity that exceeds her Actual Self), but not to stretch the imagination to breaking point.

Accompanying reality negotiation is another psychological 'game' that operates within the limits of veracity: the popular maternal sport of 'excuse-making', the focus of the next chapter. Like reality negotiation, excuse-making attempts to rewrite breastfeeding failure, turning it into something more socially palatable. Unlike reality negotiation, however, excuse-making is primarily concerned with appeasing not a mother's internal audience, but her external one – other people. What's the driving force? Manipulation.

# 3

# EXCUSES

'If it is important to you, you will find a way.
If not, you will find an excuse'.

Attributed to Emanuel James Rohn[286]

If mothers could be relied upon to give wholly honest accounts of why they failed to breastfeed, they would be the only truly authoritative source of breastfeeding statistics. There are, however, reasons to regard a mother's own view of her behaviour with some caution. She quite often engages in what social psychologists call 'impression management'. Studies have shown that failed breastfeeders regularly cite fictitious reasons for their failure.[287] They would prefer others to think, 'She tried her best, she's not to blame', rather than, 'She failed because she was uncommitted'. On the basis of breastfeeding failure alone, either of these interpretations is plausible. However, if the mother in question is skilful in describing her failure to others, people should draw the conclusion she desires. The mother might, for instance, mention that she had mastitis, that her baby had a poor latch, that she consulted numerous health professionals, or that her breasts were never engorged. In a hundred little ways, people can be influenced to conclude what the mother wants them to conclude.

The fact that infant feeding is understood as a 'choice' makes mothers' defensive compulsion to make excuses even more potent. Because breastfeeding is the epitome of personal involvement, the drive to defend oneself upon quitting is understandable: the greater the self-involvement implied by an act and the smaller the external justification for that act, the greater and more powerful the drive for self-justification.[288] Likewise, the more feminine an act, the more women feel inclined to make excuses in the event of failure.[289] Unlike other serious roles in life, mothering seems to be characterised by changeability and negotiation. Problematic maternal performances – like breastfeeding failure – can be retrospectively reconfigured and redefined through excuse-making. As you are about to see, a mother's tongue is quite a handy tool.

In our culture, we haven't exactly mastered the humble skill of saying 'I fucked up'. This flaw is startling – particularly in the breastfeeding context, given the ubiquity of failure. If there's one thing I've learned from my intimate connections with mothers,[290] it's never, ever to question a formula feeder. Nothing is her fault; rather, it is the fault of society, the health visitor, the bogey-man. The choice to formula feed was made not by mothers, but by their poor familial support network, uncooperative breasts and the assorted banana skins placed ready to trip them up. Formula feeders find it impossible to answer the question, 'How are you feeding your baby?' without the defensive postscript of self-justification. Excuses enable mothers to throw a bridge between the promised and the performed.

Asking a mother why she bottle feeds is akin to opening Pandora's Box. You never know precisely what you will find, but you can be sure it will unleash demons, fables of great illness and unthinkable psychiatric toll. The question, quite simply, bursts a mother's emotional floodgates. The way mothers explain their behaviour is very telling of the self-serving psychological mechanisms at play: mothers who fail at breastfeeding are more likely to attribute their failure to external sources, such as duress or luck, while mothers who are successful at breastfeeding are more likely to attribute their success to internal sources, such as ability or effort.[291] The rationale behind these framing strategies is protecting or bolstering maternal self-esteem. The failed breastfeeder aims to minimise damage to her self-image. The successful breastfeeder aims to capitalise on her success, thus nourishing her self-image. The old saying 'Success has a thousand fathers while failure is an orphan' is an eloquent way of articulating the social truth that everyone wants to be responsible for success and no one wants to be responsible for failure.

In this chapter we explore how women attempt to strategically manipulate how others (typically other women) understand their breastfeeding failure. We look at what mothers' excuses conceal as well as reveal. In doing so, I will introduce a radical notion: it is *essential* for maternal mental health – not to mention breastfeeding rates – that women take responsibility for their failure to breastfeed.

## WHAT ARE EXCUSES?

This seems like a fairly simple question, but the notion of excuse-making brings with it a cyclone of preoccupations. We can pinpoint the main contentions by referring to the first entry for 'Excuse' in the *Oxford English Dictionary*:

'VERB: Seek to lessen the blame attaching to a fault or offence'.[292]

What does this definition tells us about excuse-making in the breastfeeding context? Well, firstly we can deduce that for excuse-making to be triggered, a mother must believe she has caused 'a fault or offence'. The mere act of offering excuses presupposes moral wrong-doing. The greater a mother perceives this wrong-doing to be, the more compelled she will feel to make excuses.[293] Thus, the excuse-making mother views breastfeeding failure as synonymous with wrong-doing.

Secondly, we can deduce that after acknowledging her wrong-doing, a mother will 'seek to lessen the blame'. This implies that she believes most people fail to breastfeed because of personal blame, and wants to appear to be the exception to this rule. In making excuses, she dissociates herself with the image of other formula-feeding mothers. If she did not believe she was personally responsible, she would stop after stage 1: acknowledging that failing to breastfeed is bad.

Q: what are excuses? A: excuses are intentional actions undertaken to influence what others think about us. For post-breastfeeding mothers, this involves denying or minimising their causal role in bringing about breastfeeding failure (the Latin root of the word 'excuse' is made up of the prefix *ex* meaning 'from' or 'out of' and *causa*, 'cause').

## MAINTAINING MOTHERHOOD –
## THE ROLE OF EXCUSES

It's all very well defining what excuses *are*; the complexity begins when we start looking at how they are used. All of us have a self-image made up of several 'role identities'. For example, a woman may simultaneously be a mother, sister, wife, daughter, employee, friend and so on. Depending on the context, the 'salience' of these role identities (how central the role is to the current situation) varies, and when salience is high, the emotional stakes are high. The more salient the identity, the more intense the reaction when that identity is confirmed or refuted. In a woman's life, the 'mother' identity often predominates, particularly when she is interacting with other women. For example, when a woman is in a baby-group environment, her mother role is most salient; her role as wife or employee less so.

For most mothers, breastfeeding failure is the nakedness they dress up in a cloak of excuses. When caught undressed, mothers instinctively reach for that cloak. Because a mother's maternal reputation is so important to her status, when she believes it is threatened, she is motivated to take action and alleviate her concern. In Chapter 2, we looked at how the intensity of post-breastfeeding guilt a mother feels correlates with how highly she rates breastfeeding and how she frames it as part of her Desired Self (see page 88). Well, the greater the threat to her 'self-theory', the stronger the remedial work she now feels obliged to perform. Here's an example:

> 'I took it as a failure, because I wanted to give this child the best of everything. For me, it was a failure not to live up to my ideal'.[294]

Listen closely to a mother's excuses and you will notice that they incorporate and exemplify the internalised values she puts on motherhood. A mother's excuses have an idealised aspect – they offer up a scene that taps into her own, and she hopes the listener's, stereotypes of maternal selflessness and dedication. For mothers, excuse-making is a moral ceremony, an expressive rejuvenation and reaffirmation of maternal values. It is serious business.

## THE MATERNAL EXCUSE-MAKING PROCESS – FROM TRIGGER TO OUTCOME

Excuses, by their very nature, *presume* a prior judgement of moral responsibility – by failing to breastfeed, Mum thinks she has caused an offence. Mindful of her offence, she perceives her audience to have some sort of authority over her, akin to judge and jury in a courtroom. She cares what they think of her.[295] She fears that if people think negatively of her failure, they may think negatively of her 'personhood'. Of course, how a mother perceives others' reactions may or may not correspond to what they *actually* think. It is enough that she fears other people are making a worst-case reading of her failure. So most breastfeeding-related excuses are pre-emptive. They take place during social exchanges in which the mother attempts to defuse *anticipated* criticism. Essentially, she 'responds' to hypothetical accusations rather than actual ones. The perceived glare of publicity puts her in a state of heightened self-awareness. Excuse-making is an attempt to neutralise anticipated negative evaluations of her mothering, a strategic conversational move to prevent reprimand. The process is guided by one question: 'Given the facts available to the listener, what is the worst conclusion they might draw about my breastfeeding failure?' A mother then handcrafts excuses to block this worst-case reading and reduce the severity of her failure in the best way she can manage.

What is the worst possible interpretation a listener may make of breastfeeding failure? From a mother's point of view, it's one for which she has maximum responsibility, where she foresaw failure, freely and intentionally brought it about, without being coerced by external pressure or extenuating circumstances. Thus, the mothers in the most unenviable position are those who choose formula feeding in the first instance. As Professor Elizabeth Murphy noted in her study 'Infant feeding decisions and maternal deviance', 'Unlike those who initiate breast feeding but then change to artificial feeding, these women [the formula feeders from birth] cannot claim that their good intentions have been overwhelmed by events'.[296] Maximum responsibility results in maximum impact on the mother's maternal identity. If the circumstances involve pure choice, an audience can be fairly confident that the mother's actions reveal something about her motivation, character and disposition.[297] Excuses are mothers' attempts to distance themselves as far as possible from this worst-case interpretation.

## MILKING IT

A mother's engulfing fear of a worst-case interpretation can compel her to over-compensate by dramatising her feelings of guilt. She might crank up expressions of remorse, embarrassment or inadequacy to full volume in an effort to communicate how terribly she supposedly feels about her failure and how much she is suffering inside. She wants her private struggles to be authenticated by other people, and yet can't imagine this will happen unless she presents them in dramatic ways. It's a strategy that pays off. Her behaviour exerts a moral demand on her listeners, obliging them to repay her efforts with amnesty. When a person commits an offence, social-psychological research has shown that if they demonstrate that they have suffered because of their offence, they are viewed less negatively.[298] Over-communicating emotions of suffering more often than not taps into the sympathy reserves of the audience, compelling them to release their coveted bounty.

A mother may continue the milking process, going on and on in an attempt to explain or even apologise for her failure. A skilful 'milker' might even express her turmoil to the point of appearing manic. The audience may see no real need for the mother's apparent emotional suffering, but the mother takes no chances. The more extreme her story, the greater the implied dedication to her child – and the easier it is to get carried away with her show, unable and unwilling to suppress her spiralling emotional response. Such is the passion of this performance, you could roast a marshmallow on her forehead. Observe this pitiful hyperbolic display and it's obvious that it serves not only a communicative function but also a tension-release role.

A mother's willingness to initiate her own castigation by overstating and overplaying the case against her has another benefit: her apparent lack of self-control burdens her audience with the task of cutting the self-derogation short. In doing so, the audience, abiding by its moral obligation to keep the interaction running smoothly, minimises the magnitude of her failure. This typical outcome is a perfect illustration of how excuses serve a mother's personal as well as social needs and goals.

But, before you believe the 'milking it' routine is a mum's free-for-all sympathy buffet, it's not. Even the kind, tender, feminine emotion of sympathy has its limits. To maximise returns, a mother must adopt a milking strategy that is suitably dramatic yet mindful of the audience's sensibilities. If the audience is a regular acquaintance, repeat performances are seldom necessary – one or two curtain calls at various meetings should do the job. This is because the regularity with which one recites one's breastfeeding plight tends to affect sympathy in a curvilinear fashion (see diagram below). Audiences award markedly sparse sympathy for a very short, vague one-off explanation ('Oh, breastfeeding wasn't for me') yet also for very long, elaborate and repeated recitals ('My baby had jaundice, then I got mastitis, my cat died and my husband left me'), so a skilful milker aims for a performance that slots between the two extremes. If the mother is partaking in a public recital: less is more. Western emotional standards treat public emotional displays as less authentic than private ones.[299] If a mother recites her story at every meeting, sympathy margins can erode, leading the audience to ignore or even resent her.

It's not an easy ride for the audience, either. In fact, being an audience member is just as burdensome – if not more – than being a sympathy-seeking mother. She (or he, but it's invariably a she) must determine the right amount of sympathy to award, being careful not to dish out too

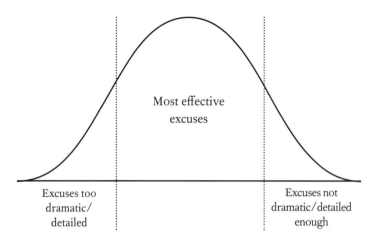

*Figure 3: Excuse Effectiveness*

much or too little. This finely balanced exercise necessitates a series of delicate judgements. Factors in determining how much sympathy to serve up include: the merit of the mother's performance (both her dramatic retelling of her story and her role in the narrative), the setting of the retelling, time constraints, and the audience's current circumstances relative to the mother's.[300] If the audience also happens to be a fellow failed breastfeeder, she will be particularly prone to sympathy fatigue, having instigated this charade many times herself. The excuse-making exchange certainly is an uncomfortable and mentally exhausting game for both parties. After her performance, a mother waits on tenterhooks to see if an accolade is forthcoming; the sympathiser fumbles around for the perfect pity prize. Both are left wishing the subject had never arisen.

Are you beginning to see how excuse-making, far from being an easy road to redemption, is actually a cognitively taxing business? And we haven't even considered the dress rehearsals! Before taking her show public, a mother engages in mental simulations in which she presents her excuse to a hypothetical audience and anticipates their hypothetical reactions. The possibility that an initial attempt at an excuse might be met with a lukewarm reception can prompt the preparation of an alternative or back-up excuse.[301] In this sense, Mum's behaviour is not unlike that of an actor trying out costumes or accents before going on stage. When she is as confident as she can be that her script is acceptable, a mother will give a tentative public performance. She will 'try out' various excuses on different audiences to see which is most effective, searching, ideally, for the one that presents her breastfeeding failure in the most palatable way for this audience. She might not win an Academy Award, but the BAFTA is in the bag.

## SELECTING THE SCRIPT – A MENU OF EXCUSES

Excuses in the post-breastfeeding context fall into two main categories. They are either external to the mother and hence uncontrollable ('My baby wouldn't latch'), or internal but uncontrollable ('My breasts wouldn't produce enough milk'). Many flavours of excuse nestle within these categories. When putting together their dish, mothers choose one or more flavours according to taste. For entertainment and education, let's examine the menu. Black pepper, anyone?

### The Anatomical Excuse

*Category:* internal and uncontrollable
*Efficiency rating:* 10/10

Women who genuinely cannot breastfeed – the non-choosers – have no reason to dwell on how their outcome stacks up against other mothers, and since they did not choose it, the outcome is not a measure of maternal success or failure. The genuine non-chooser arouses sympathy and empathy. This is an attractive prospect for any struggling *chooser*, hence the influx of mothers choosing to cite anatomical issues ('I couldn't produce enough milk') as the root of their failure. In fact, breast milk insufficiency is one of the most common reasons given by mothers in most cultures for terminating breastfeeding and/or introducing supplementary feeding.[302] The disingenuous inference we can make from this scary statistic is that most women seemingly have broken breasts. Of course this is not a tragic error of evolution, but rather a self-serving fabrication.

As a tactic to excuse breastfeeding failure, the Anatomical Excuse is the undisputed heavyweight champion. It derives its power from the occasionally inconvenient (but this time very convenient) involuntary nature of human anatomy. You see, two words sum up breastfeeding potential: *can* and *try*. There must be some degree of each for success to be achievable. Mothers love the anatomical excuse because they can focus on one of these words in order to render the other irrelevant. The rationale is that faulty anatomy is an ability constraint that directs attention away from psychological constraints.[303] When she uses the Anatomical Excuse, a mother constructs a barrier between her maternal character and her failure to breastfeed. She does not challenge the fact that she failed to breastfeed; rather, she attempts to show that she was in no way personally responsible for that failure. By blaming a relatively uncontrollable cause (physical anatomy), a mother draws attention away from controllable causes (motivation and intention). Mum may, for instance, claim that her milk suddenly 'dried up' or never came in at all. Most mothers prefer to claim that they had milk, but that their breasts did not produce enough of it. Their breasts were 'faulty'. Their rogue anatomy acts as a convenient, technically plausible and socially acceptable smokescreen.

The Anatomical Excuse works because we tend to put failure into one of three distinct camps:

1. Defective skill or ability (Mum not able).
2. Insufficient care or effort (Mum not dedicated).
3. Improper intentions (Mum not sincere).[304]

Mothers who experience failure because of lack of competence (those in the first camp) are generally not blamed for their errors. Those in the second camp (who have the competence, yet make a half-hearted attempt at performance) are generally held to account – they have failed not because of lack of ability, but lack of concern. The most serious kind of failure is deemed to lie at the door of camp number three. Failure due to 'improper intentions' reflects a mother's moral character. Clearly camp 1 is the most desirable residence from a mother's point of view, and the Anatomical Excuse is perhaps the only excuse that can claim an unquestionable stronghold in this camp.

So efficient is the Anatomical Excuse that, paradoxically, mothers using it can even lie by telling the truth! For instance, Mum can claim that her breasts did not produce enough milk, but refrain from mentioning that she did not give them the requisite stimulation. Thus, while effectively telling the truth, she claims a much smaller personal contribution than is appropriate in reality. Very efficient. If Mum could high-five herself, she would.

Yet despite her pleas, it is statistically unlikely that she had malfunctioning mammaries. On the contrary. Amy Evans, a paediatrician and medical director of the Center for Breastfeeding Medicine in California, has insisted that no more than five percent of women have underlying medical conditions that may prevent or hinder lactation.[305] Italian paediatrician Carlos González summed up the rarity of true lactation failure in his book *Breastfeeding Made Easy*[306] when he explained that a woman has more chance of winning the rollover lottery than suffering from hypogalactia (insufficient secretion of milk), and more chance of marrying a prince than of suffering from congenital prolactin deficiency.[307] Herein lies the dirty secret behind the Anatomical Excuse: even if a mother was not directly responsible for the failure, she was probably indirectly responsible. Causality can be complicated, involving long, complex links between origin and consequence. A mother may indeed have insufficient milk supply, but this state is likely to have been cultivated by her own actions – by introducing formula, refusing to feed on demand or introducing a dummy. Claims of innocence fade into excuses as such causal linkage emerges.

What's more, mothers' abuse of the Anatomical Excuse has implications that reach further than Pinocchio's nose ever could. The widespread exploitation of this excuse firstly creates a cultural rule of thumb: the tendency to automatically regard breast malfunction as typical or representative of the breastfeeding experience. Secondly, it means that mothers who do not cite anatomical issues are vilified more readily. A third result is that mothers without anatomical issues who succeed in breastfeeding have their success attributed to good luck rather than effort. Everyone is hurt, except the excuse-making mother.

### The Mitigating Excuse

*Category:*        internal and uncontrollable
*Efficiency rating:* 7/10

This perhaps more inconspicuous excuse strategy involves a mother accepting fault, but rejecting responsibility. The Mitigating Excuse permits a mother to admit failing at breastfeeding and (unlike the Anatomical Excuse) also admit that her own actions in some way caused that failure. But here's the crucial component – she was not as responsible for the failure as it might appear. At the core of this excuse is a mother's attempt to persuade people that she was not free to act as she wished. The Mitigating Excuse can be exemplified by the declaration, 'I failed, but I couldn't help it; I had no choice'.

The mother may concede that she failed to breastfeed due to lack of effort, but defends this by introducing mitigating circumstances: postnatal depression is a prominent example. The Mitigating Excuse is a form of moral disengagement. It is exemplified by a process of convincing others that ethical standards do not apply to oneself in a particular context. By citing a force other than will, a mother argues that her intentions do not account for what occurred. Instead, the message is that her intentions were caused by other forces. Publicising your handicaps is a very effective means of image-enhancement. Social psychologist Steven Berglas has called it 'downward self-promotion'.[308] Mum typically asserts that her performance was inconsistent with her usual behavior, and that she had diminished responsibility by virtue of her vulnerability. By claiming powerlessness and mental incompetence, a mother can give the impression that she could no longer function effectively in order to breastfeed. These extenuating claims release her from the moral responsibility tied up in the obligation to breastfeed. This type of excuse is particularly seductive because we all feel vulnerable to some extent during the post-natal period. The audience readily accepts the mitigating circumstances as plausible, a temporary character flaw for which the misfortune of breastfeeding failure is retribution enough. This 'characterological blame'[309] frames the scenario as the mother being affected by, but not producing, her breastfeeding failure.

Citing postnatal depression is tactically impressive. Depressive symptoms have manipulative utility: they can control and direct the responses of others. Cultural concepts of mental illness are closely intertwined with the notion that people are 'victims' and not fully responsible for the symptoms that cause them suffering. The guarantee of sympathy is attractive. Studies have found that even patients of serious mental illnesses are capable of using their symptoms in a strategic fashion in order to achieve secondary gains.[310] And the gains are plentiful. In the Mitigating Excuse, blame is attached to a 'self' that no longer exists or has changed so much that the audience does not need to be concerned about it happening again.[311] Thus a mother's current 'competent' self is split from her past 'incompetent' self. The competent self continues beyond the failure; the incompetent self is left behind, discredited by the mother as a moment of alienation from her true self. Strictly speaking, the more a mother can successfully argue mitigating circumstances, the more she can establish that her breastfeeding failure is not an expression of her moral character.

To exploit this strategy to its fullest, some mothers pimp it up with exonerative moral reasoning, emphasising their view of the larger, more positive consequences of their actions. An example is the mother who claims ceasing breastfeeding aided her recovery from postnatal depression and consequently helped her bond with her baby. This tactic can be exemplified by the mantra, 'Happy Mum, Happy Baby'. Here, the mother prioritises her own preferences but *disguises* them as loyalty to her baby. Professor Elizabeth Murphy of the University of Nottingham has a handle on this game:

'Asserting her own needs risks undermining her claim to responsible motherhood. However, she overcomes this by presenting her own welfare as indivisible from her child's. If she is not happy with breastfeeding, her child will not be'.[312]

Another common example of the Mitigating Excuse is a caesarean delivery. There is no reason a caesarean should prevent breastfeeding. In fact, once breastfeeding has been established, birth experiences do not have a lasting effect on breastfeeding duration.[313] There is an inverse correlation between caesarean rates and breastfeeding rates:[314] the higher the c-section rate, the lower the breastfeeding rate. However, this has less to do with the method of delivery than with people's false preconceptions of c-sections as a barrier to breastfeeding. For instance, the false assertion that the act of breastfeeding itself would cause further pain or inconvenience.

Yet another excuse is that a mother's medication is incompatible with breastfeeding; this from the mother who didn't bother to find out[315] whether there were alternative compatible medications (likely, yes). Then there's the mother who claims 'extreme exhaustion'. Here, we see that reduced states of competency are not created equal, and vary in terms of their power to excuse. The degree to which a Mitigating Excuse is successful is influenced by the strength of the excuse and the commonly held beliefs of those listening to it. It is one thing for a peer group of mothers to accept mental illness as a plausible explanation for breastfeeding failure; it is quite another to give amnesty for everyday visceral factors such as tiredness or lack of sleep – to which the vast majority of mothers are exposed. After all, we tend to under-weigh or even ignore visceral factors experienced by other people.[316]

*The Duress Excuse*

*Category:* external and uncontrollable
*Efficiency rating:* 6/10

With this excuse, we switch our focus from internal to external causes – and this is where the efficiency of excuses begins to drop markedly. Because of the undeniably physiological nature of breastfeeding, mothers can never totally shift the locus of blame to an outside source; it is impossible for a mother to completely detangle herself from the act. So her goal becomes to move the blame from a very threatening internal source ('I failed because I was uncommitted') to a less threatening external source ('I failed because I was pressured to quit'). The Duress Excuse, even when executed skilfully, cannot produce an absolute shift from an internal to an external cause, only a relative shift.

Duress is a very popular strategy, albeit weaker in comparison to anatomical and mitigating excuses. Like the Mitigating Excuse, it allows a mother to claim reduced freedom of decision. But with the Duress Excuse, she pins the blame not on an internal impediment, but on external coercion. She shifts some responsibility for breastfeeding failure from herself onto other people. While her failure to breastfeed was brought about by free choice – without choice there can be no responsibility – a mother who cites duress dilutes her responsibility to the point that she is regarded more as a victim than an autonomous adult.

The alleged coercion can come from a variety of sources: family members, friends, employers and health professionals are all common scapegoats.[317] Consider the popular claim that another person, usually a health professional, has intervened in the breastfeeding process, perhaps by pressuring the mother to switch to formula. In this scenario, there is no doubt that the mother was the proximate cause of her failure (she made up the bottles and gave them to her baby), but because of the duress involved, Mum implies that she should be assigned only minimal personal responsibility and no blame – that she was an insignificant part of the causal chain. Blaming others in this way can have a cathartic effect. Never underestimate the sense of relief that comes with passing the buck.

The mother opting for the Duress Excuse is painting herself as a victim of circumstance. She is a victim of others' decisions. The excuse is her own Shakespearean tragedy and curiously bears sod all resemblance to anyone else's version of events.[318] In her narrative, as far as potential perpetrators go anyone is fair game; even toddler siblings are acceptable scapegoats. Case in point:

'Every time I sat down to breastfeed, our eighteen-month old son was trying to climb on my lap. He was too demanding.... After three weeks he began to get into things. Then I went back to work and it was just too much; he began to hit and bite the baby when I was breastfeeding. He's much better now that he can hold the bottle when it's time to feed'.[319]

Despite its low efficiency rating relative to the Anatomical and Mitigating Excuses, the Duress Excuse has two major assumptions advantageous for mothers who use it. The presence of external pressure firstly implies that anyone in the same situation would have behaved as the mother did; secondly it suggests that the mother behaved differently to how she normally would. Both assumptions reduce her personal maternal responsibility and in turn place the responsibility on the external pressure. They also raise the distinctiveness of her failure, implying that it was limited to one narrow space in time.

Before you reach for the bunting, it's not all good news. The Duress Excuse carries with it a paradox of responsibility. This may seem an ill-fitting notion because generally excuse-making is designed to delimit responsibility. Nonetheless, by using the Duress Excuse the mother implies that she now recognises the objectionable nature of the external coercion that led to her downfall. This awareness places the onus of responsibility on her to take steps to eliminate the need for Duress Excuses in the future. Bummer.

## The Higher Loyalties Excuse

*Category:*          external and uncontrollable
*Efficiency rating:* 5/10

If a mother wishes to present her excuse in such a way as to make her formula-feeding choice appear principled – ethical even – she can invoke the Higher Loyalties Excuse. This excuse requires crocodile tears, balls, a diploma in morality and a degree in acting. Typically, a mother using the Higher Loyalties Excuse will select her script from three of the most popular and objective moral principles: justice, benevolence or pragmatism.[320] She may claim 'justice' by asserting that she chose to formula feed so that her husband could do his share of the feedings, a popular tactic showcased by this mum:

> 'I think it is important for my husband to be able to feed it…. I don't think I could stand being tied down to every single feed. At least my husband can feed him at weekends and nights. We both seem very tired and I just can't imagine having to feed him every time'.[321]

Alternatively, she may claim 'benevolence' by arguing that her breast milk was inadequate for her baby's needs. By switching, she was acting in baby's best interests. Pleas of 'pragmatism' can be invoked by citing a return to employment[322] or 'needing' to go on a family vacation, the stress of which, she argues, would prevent her from breastfeeding. In defending their choice to formula feed, mothers can claim they did what was right for everyone concerned. In other words, they assert that they struck a balance between their own rights, their baby's rights, their husband's rights and the rights of the rest of the family. That's a hell of a lot of rights. Yet striking a balance is a woolly and platitudinous thing to do. Such talk is empty unless it explains what balance has to be struck and why. It also fails to recognise that often what's needed is a radical rebalancing of priorities. The apparent reasonableness of balance blinds us to the fact that sometimes one set of concerns just overrides the other. Consider the balance between the needs of a baby and older children. In the abstract, there is some truth in this claim. But in specific areas, such as the baby's lifelong health, the right balance often means tilting the scales entirely to one side for a finite period of time.

In the Higher Loyalties Excuse we see mental gymnastics of Olympian standard. The mother attempts to turn 'good mothering' into an altogether different notion – with self-interest at the core. We see a 'good mother' morph from 'one who breastfeeds' into the purposely vague 'happy mother' or 'working mother' or 'confident mother' or, if Mum is feeling particularly cheeky, a combination of all three.[323] When a mother uses the Higher Loyalties Excuse, she doesn't deny her breastfeeding failure, but asks an audience not to hold her fully responsible because it occurred with good rather than bad intentions. The Higher Loyalties Excuse exploits the idea that people who do bad while trying to do good are usually viewed more favourably than those who intend to do bad.

### The Redefining Standards Excuse

*Category:*          external and uncontrollable
*Efficiency rating:* 3/10

When a mother senses that her breastfeeding failure will be interpreted as sub-par because of external standards, she may adopt the ambitious strategy of going to work on the standards themselves. In order to generate a more palatable picture of her efforts, a mother attacks mainstream breastfeeding standards and then customises them to fit her own performance. So, for instance, she may first try to convince the audience that the NHS recommendation of six months' exclusive breastfeeding is 'too unrealistic'. If she's done her research, she may bolster this assertion by drawing attention to the low number of mothers who reach the aforementioned standard.[324] Next, she may argue that simply breastfeeding for the first few days is sufficient, on the grounds that, 'Colostrum is what's really important'. This new, trivialising frame of reference is designed to reduce the factual importance of breastfeeding. The motive is to reshape standards so that they actually define the mother's performance as a success.

The flexibility of this excuse means it can be used both retrospectively and anticipatorily. The excuse, however, has a low efficiency rating because it is primarily self-soothing – it doesn't convince her audience, unless Mum can somehow produce credentials to outshine those of the NHS or the World Health Organization.

### The Embedded Excuse

*Category:*          wildcard
*Efficiency rating:* 4/10

If there is a 'benefit of the doubt' to be garnered, many mothers will opt for the Embedded Excuse. This type of excuse is a two-pronged strategy employing 'diversion' and 'splitting' tactics. Here, the mother acknowledges that her breastfeeding failure constitutes a sub-par mothering performance, but suggests that it really should be seen as one relatively minor negative event in the context of much broader competence. She diverts attention to her good points, splitting her breastfeeding failure from her otherwise good performance at mothering.[325] For instance, a mother diverts attention from the implicit health risks of formula by asserting that, 'As long as my baby is fed, clothed and loved, that is all that matters'. The mother effectively hides her failure within the crystal white sheets of an alleged bed of competence.[326] The excuse is often given in response to questions the mother really does not want to answer, 'Did you breastfeed?' perhaps being the most salient. The embedded excuse is a type of 'bullshit' response that does not directly answer the question. As philosopher Harry Frankfurt comments, a typical bullshitter:

'...does not reject the authority of the truth, as the liar does, and oppose himself to it. He pays no attention to it at all. By virtue of this, bullshit is a greater enemy of the truth than lies are'.[327]

### The Blame the Victim Excuse

*Category:*  external and uncontrollable
*Efficiency rating:* 3/10

Perhaps the most controversial yet widely used excuse is to 'blame the victim'. Mum may blame the baby for sleeping too much or not sleeping enough; for feeding too much or not feeding enough. This example of the latter is taken from an interview in which a mother was quoted blaming her premature baby:

'He was too weak. His little heart was weak, his breathing weak, I didn't have a choice. I was feeding five minutes per breast, then I had to stop and quickly give him bottled milk'.[328]

When faced with situations they do not understand or know how to control (pain, leaking, poor latch, perceived hunger, weight loss), it is common for mothers to conclude that the baby did not like breastfeeding.[329] They declare that their babies were particularly hungry and their demand for milk too high.[330] Similar to those using the Higher Loyalties Excuse, 'blame the victim' mothers claim that quitting was in the baby's best interests and that a good mother is one who recognises when breastfeeding is not working out.[331] However, as one scholar has had the gumption to point out, even the fussiest of babies cannot logically be the culprit of breastfeeding failure; it is mothers whose own characteristics inhibit them from coping who are the 'true culprit'.[332]

### The Justification

*Category:*          internal and controllable
*Efficiency rating:* 0/10

For mothers unable or unwilling to cut the ties that bind them to their poor breastfeeding performance, the only strategy left is to lessen the negativity of the performance itself – through justification. Justification is not technically an excuse. This distinction is important. Excuses are used when a mother wants to deny responsibility for formula feeding, but acknowledge the implication of harm. Justification, on the other hand, is used when a mother wants to acknowledge her responsibility for formula feeding but deny the implications of harm. Unlike excuse-makers, mothers who use justification do not concede that formula feeding is undesirable. Instead, they engage in redefinition strategies. They directly minimise their failure to breastfeed by denying that their baby is in any way a victim.

Often, when a mother takes a justification approach she is really participating in an elaborate fantasy. In order to pacify her guilt, she attempts to persuade herself that her breastfeeding failure is inconsequential. This is particularly obvious in mothers who set out to breastfeed in the first instance. Freud labelled such behaviour 'reaction formation'[333]

– an attempt to deny one's true emotional state by taking on the opposite emotion. The rationale is that if one can argue that formula feeding is not a reprehensible act, in theory Mum's reputation should not be damaged. Justification allows mothers to convince themselves that what they did was the best thing they could have done. It blurs the discrepancy between rational thinking and self-serving fantasy.

The justifying mother may garnish her dish by throwing in a red herring or two. A red herring is essentially a diversion tactic. The phrase stems from the 17th century, when escaping criminals would drag strong-smelling red herring across a trail so that pursuing blood-hounds would lose the scent.[334] In the same way, a formula-feeding mother may differentiate formula use from more undesirable nasties, such as fast food, early weaning, poison or even child abuse. Such topics are, of course, red herrings.

A skilful justifier can even transform her failure to breastfeed from something negative to something positive; then, instead of feeling guilt or shame, she can take pride in being responsible. She describes formula feeding as less (or not at all) as harmful as it might appear from a worst-case interpretation: 'My child is advanced and bottle fed; it must be extra vitamins they put in formula'. Psychology scholars call this 'selective perception', a phenomenon in which individuals pay attention to cues they think support their argument and ignore those that do not.

The irrevocable nature of a mother's failure to breastfeed fuels her urge to choose justification over excuses. Idiotically, the more permanent a decision, the more certain people tend to be that it is correct.[335] The urge to justify formula feeding is made even more powerful by the implication that using it harms babies. The more costly a decision and the more permanent its consequences, the stronger both a mother's cognitive discomfort and her need to reduce it by over-emphasising the good things about her decision. This is why it is unwise to ask a formula feeder for infant-feeding advice – particularly a new convert. That person will be highly motivated to convince you that formula feeding is the correct choice.[336]

In their book, aptly titled *Mistakes Were Made (But Not By*

*Me)*, Carol Tavris and Elliot Aronson described justification as more powerful and more dangerous than standard excuse-making:

> 'Mindless self-justification, like quicksand, can draw us deeper into disaster. It blocks our ability to even see our errors, let alone correct them. It distorts reality, keeping us from getting all the information we need and assessing issues clearly.... It keeps us from letting go of unhealthy habits. It permits the guilty to avoid taking responsibility for their deeds. And it keeps many professionals from changing outdated attitudes and procedures that can be harmful to the public'.[337]

So why the zero efficiency rating? Well, apart from technically not being an excuse, justification is perhaps the most ill-received explanation strategy. It has even earned the label 'aggravating' tactic from social psychologists, since it often leaves an audience with the feeling that a mother is both unrepentant and fully responsible for the offence.[338] Trying to make an offence seem trivial can be perceived as unethical, irresponsible, ignorant and inappropriate. Mothers who use other types of excuse-making strategies are seen as more remorseful than the justifying mother.[339]

## PICK 'N' MIX – USING MULTIPLE EXCUSE STRATEGIES

In some circumstances, a mother may feel that a single excuse is not quite sufficient to persuade her audience, and so opts for a combination. However, like choosing a pick 'n' mix selection in the sweet shop, this tactic is only beneficial if the chosen excuses complement one another. You're not going to put crisps with flumps, but flying saucers – yeah, bring it on. Likewise, a Higher Loyalties Excuse (see page 125) is the perfect companion for a Mitigating Excuse (see page 121), exemplified by the assertion, 'I had postnatal depression and my husband couldn't cope, so I needed to focus all my energy on getting better to save my marriage'. Similarly, a Duress Excuse (see page 123) complements an Anatomical Excuse (see page 118), exemplified by the assertion, 'My milk never came in and the health visitor said I must formula feed or my baby would fail to thrive'.

It is also possible that particular excuse combinations could interfere with each other as well. Like the crisp-tainted flumps, a Justification (see page 129) would be ill-placed alongside a Duress Excuse, as exemplified by the assertion, 'My doctor forced me to breastfeed because my baby was losing weight, and anyway, formula feeding is just as healthy as breastfeeding'.

### The Baby Group – aka the Theatrical Stage

You may have noticed dramaturgical words like 'audience' and 'script' popping up throughout this chapter. They aren't intended as sarcasm, but rather as a tool to aid comprehension. Thinking of mothers' excuses as theatrical performances is a dynamic way to understand them, and the analogy of life and the theatre mirroring each other is an old one. Shakespeare opined that 'all the world's a stage'.[340] Plato spoke of the 'great stage of human life'. The analogy helps us understand the interaction between mothers – and in particular, their excuse-making behavior – in holistic detail. Mums possess scripts; they perform roles that symbolise how they wish to appear to others; they select words and gestures to illustrate that character, perhaps even throwing in a relevant prop. A quality performance can bring praise, esteem and affection. A poor performance might end the show, bringing criticism, rejection, disrespect and a bad review. Then, there is the backstage area, where mothers can chill and loosen up, out of sight of the audience.

The baby group environment provides the most obvious audience in many mothers' lives, a stage where mums are 'on' to their peers. Feel free to replace the words 'baby group' with any maternal gathering in which the shared focus of attention is motherhood; the dynamics will be largely the same. I have chosen to refer to baby groups because they are one of the most popular gathering points for mothers of infants. In a recent UK study of 2,000 new mothers,[341] nearly half the women questioned said they made friends at baby groups, while a fifth said they kept in touch with mothers they met at antenatal classes. By their nature these maternal gatherings are emotionally charged. In fact, prominent sociologists have for decades noted that the act of gathering is a powerful stimulant, generating a 'sort of electricity' from mere closeness.[342] Four in ten of the mothers in the aforementioned UK study said they admitted feeling more comfortable sharing intimate and personal information with women they had just met, including saucy details of their post-baby love life. Almost 80 percent have poured their heart out, sharing concerns about being a good mum and the guilt of whether to go back to work after maternity leave. Other discussion topics include sleepless nights, nappies, baby ailments and, of course, the biggy – breastfeeding.

In the intimate boiling pot of the baby group, each and every participant has something in common: motherhood. Presenting a 'competent mother-self' is paramount to the transaction. The evaluative pressure of the baby group environment forces each mother's insecurities to the surface: about her mothering accomplishments, about her commitment, about her status. Twisting the truth via excuse-making is a way of answering these insecurities.

During these meetings, babies are compared for weight, motor skills and cognitive ability, and when one fails to measure up to the threshold set by the group, the mother will formulate an excuse to defend the poor performance. To use a common example, discovering that her baby is on a very low centile for weight gain may prompt a mother to attribute her baby's size to genetics. In this sense, excuse-making allows mothers to navigate social situations in which they feel they don't quite measure up. If a mother fears she doesn't embody the qualities she suspects are expected by the group, she can substitute fact for a fiction that does. This process is aided by the fact that the image she makes through excuse-making is one she admires. In group contexts, the urge to impress easily trumps commitment to honesty. The barriers against deception are fragile, and the psychological pressures nudging mothers towards excuse-making are powerful, as Susan Douglas and

Meredith Michaels whinged in their book *The Mommy Myth*:

> 'Intensive mothering is the ultimate female Olympics: We are in powerful competition with each other, in constant danger of being trumped by the mom down the street'.[343]

Susan and Meredith were justified in their twisted panties. Maternal encounters involve a great degree of mutual evaluation. Mothers use each other as social mirrors, which puts psychological pressure on all involved. When mothers are judged, they – like everyone else – naturally want to be judged positively. Even if a mother has no interest in generating and maintaining friendships with the other mothers in the group, the drive to maintain self-esteem endures. The need to protect her stature, even in the eyes of mere acquaintances, can be intense.

To turn up the heat further, not only do mothers come face to face with each other at baby groups, they have to do so with their babies in tow. Since babies shoulder most of the consequences of a mother's infant-feeding choice, they are effectively the victims in the situation. The 'salience' of the victims to the audience – were it not for the babies there would be no baby group – is a driving force, triggering a mother's urge to fire up her excuse-making arsenal. The closer in view the 'harm', the harder mothers have to work to restore their maternal reputations.

An alternative to launching into excuse-making is to nudge the door open subtly by offering fleeting evidence. A purposeful slip, such as 'Baby is due his bottle soon', can make others aware of one's feeding status and excuse-making intentions. This approach, if executed in a nonchalant tone, has another benefit: by admitting her failing in a matter-of-fact way, the mother sets up the atmospheric assumption that those present should be indifferent about the topic while discouraging them from losing face by showing they are not.

Breastfeeding mothers, too, can nudge the door open by the simple click of a bra strap. Normally this occasions no explicit comment, yet the heightened, narrowed awareness causes a tacitly tense atmosphere accompanied by hallmark signs of discomfort from all present – fixed stares elsewhere, stifled conversation, feigned humour and awkward solemnity.

## TRIBAL TOGETHERNESS

Despite supposedly being social creatures, we humans are very discriminative when it comes to whom we share our space with. We tend to seek out opportunities to 'be ourselves', gravitating towards relationships that increase the likelihood of receiving 'self-confirmatory' feedback.[344] Other mothers who share our infant-feeding choice create a circle of lament to which we can withdraw for moral support. By coming together, mothers reaffirm their selfhood and feelings of solidarity.

In environments where formula feeders dominate (that'll be most, then), the topic of breastfeeding is not, as one would expect, the elephant in the room – far from it. Feeding time at the baby group for instance, sees formula-feeding mothers pull out their bottles in unison. Then, while their babies regurgitate their meals, the mums regurgitate the scripted woes that brought them to this point. At this stage in the proceedings we observe a miraculous coincidence: not a single mother was responsible for the decision to formula feed. Everyone has excuses.

Many formula feeders, particularly in the early days of parenting, stew in a relationship built on shared biographies of suffering. They seek out and latch onto other 'sufferers'. As one mother explained, 'I felt comfortable with people who'd suffered a little bit of what I'd suffered, mainly bottle-feeders who'd done so because they'd tried breastfeeding and it hadn't worked'.[345] This community of hardship leads to an interesting chain reaction. The self-disclosure of one mother is seen to demonstrate a trust that prompts other mothers to reciprocate with a comparable amount of self-disclosure.[346] Each mother chooses which details of their infant-feeding biography to disclose to the group and which to conceal. The presentational behaviour of one mum sets the tone for the presentational behaviour of the others, and vice versa. It is a finely orchestrated waltz of revealing and concealing, emphasising and downplaying. Emerging from this conversational dance comes a type of inverse pride: 'My misfortunes are even bigger than yours'.

However, rather than lose themselves in the grip of competitive suffering and begin to question each other's fictions, formula-feeding mothers share an understanding. This tacit contract stipulates an acceptance of each others' excuses without question, a type of goodwill that one mother extends towards another, 'Don't out me and I won't out you'. Such colluding groups of people led one of the daddies of social psychology, Erving Goffman, to label them 'performance teams' because they cooperate in staging a single routine.[347] He noted:

> 'Persons who are brought together by affinal ties are brought to a position from which they can see behind each other's front; this is always embarrassing but it is less embarrassing if the newcomers have themselves been maintaining the same kind of show'.[348]

Before a group newcomer feels like a legitimate member of the clan, she becomes hyper-observant of the mannerisms, symbols and rituals of this collective.[349] Then, gradually, as she puts on the same performance, intra-group bonding solidifies. At this point, members may divulge 'inside secrets' – unsavoury facts, such as that they just didn't like breastfeeding. So the front maintained before 'outsiders' is not always maintained within the group. A certain degree of relaxation becomes possible. Indeed, when alone as a group, away from 'the other team', both formula feeders and breastfeeders can unwind and may engage in what Goffman has labelled 'staging talk'.[350] Essentially, discussions arise about techniques, props, positioning and other equipment that help the mothers engage in their choice of feeding method. Formula feeders debate the merits of one formula brand over another, and whether you *really* have to boil that bothersome water. Breastfeeders swap recommendations for the latest nursing fashion or breast pump. Useful gossip spreads faster than a runny nose in a nursery school. Both teams discuss the merits and demerits of various concealment tactics, 'post-mortem' stories are shared in which embarrassed wounds are licked and morale is massaged, ready for the next public performance. This is the backstage arena, where mothers feel free to be themselves and let down their facade.

## THE MOTHER AS CHAMELEON

Once an excuse is preferred or becomes available, a mother continues to evaluate its efficacy – she may change or modify the excuse depending on its perceived effectiveness. She uses the responses of her audience as a guide to help her determine what she can legitimately claim about her breastfeeding past. In this way, she presents her 'failure narrative' in different ways within different social situations and in response to different people. It is as if she presents 'edited' versions of her script to different audiences. This is because varying social circumstances impose varying demands; excuses that make the desired impression at baby group may not do so in another situation. Mothers temper their excuse-making when in the presence of a someone – for instance, a close friend – who can invalidate the excuse.

Let's use another analogy to understand this chameleon-like behaviour: the centuries-old notion that a person dons a mask for her audience. The derivation of the words 'person' and 'personality' can be traced to the Latin word *persona* – the mask an actor wears in performance. Thus, a mother wears a different mask when speaking to health professionals than when interacting with peers. Indeed, the number of masks a mother may put on is as varied as the environments she inhabits. Take the health professional. Mothers choose excuses they believe fit the situation as her audience (here, the health professional) sees it. Presuming the professional has 'expert' knowledge, the mother tailors her dialogue accordingly, moderating or even avoiding excuses all together.[351] So instead of choosing the popular route – the anatomical excuse – she may cut her losses and head straight for justification.

## A DIAMOND IN THE ROUGH

Sometimes chameleon mum can unknowingly find herself in the presence of an altogether different and much rarer breed of chameleon: a stealth species of individuals capable of invalidating her excuses. This is the veteran breastfeeder, or as I call her, the diamond in the rough. As a holder of extensive personal breastfeeding experience, the veteran breastfeeder can spot cracks[352] in an excuse-making script with impressive accuracy. The veteran breastfeeder may be inclined to discount appeals to luck when, in her experience, breastfeeding is clearly effort-related. She is likely to regard failure to breastfeed more seriously than others and therefore to have taken extra precautions herself to prevent it. If it appears from another mother's excuses that she did not do this, the excuse will be rejected by the breastfeeder – at least internally if not publicly – and she may feel offended and resentful when the excuse-maker laments over minor troubles.[353]

This scenario is exacerbated by the unfortunate fact – for the excuse-making mother – that common sense takes a vacation in the presence of a breastfeeder. Ironically, once the breastfeeder reveals her feeding creed, her mere presence triggers the excuse-maker to launch into a lengthy presentation of her failure narrative, despite the very real possibility of having her excuses debunked by the breastfeeder. Why does the formula feeder do this so passionately, yet so mindlessly? Her motivation stems from the relevance and importance she attaches to breastfeeding. In other words, the formula feeder launches into a defensive speech precisely because breastfeeding hits a personal nerve. And the rawer this nerve, the more elaborate her speech.[354] The excuse-maker doesn't distinguish between the person to whom she owes much information and the person to whom she owes very little – her life history is what you're gonna get. Indeed, the unsuspecting breastfeeder need not request such information – she almost never does – rather, the mere sight and smell of a nursing mother rouses an overwhelming, almost carnal, drive in the excuse-maker to perform her excuse-giving ritual. This is common formula feeder behaviour. At the mere click of a bra strap, every formula feeder within a mile radius launches into her excuse repertoire.[355]

## IS MATERNAL EXCUSE-MAKING WELL RECEIVED?

The omnipresence of post-breastfeeding excuses begs the question: are such excuses well-received? The answer hinges on two characteristics of the audience – their cognitive and personal biases. Let's get the intricate cognitive stuff out of the way first.

### Cognitive bias

To understand what goes through someone's head when in earshot of an excuse-making mother, it helps to see everyone as an amateur detective. When faced with a bottle-feeding mother, people instinctively experience Sherlockian internal thought processes; we are naturally drawn to search for explanations:[356] 'Is that breastmilk or formula in the bottle? Why did she fail at breastfeeding? Did she intend to fail or was it accidental? Is she embarrassed? Oh God, can she see me looking at her? Better look away....'

Whether we admit it or hide behind a faux-supportive guise of indifference, most of us feel compelled to understand a mother's bottle feeding by trying to 'find' appropriate clues in her characteristics. Such instinctive deduction is part of our human character. It's how we try to confer 'stable meaning' on our social surroundings. We ponder the mother's motives in bottle feeding, then we wonder whether these motives suggest more enduring traits, values, beliefs and attitudes. Labelling in this way is comforting, it enables us (so we think) to navigate our social realm with more confidence. Once we have labelled a person, we feel better able to deal with her because we can draw upon our stock knowledge of the label we have stuck on her.

Central to this deduction process is a set of 'cognitive biases' we all share. One of the first biases – igniting major ass-pain for the excuse-making mum – is our automatic assumption that 'she could have done otherwise'. We have a tendency to attribute other people's behaviour to internal disposition, such as personality traits, abilities and motives, as opposed to external situational factors. This is known in the psychology business as 'correspondence bias'. This bias is so pervasive that some psychologists have got all excited and called it 'the fundamental attribution error'. It happens like this: when it becomes obvious to us that a mother is not breastfeeding, we automatically assume her failure occurred due to her internal characteristics. We tend to process the mother's story backwards from effects, through action, to inferences about her personal disposition.[357] So, we start by looking at the final effect (baby is not being breastfed) and work backwards from there, ultimately ending with the mother as the prime cause. Our first instinct is to imagine lack of commitment or lack of ability – particularly when we have little or no first-hand information about the circumstances affecting the failure, as is often the case. We view the *behaviour* as something that calls for explanation rather than the *circumstances*. The notion that circumstances can cause action is too abstract and derivative for us;[358] 'correspondence bias' is our cognitive starting point.

This is problematic for the excuse-maker, because she is inclined to blame her failures on external circumstances. But circumstances like having to return to work or developing mastitis don't automatically lead to breastfeeding failure. Nor does having a baby with colic, an unsupportive husband or postnatal depression. These excuses are hard sells for the mother. If we notice even a hint of choice in her dialogue, we will hold her accountable.[359] So, even though we don't completely disregard a mother's situational claims ('My husband left me', 'The health visitor bullied me'), we see them as much less influential than her behavior.[360] Our bias towards seeing the mother's failure as the result of an internal fault is in direct tension with the mother's bias – she believes her failure stems from external fault. And the bad news for Mum doesn't end there: even when the audience is a fellow mother who herself failed at breastfeeding, she will still succumb to the bias.[361]

What about those close to the mother – her husband, parents, friends and others who may have witnessed the scene of the crime first hand? Do their direct observations counter their innate human tendency towards confirmation bias? Surely being part of the action guarantees a more realistic assessment of the situation? *Au contraire, mon amie*. Amazingly, close observers of a mother's struggles also tend to overplay her culpability while downplaying circumstantial influences. One reason is that a mother's nearest and dearest are distracted by their own actions – helping with the housework, marvelling at the newest family member, buying gifts, liaising with health professionals – all that new baby jazz. In fact, observers who are distracted or engaged in multitasking actually show *even greater* correspondence bias![362]

It's not looking good for our excuse-making mum. Fortunately for her, another cognitive bias springs to her aid – the 'truth bias'. We all have a default belief – a presumption – that we are being told the truth and are not being deceived.[363] It works like this: rather than objectively judging the honesty of everyone we interact with (bothersome and cognitively taxing), we automatically assume people are telling the truth. In the absence of a compelling reason to suspect they're lying, the thought never occurs to us. How many times do you count the change you're given at the supermarket? Truth bias is a powerful yet unconscious cognitive rule of thumb, and it serves excuse-making mothers well, allowing them to evade their audience's awareness radar. The fact that the excuse-making mum is reporting what happened, rather than someone else, strengthens the process. Normally, the audience has few objective criteria for determining the truthfulness of her explanations, especially when these explanations appear to fit the nature of breastfeeding failure.

This advantage, however, is short-lived. One way an audience tries to gauge the truthfulness of a mother's account is to look at its 'distinctiveness'. Was her failure a one-off, or is failure a reoccurring trend in her maternal script? Mothers perceived as performing poorly in other mothering tasks (alongside breastfeeding) are judged more harshly than those for whom breastfeeding failure is but an isolated blip. In other words, the higher the incidence of failure in the mother's life, the greater the degree to which she is likely to be held responsible for it.[364] This sounds disastrous for the mother –

and it is. Get this: even if information about the mother's other parenting performance is not available, an audience is inclined to make implications that would be predicted if it were. So when we see a mother bottle feeding, we assume she must take 'short cuts' in other areas of parenting.[365] People use 'causal schemas'[366] – a type of mental shorthand – for ascertaining responsibility.

The strength of our inclination to blame mum is understandable when you consider that it's impossible for a mother to be a passive participant in breastfeeding. Her behaviour is much more 'salient' than the context or situation in which it occurs, and we are naturally driven to assign salient factors a more causal role in events than non-salient factors.[366b] The most salient factor in breastfeeding failure – the mother – forms an anchor in our judgement process. We then attempt to adjust our judgement in light of the mother's circumstances, but we're rather crap at this adjustment process. We tend to be over-conservative – we pin everything on her internal character, giving little thought to her external scenario – so our adjustments turn out to be insufficient.[367]

### Personal bias

'Others don't judge your actions in a vacuum but interpret them through the lens of their own experience'.
Sheena Iyengar, 2010, *The Art of Choosing*[368]

When does another person's behaviour trigger an emotional response in us? When, for whatever reason, that behaviour makes us feel better or worse about ourselves. When mothers start talking about infant feeding with one another (particularly if they are not firm friends), they are not just trying to get through a coherent conversation, they are trying to figure each other out. When they enter the conversation, each mother may be positively or negatively biased in how she perceives breastfeeding failure. Positive bias is an ally to the excuse-maker, but negative bias is problematic.

'What would I have done in her situation?' is a question we ask ourselves when we hear excuse-making. Our answer to this unspoken question becomes the starting point for the judgement process, creating a bias in the way we judge the validity of the excuses presented to us. If a mother behaved as we did (or as we think we would), we are more likely to attribute her behaviour to circumstance. However, if the mother behaved in a way we wouldn't, we instinctively accredit her behaviour to her personal disposition.[369] We judge her personally. This process is directed by two emotional needs – and we all share them to some extent. Firstly, our innate human desire to see the mother get what she deserved.[370] Secondly, the desire to avoid the possibility of being blamed for a transgression ourselves. These needs may sound perplexing; to understand them it helps to consider the way in which mothers are intermeshed; they inhabit a social matrix in which their outcomes are invariably linked.[371]

A mother learns how to view herself by interacting with her maternal peers. In exchanges about infant feeding, every mother has a personal stake in the outcome of the discussion – a degree to which the behaviour being explained carries positive or negative consequences for her.[372] This is because every mother carries her own breastfeeding baggage. Whether she used formula from the start and failed to try breastfeeding; whether she tried and failed; whether she allowed her child to self-wean or not; whether she adopted an older child and so missed out on the breastfeeding experience – the breadth of possible breastfeeding experience is infinitely diverse. To understand how mothers respond to each other's excuses, we need to look at which stage they are at in their respective breastfeeding journeys. Take, for instance, a mother's excuse that her baby wouldn't latch. This declaration is as important for what it denies as for what it asserts. The scenario of a baby refusing to latch denies the mother responsibility while asserting that refusing to latch is a characteristic of babies. A pregnant mother, on hearing this excuse, will withhold harsh judgement for fear that she will find herself in the same situation with her own baby in the near future.[373] A novice breastfeeding mother will also withhold harsh judgement for fear that she too may fall into the situation described by the excuse-maker. In both examples, the reaction of the listening mother is dependent on her desire to minimise her own personal threat. She frames the excuse as a credible threat to her own efforts, a possible fate to be wary of.

Thus, listening mothers can be wholly rational judges of another mum's excuses *only* if they can be confident that they will never be in similar circumstances. If, however, they believe that they might some day find themselves in the same position, their analysis becomes tainted. In the case above, the level of responsibility attributed to the excuse-making mother by the listening mothers depends on how similar they think they are to her.[374] A veteran breastfeeding mother is much less inclined to accept excuses as plausible because her extensive experience of successful breastfeeding distinguishes, and thus distances, her in terms of character and behaviour from the excuse-maker. If, on the other hand, the listener considers herself to be similar (and therefore likely to make the same mistakes), the excuse-maker's responsibility is minimised, and the listener may even jump in and offer an account for the excuse-maker that resembles what she would prefer to say for herself.

Audiences composed of friends and regular acquaintances are particularly active co-conspirators in this regard. Their meetings are fertile grounds for mutual ego-propping. The more linked mothers become, the more likely they are to assist one another with excuses, thereby defending their own identities. In this way, the excusing process involves each participating mother actively negotiating the outcome of the exchange. The mothers shift and shape themselves in relation to the unfolding encounter. In essence, when they accept each others' excuses, mothers are partaking not only in a form of solidarity, but also in self-protective denial.

## KEEPING MUM –
## THE FEMININE ILLUSION OF INGRATIATION

Another asset to the excuse-maker is the fact that listeners – particularly female ones – go to great lengths to preserve themselves and others from embarrassment. Most women when hearing a mother's excuse will publicly condone her while privately condemning.[375] They choose to accept the excuse-maker's account outwardly, even if not internally. They conceal their scepticism behind textbook statements of sympathy. This behaviour is itself a form of deception, albeit a very widespread one. We are all actors in a social masquerade, reluctant to deliver feedback that is unpleasant for the recipient mum. Social psychologists Abraham Tesser and Sidney Rosen[376] termed this (ironically for our purposes) the 'Mum effect'. It refers to people's predilections to 'keep mum' about negative feedback. Indeed, an audience is often less interested in the mother's veracity and more concerned with maintaining an ongoing interaction and 'keeping the peace'. This explains why an excuse will often be met with a no-reaction reaction!

Keeping mum is particularly prominent among women because, on average, women spontaneously empathise to a greater degree than men. Empathising in this sense involves reading the emotional atmosphere between people and sensitively negotiating the interaction so as not to hurt or offend. In other words, women are better at judging when it would be better to suppress showing an emotion, so as not to hurt the other person's feelings. This intuitive grasp of emotions extends to women's superior sensitivity to facial expressions and other non-verbal communication, and their talent at picking up on subtle nuances.[377] Some neuroscientists believe that the brain circuits of women, in anticipation of retaliation, instinctively attempt to hijack the inclination to criticise others. They maintain that the female brain has a strong aversion to conflict, triggered by fear of angering the other person and losing the relationship.[378]

Gender aside, rare is the audience that asks questions, refuses to accept excuses or challenges them. To take the wind from another person's sails often results in one participant in the exchange being disliked. Therefore listeners adopt a simple tactic – merely keeping mum. Both excuse-maker and excuse-receiver want to bring the dialogue to a rapid and mutually agreeable close. Most people prefer solidarity to conflict and disagreement; they help each other out with trust and tact. This behaviour may appear altruistic; however it is often conditional upon the expectation that it will be applied to us in return.

In conversation, mums readily mirror opinions to avoid disagreement and demonstrate similarity, often at the cost of truth. Part of the reason is the old nutshell we cracked in the previous chapter: guilt. Maternal guilt radiates from the excuse-maker, and guilt is a contagious emotion. Just as it has an intrinsic tendency to encourage excuse-making, so there is a tendency for the audience to another's guilt to formulate excuses for the guilty party. A member of the audience may, for instance, help the excuse-making mother by making some light comment and tossing in a justifying remark such as, 'Yeah breastfeeding is hard, there's no shame in quitting' or the cringe-worthy, 'Happy Mum, Happy Baby!'. Such comforting tactics are particularly prevalent among women, who are said to use 'socially enabling' language more frequently than men.[379] In fact, the mother's guilt vis-a-vis her audience also evokes guilt on the audience's part – for its inevitable role in the mother's painful feelings.

This is hardly surprising in our gendered culture, where women are expected to take care of other people's emotions.[380] Sympathy and nurturing are the social script women are expected to adhere to in order to elevate the mood, feelings and status of others. As feminist scholars Susie Orbach and Luise Eichenbaum put it, 'A woman's emotional tentacles seek out the precipices in life's emotional terrain'.[381] From early in life, females are directed to be aware of the feelings and needs of others. Empathy becomes the grammar of female social conduct. We can see the natural fruition of this in women's speech, which tends to be more cooperative, more reciprocal and more collaborative. In other words, it is a socially-binding process. Women are more likely than men to express agreement with each other, make softer claims and use more polite forms of speech. When women disagree, they are more likely to soften the blow by expressing their opinion in the form of a question rather than an assertion.[382] A typical female audience lets a mother know that they don't regard her failure to breastfeed as particularly undesirable and won't hold it against her. Such ingratiation greases the wheels of maternal interaction. However, it also plays into the hands of the excuse-maker, reinforcing her behaviour and encouraging future excuse-making exchanges. In this sense, the excuse-making mum and her audience actively collaborate to enable Mum to succeed in her goal: preserving her image and reassuring her ego.

## WHEN EXCUSES GO RIGHT

Nothing enables mothers to cleanse their reputations more thoroughly than a well-staged excuse. Indeed, research has shown that mothers have pretty accurate ideas about what's likely to be deemed a 'good' excuse by others,[383] so they're already wearing decent running shoes for this race. Since people – those with ovaries in particular – loathe to dish out negative feedback, any feedback given is highly likely to be positive,[384] and mothers, being human, are apt to lap it up.[385] In fact, we are all predisposed to interpret even ambiguous or non-existent feedback – a blank stare or changing the subject – as positive![386]

In this light, excuses are therapeutic. They dilute maternal guilt and give amnesty. Why is excuse-making so widespread among post-breastfeeding mothers? For the simple reason that on so many levels excuse-making 'works'. Excuses arouse sympathy and the related emotions of pity and compassion, particularly when recited to a female audience. Mothers use excuses because their usefulness is reinforced either by a positive outcome or the avoidance of a negative outcome. Is it any wonder so many mothers give up breastfeeding when they can be confident that they have a safety net of excuses to fall back on?

Excuse-making in a bottle-feeding culture is more or less fully socially prescribed and scripted. In the Deception chapter, we explored the extent to which a mother believes her friends and family condone breastfeeding and found out it's an accurate prediction of her own motivation. Well, guess what? The same goes for excuse-making. If a mum has witnessed her own homies excuse-making to make their breastfeeding failures more palatable, she will be more energised to do the same.[387]

## WHEN EXCUSES GO WRONG

'Deny someone truth, and you deny their humanity'.

Ian Leslie, 2011, *Born Liars*[388]

At best, excuses make it difficult for others to relate to us. At worst, they provoke hostile social reactions, destroying trust and confidence between people.[389] Excuse-making is profoundly insulting to an audience because it presupposes the gullibility of those listening to the excuses.

> 'One mom defends her right to bottle-feed her baby without judgment. We're with her. But then she tests our theoretical tolerance by giving her reasons...'

...snarked online feminist magazine *Jezebel* in an article entitled 'Not Breastfeeding Is Fine, But What About Her Reasoning?'.[390] Indeed, excuses seek to manipulate, to arouse certain behaviour (praise rather than blame), emotions (pity rather than anger) and motivations (altruism rather than aggression). Mothers use excuses to manipulate the way in which their relationships with other mothers will be defined and their status in those relationships.

A major problem for excuse-making mothers is that when reciting their script, they give and receive multiple signals – many unintentional – that indicate they are breaking the rules. Erving Goffman, dubbed 'the most influential American sociologist of the 20th century', distinguished between two principal dichotomous signals we emit when interacting with people: the expression we *give*, and the expression we *give off*.[391] These types of signal are quite asymmetric. We can manipulate the former at will, chiefly through our verbal assertions. The latter form our Achilles's heel: we seem to have little or no control over these signals because they mostly come from the expressions we give off. When a mother is excuse-making, she is only aware of the former signals (her stream of communication), but the latter (her expressions) are often a more accurate reflection of reality. So when a mother claims (verbally) that her infant's health is her highest priority, she can negate this message in the same breath by pulling out a bottle of lukewarm water and proceeding to add formula powder. Just as in music, where a single note can discredit the tone of a whole performance, this slip can undermine the mum's façade. She may then dig her hole deeper by using a cushion to prop the finished potion at her babe's mouth. The lack of coherence between the mother's verbal excuses and her physical actions reveals a crucial discrepancy between her socialised Ought-to-Be Self and her flaw-ridden Actual Self (see page 88). Actions speak louder than words.

However, words can be similarly telling. Notice the off-key note in the otherwise stellar performance of this mum:

> 'It was hard. It is our first baby, and it was hard to get on the same wavelength as the baby. My husband's mother kept wanting to give her water. She was afraid she would get dehydrated. At one point she was very upset that she never got to feed our daughter. She was sure I was starving her because she ate so often. Me and my husband had a big fight over that. So I stopped pumping at work so she can feed her. It was a hassle to pump at work anyway.'[392]

Did this mother quit because she was under duress from others? Or because breastfeeding 'was a hassle'? A large amount of ambiguity jeopardises the believability of the excuse.[393] Being economical with the truth – in other words, selectively withholding information with intent to deceive – is a common way for mothers to edit their failure narrative. For instance, mothers may proclaim they tried very hard to breastfeed, but neglect to mention that they only tried for three days. Or they may say they had insufficient milk, but not mention that they sabotaged their milk supply by supplementing with formula. Many of these mothers 'leak' tell-tale signs of deceit. For instance, they may be vague about details and make extraordinary claims such as, 'My milk suddenly dried up'. Their dialogue often involves faulty reasoning or exonerating moves. If the excuse contains elements of truth, they over-emphasise them. Then, if the logic is challenged, a mother is likely to defend it with an emotional intensity that suggests her feelings of self-worth are at stake.[394]

The passion with which a mother recites excuses masks a deep-rooted fear of others discovering her character flaws; discovering that she is indeed responsible for her failure. This fear is wise: empirical research[395] has revealed that most people in most cultures consider ability and effort to be the main determinants of achievement. And it would appear that women's harshest critics are other women: they have been shown to value effort more highly than men[396] and to regard intrinsic qualities, such as a parent's love, as explanations for parental success or failure.[397] Against this backdrop, poor excuses backfire. Often excuses are deemed poor when they can be controlled by the mother and changed by her actions ('I had to return to work and didn't want to express at the office').

Not only do poor excuses fail to create the intended impression, they can have the opposite effect: the dishonour accompanying them can also accompany Mum like a shadow.[398] Blaming, for instance, is one of the most transparent and relatively offensive of excuses. To use an analogy: as excuse strategies go, blaming is a rusty sword that fails to perform the task it was designed for while giving the holder a nasty case of tetanus. The major snag with blaming is that, rather than eliciting sympathy, it risks arousing disdain because Mum appears neither to accept responsibility nor show remorse.[399]

Moreover, whether or not a mother has failed to breastfeed in the past constrains the usefulness of excuses relating to current breastfeeding.[400] If a mother has a 'track record' of bottle-feeding babies, it is harder for her to excuse her present failure to breastfeed.[401] Breastfeeding failure is a common denominator in her life story; one more failure is consistent with, and strengthens, this chain of events. Knowing this, many mothers who have failed to breastfeed in the past don't even attempt to excuse their behaviour. Instead, they move direct to justification. Their dialogue is often tinged with defiance: 'It doesn't matter what you say to me I've got a very healthy child who hasn't in any way been affected, as far as I can see, by not being breastfed, and I am not doing it,' spat one mother regarding her choice to jump straight to formula with child number 2 after failing to nurse child number 1.[402]

Blinded by the spotlight of past failure, mothers may attempt to wheedle their way out of their current moral predicament. Some wannabe contortionists even use past failure to excuse present failure! Professor Elizabeth Murphy[403] discovered this façade when she interviewed mothers and found them using 'sad tales', which she described as 'a selected (often distorted) arrangement of facts that highlight an extremely dismal past, and thus "explain" the individual's present state'.[404] Unfortunately for these mothers, because failure has been a consistent narrative in their parenting, people are more likely to attribute it to their personal characteristics.

Wait, it gets worse! If a mother has a clean slate, 'situational' reasons for her failure to breastfeed that would normally be seen as compelling explanations, are ignored. With this type of mother, they are ignored.[405] So, if a mother formula-fed her previous children and failed to breastfeed her current child, the skeletons in her closet ensure the blame lingers (and even intensifies), regardless of how unsurmountable her present challenges may be. Whether they are aware of it or not, listeners form a naïve hypothesis – a tentative theory – of why Mum keeps failing: she just doesn't like breastfeeding or isn't dedicated enough or didn't try, to quote common suspicions. This sets the listeners's radar on red alert for any information, no matter how tenuous, in Mum's story that can confirm this hypothesis.[406] Sometimes listeners even fantasise beyond the information given, in order to confirm their suspicions.[407]

By now, you'll have figured out that, as a general rule, folk don't take kindly to excuse-makers. We are more likely to evaluate them harshly compared to non-excuse-makers who experience the same failure.[408] As it was concluded, somewhat indelicately, in one study, 'Excuse-makers risk being seen as deceptive, self-absorbed, and ineffectual; they are viewed as unreliable social participants with flawed character'.[409] When someone messes up, we expect her to take personal responsibility for her actions.[410] 'I quit breastfeeding because I didn't like it' is a great, if extinct, example of a mother adhering to this expectation.

In lieu of such honest confessions, the actual *public* backlash that excuse-makers face is minimal. At worst, the excuse-making mother is met with a raised eyebrow or a seemingly innocuous why question. Mostly, however, her excuses are responded to with expressions of sympathy or compassion. Yet, if people dislike excuse-making so much, why respond to it with 'pro-social' gestures?

Excuse-making mothers are seldom publicly reproached thanks to a particularly feminine social weakness known as 'face-saving'.[411] I'm not talking about swapping acne-busting tips; 'face', in this respect, is the 'social commodity' granted by others, the advantage or value akin to personal dignity.[412] If one mother were to threaten the face of another – for instance by asking uncomfortable questions – she risks retaliatory attacks on her own face. When studying this behaviour, social psychologists have coined the twee term 'politeness theory' to describe the simple notion that 'it is generally in everyone's best interests to maintain each other's face'.[413] Listeners, particularly those who anticipate future interactions with the excuse-maker, feel compelled to save her face.[414]

## COLLATERAL DAMAGE – FUELLING THE CULTURE OF FAILURE, ONE EXCUSE AT A TIME

If you've been alive over the last few decades you will probably have made the following observation: everyone appears to be failing at breastfeeding. Now if everyone is failing, the assertion is that the averseness of failing should somehow be lessened. Because everyone does it, failure almost seems acceptable.[415] Ian Leslie described this legitimising effect in his book, *Born Liars*:

> 'The lie you tell to maintain your reputation might have a knock-on effect if it reaffirms the belief of others in the room – who may privately think the same thing as you – that the "correct" social behaviour is to say otherwise. An accumulation of these small lies can lead to large public lies, enabling the perpetuation of outmoded social practices long after people cease believing in them'.[416]

To further illustrate the legitimising effect, let's briefly revisit a concept we explored in the Deception chapter – the Culture of Failure, see page 79 – and look at how excuse-making relates to this culture. Remember that because breastfeeding failure is more visible in daily life than breastfeeding triumph, mothers systematically underestimate their chances of succeeding. They succumb to an illusion and mistake how sizable the biological probability of success really is. This underestimation becomes especially pernicious when they encounter a breastfeeding challenge themselves. They soon discover similarities between their current challenge and the stories of failed breastfeeders, and are tempted to mark these as indications of their impending doom. The risk of not having enough milk is prominent in our culture. Success is not. Unfortunately, negative information – like milk-deficient sob stories – has more impact than positive information, and people 'process' it more thoroughly.

It's easy to see how the consequences of excuse-making extend far beyond the excuse-making mother. Excuses affect our social structure by inflicting widespread damage to mothers' confidence in their own bodies, in each others' integrity, and in society's confidence in mothers. Mums assess the probability of failure based on the ease with which they can bring these thoughts to mind. The number of mothers failing at breastfeeding and promulgating excuses strengthens the illusion of a generation of broken-breasted women and breast-evasive babies. The Culture of Failure makes it easy to imagine what can go wrong and have a foggy and incoherent perception of what can go right. The ability to easily imagine how failure might come about leaves women convinced it will happen. Many mothers hide from the possibility of real success in their preconceptions about the inevitability of failure.

Think about it: people who believe they cannot accomplish a goal work less hard and quit earlier than those who do. In this sense, pervasive excuse-making fashions a universal state of maternal helplessness. Would-be mothers form a false preconception that breastfeeding is, for the most part, a matter of luck; that women's bodies regularly malfunction. They become firm believers in Murphy's Law: anything that can go wrong *will* go wrong. Because they are always shadowed by the likelihood of failure, they learn, at best, to 'ironise' their wishes. They say they will 'try' to breastfeed. They will 'give it a go'. For those mums who don't buckle pre-pregnancy, most of them encounter a breastfeeding issue and give up because failure is imminent – it must be, all their friends failed. It looks like their bodies, too, have malfunctioned.

As we saw in the Deception chapter, feeling confident about succeeding is an important variable with regard to who will attempt (and succeed) to breastfeed. For more insight, consider that in one study a team of researchers[417] found that maternal confidence was the most significant of 11 psychosocial and demographic factors affecting breastfeeding duration. Women with low breastfeeding confidence were three times more likely to give up compared to very confident breastfeeding women. A different team of researchers in another study[418] found that 27 percent of women with low confidence in the prenatal period discontinue breastfeeding within the first postnatal week compared with only 5 percent of highly confident women.

Propagandising excuses lower the confidence of would-be breastfeeders everywhere. Take the typical pregnant mother. When she contemplates breastfeeding, she thinks about the probability of failing, and more importantly, the possible causes of her 'hypothetical' failure – and formula feeders are all too willing to supply numerous causes for her to consider. If, on hearing their countless and varied excuses, she internalises them, she will have little confidence in her own likelihood of succeeding. She may even decide not to bother trying to breastfeed at all, and in turn avoid people attributing her failure to her ability, which is never tested. In one study, a pregnant mother shared her worries:

'I've known too many people say, "Oh yeah, I'm only giving my baby breast milk", and you find that they reckon two or three days later they just couldn't do it. The baby just couldn't take the milk or couldn't take the breast at all. So obviously you've got to keep an open mind.... You never know what's around the corner. No one can predict the future'.[419]

In other words, the culture of failure manifests itself in women underestimating the control they could, in fact, exert in their breastfeeding journey – they expect uncontrollability where, in fact, controllability exists. Women immersed in this culture are needlessly pessimistic with regard to their breastfeeding potential. This is important because while expectations are intangible, their effects are quite real – they have the power to change everyday life. Expectations alter the biochemistry of the brain and thus the whole body. We see this in the placebo effect – some pills and therapies that are unlikely to improve health miraculously do so anyway. If breastfeeding advocates are to be successful (and there are tips to support them on page 67), they need to raise mothers' expectations of themselves. In doing so, they will raise maternal motivation. At present, the optimistic voices of breastfeeding advocates are being drowned out by the torrential noise of excuse-makers who vastly outnumber them.

## INTERNALISATION – BELIEVING YOUR OWN EXCUSES

'Excuses are self-serving explanations, or accounts, that aim to reduce personal responsibility for questionable events, thereby disengaging core components of the self from the incident. Their goal is to convince audiences, often the actor included, that a questionable event is not as much the actor's fault as might otherwise appear to be'.

Barry Schlenker, Beth Pontari and Andrew Christopher, 2001, *Excuses and Character*[420]

As the quote suggests, there is much more to excuse-making than reducing your own responsibility and other people's condemnation. Excuses are often used, particularly by mothers, to protect themselves from the low self-esteem that accompanies attributions of failure. Excuses solidify a mother's 'reality-negotiation process'.[421] We looked at this largely internal thought process, a type of orchestrated self-deception, in the Guilt chapter. When a mother is performing her excuse-making routine, she is performing for the benefit not only of an external audience, but also for herself, the ultimate internal critic. She becomes her own audience.[422]

The excuses she verbalises may make her feel better about herself; indeed, studies have found that, initially, excuse-making enhances self-esteem.[423] But in order for this to occur, Mum must come to believe her own rhetoric. This raises the question: can a mother who starts with the goal of fooling an audience actually end up fooling herself?

Undeniably some, if not most, mothers do come to internalise the victim role they carve for themselves through excuses. In fact, they are predisposed to do so. A mother gets comfortable in her new role and comes to value the rewards the role generates, be those sympathy, escape from responsibility or reassurance from others. At first, she is aware of her excuse-making ploy, but as she develops a protracted narrative and employs the same excuses, over time their performance becomes a habit. Then, like most habits, the excuse-making gradually recedes from awareness. Explanations are relabelled as reasons rather than excuses although their content remains substantially the same.[424] Unless this façade is brought to a mother's attention, it limbos quite elegantly under her radar. Essentially, she is wearing a mask that represents her Desired Self – the role she could feasibly live up to, if only she had made different choices. In the end, this role becomes second nature, in part because it masks her Actual Self – a role she is forever trying to escape.

It is not difficult to see how this internalisation process unfolds. Self-deception is cemented by excuse-making. In the words of the Greek philosopher Demosthenes, 'There is nothing easier than self-delusion. Since what man desires, is the first thing he believes'. Take the mother who cites pressure from her doctor as the reason for quitting breastfeeding. Even though she knows the pressure was not as great as she is making out, over time she internalises her public statement and comes to believe privately that it actually describes the facts. Any memories of an element of pressure, albeit weak, further strengthen her internalisation. Then, as she becomes reliant on this narrative to excuse her breastfeeding failure, her memory becomes warped in its service. She remembers only the confirming examples of her blamelessness and forgets dissonant instances in her active engagement in the chain of events that led to the failure. Most of us are programmed to search for reassuring truths in this way. As psychologists Carol Tavris and Elliot Aronson have noted, 'When a story is repeated often enough, it becomes so familiar that it chips away at a person's initial scepticism'.[425]

However, when a knowledgeable audience is involved, there is – in theory at least – less opportunity for such self-deception. A midwife or even a husband who closely witnessed the events leading to the failure can invalidate the mother's story quite readily. This seldom occurs because, as I explained on page 152, people are generally protective of the public face of others. Instead, they give the impression of accepting the mother's account as truthful – and this makes the mother even more likely to internalise it. Even though the account does not perfectly reflect the mother's initial (private) view of how her failure occurred, its acceptance by key figures in her life leads her to think that the account accurately describes the situation. A mother may start to believe that perhaps she really *didn't* have enough milk. After all, her baby was constantly at the breast and often unsettled. It doesn't matter that these symptoms could have a virtually limitless list of other explanations. Having insufficient milk suits her narrative. In this way, she becomes estranged from herself.[426] Kathryn Schulz, in her book *Being Wrong – Adventures in the Margin of Error* describes the conflict people experience between feeling their wrongness and feeling their rightness:

> 'Upon retracing our steps to discover where we erred, we find that the path we took still feels both sensible and defensible, and we start making excuses almost despite ourselves. (We've all had the experience of saying, "Look, I'm not trying to justify what happened, I just want to explain it" – only to realize, in a very short order, that we are justifying left and right). Here, too, wrongness reveals its fugitive nature: it's as if, once we can explain a mistake, it ceases to feel like one'.[427]

Thus, a mother's internal perspective of her breastfeeding experience can dramatically shift over time. Mothers, exercising hindsight weeks after their failure, are more likely to remember situational causes than their personal disposition at the time.[428] Combine this with *wanting* to believe her own excuses, and it's easy to see how a mother's memory can actually be 'reconstructed' through excuse-making,[429] with a single excuse prompting a domino effect of cognitive restructuring. For instance, if a mother claims she was bullied into quitting breastfeeding by a health professional, this cognition may not align with her existing perception of herself as a strong-willed person. Consequently, she alters her self-perception in order to lend integrity to her behaviour. Sadly, in this scenario a depressive effect can result.[430] Thus is revealed the often dark personal inheritance of excuse-making.

## EXCUSES – A POISONOUS PERSONAL LEGACY

Excuse-making, like guilt, is the legacy that lingers. Excuses are self-affirming and self-renewing. Their immediate benefits are much more attractive than the long-term negative consequences – which are numerous. Taking personal responsibility is an invaluable gift that only we can give to ourselves. By taking personal responsibility for failure, mothers can mentally nourish themselves. Yet this is a radical notion. Why? Because on the face of it, excuse-making *appears* to be self-protective. It is easy to assume (and there is plenty of empirical evidence to suggest) that the non-reflective mode of living facilitated by excuse-making is more compatible with psychological well-being; that focusing on one's mistakes is a recipe for lower self-esteem. Indeed, an Arab proverb states that you should write the bad things that happen to you in the sand; that way, they can be easily erased from your memory.

However, although excuses can buy some breathing space, they do not, in themselves, correct any underlying problems. In the previous chapter we examined how a mother must find a way to assimilate her breastfeeding failure into a positive view of herself in order to stop guilt from eroding her self-esteem. In this sense, excuses are a reality-negotiating vehicle for sustaining the illusion of positive image. The process invariably involves Mum being economical with the truth – both to others and to herself. This strategy creates a paradox:

by twisting reality, Mum often damages, rather than protects, her self-esteem in the long run. This is because 'accurate reality perception' is a key ingredient for mental health.[431] As psychologist Marie Jahoda[432] put it, 'Mentally healthy perception means a process of viewing the world so that one is able to take in matters one wishes were different *without distorting them to fit these wishes* [my emphasis]'.

Bending the truth via excuses causes what may be described as a 'twinge of distress' – not necessarily in the listener, who may be ignorant of the façade, but in the excuse-making mother herself, making her feel worse than she did before she made the excuse. Sometimes the resulting feeling is a shade of guilt; sometimes it is a feeling of being less connected to the person being deceived. This darkening of mood often lasts even after the conversation has returned to honest realms. The consequence is what Bella DePaulo, a psychology researcher at the University of California, has coined an emotional 'smudge' on the interaction.[433] Another shrink, Helen Lynd, acknowledged the smudge, and went on to describe the process of excuse-making as self-harm:

> 'There is a particularly deep shame in deceiving other persons into believing something about oneself that is not true. No one else knows of it; one has lied to oneself'.[434]

For a mother, making excuses may feel good initially, but the behaviour is counter-productive in the long run. Her public descriptions of herself and her circumstances can affect what she later comes to believe privately.[435] Like most people, mothers have a drive to see themselves as consistent, comprehensible individuals. It follows that success increases and failure decreases the perceived probability that she will be successful in the future. The causal narrative that a mother gives to explain her breastfeeding performance can help or hinder her future breastfeeding efforts. Her expectation of future breastfeeding success not only reflects her past breastfeeding performance, but is influenced by the explanation of why she performed that way then. The choice to excuse-make can impact not only on those listening, but on the mother herself.

It is dangerous territory.

We can see just how self-harming excuse-making can be when we look at the mother who attaches an anatomical excuse to her breastfeeding failure. In this scenario, the mother's friends and family (and often the mother herself, if she has bought into her own excuse) anticipate her anatomical difficulties remaining in place, and so expect breastfeeding failure to recur with subsequent babies. Here, we see the long-lasting and serious consequences of anatomy-related excuses. By their very nature, they are irreversible. A paradox of reflexivity occurs in which the mother inadvertently undermines her pool of future options. Where breastfeeding is concerned, she is locked in chronic helplessness. This disabling emotion easily leaks through to other areas of life. It presupposes hopelessness. The mother's excuse-based inability to accept responsibility alienates her not only from other people, but also from herself. It makes it impossible for her to engage in any process of constructive improvement.[436]

The same fatalistic burden applies, in varying degrees, to *all* excuses for breastfeeding failure explored in this chapter. When a mother covers up poor commitment with excuses, she is confronted sooner or later with the realisation that if she successfully breastfeeds at some point in the future, theoretically she could have successfully breastfed before. This is a tough pill to swallow. Consider also instances where a mother used her lack of belief in the credibility of breastfeeding to justify her actions. Once she has proclaimed that she doesn't believe in the virtues of breastfeeding, it becomes more difficult for her to make a serious investment in breastfeeding in the future without losing face. Erving Goffman has aptly called this 'in-deeper-ism'.[437] Carol Tavris and Elliot Aronson[438] called it a 'process of entrapment': the route of action – justification – further action increases a mother's commitment to an initial undertaking and ends up taking her far from her original intentions or principles. By using excuses, Mum surrenders her responsibility, and with it her freedom.

To explore the concept of surrender further, let's take two examples from outside the breastfeeding domain, but still in the sphere of health: spinal injury and breast cancer patients (trust me, I'm going somewhere with this). In a frequently cited study, two psychology researchers[439] investigated the coping behaviour of individuals who had become paralysed after spinal cord injuries during accidents. They found that those who blamed other people or other external factors for their accident adapted comparatively less well to their handicaps than individuals who 'blamed themselves' for the accident. Another study[440] reported that breast-cancer patients who believed their cancer was caused by controllable factors such as 'dieting' or 'negative attitudes' coped better with their misfortune than those who attributed the illness to uncontrollable causes.

These studies echo what we explored in the Deception chapter: maintaining a level of 'control' has a positive influence on how people cope with stressful life events. If we consider breastfeeding failure to be a stressful life event, we see that if mothers took responsibility for their actions (or inaction) they would be able to cope better subsequently. When a mother regards her own actions (such as lack of effort) as responsible for her poor show, she responds first with feelings of inferiority, and then with motivation to improve herself. However, if the same mother attributes her breastfeeding failure wholly to perceived unfair causes, anger and resentment predominate.[441] These feelings can sabotage her future efforts, distracting her from beneficial acts like preparation and self-improvement. Taking personal responsibility means retaining control and generating hope. Effort is a fluid condition; it is subject to change in the future, and consequently the outcome of that effort is also subject to change. While excuse-making provides short-term protection to a mother's self-esteem, taking personal responsibility provides long-term protection to her well-being. Unhappiness and depression are inversely linked to one's ability to foresee change and retain hope.[442]

In other words, attributing breastfeeding failure to uncontrollable factors, whether internal (breast malfunction) or external (employment constraints), implies that failure will reoccur in the future, whereas attributing breastfeeding failure to variable causes (effort, motivation, determination) gives rise to 'hope' for the future ('I can try harder next time'). It is a healthier, more adaptive response because it allows Mum to change her behaviour in future circumstances.[443]

This has been a mammoth chapter, but that's what you get when you tackle an excuse-riddled domain like breastfeeding! To sum it up: mothers are under both external and internal pressure to project a favourable image of themselves as dedicated, conscientious, moral and so on. They craft post-facto excuses that they believe will express and maintain these qualities in the face of factual information that threatens them. However, in as far as they are designed to be protective devices, excuses are largely impotent. If a mother is already uncertain or doubtful of her credibility in the first place, excuses merely serve the thinly veiled social function of saving face. The newly quitted mother often feels torn in two directions: she feels some alienation from other formula feeders, unable to identify with them fully at this point, while at the same time suffering feelings of disloyalty and self-contempt about breastfeeders, the group she is passing out of. The gnawing misery that successful breastfeeders prompt in failed breastfeeders is the focus of the next chapter.

# 4

# ENVY

'People hate those who make them feel their own inferiority'.
Lord Mahon, 1845, *The Letters of Philip Dormer Stanhope,*
*Earl of Chesterfield*

Envy. Gotta love envy. If there were such a thing as an
Emotional Oscars, envy would win an award for the emotion
most likely to be routinely denied, disguised, repressed or relabelled. Admitting that one is envious is akin to declaring
one's inferiority. This dark, intense, implacable and irrational
emotion is painfully private and publicly feared. Women's
envy, in particular, is all pervasive yet deeply unfashionable.
It is characterised by tension and torment. The begrudging
nature of envy stems from a preoccupation with one's own
limitations and defects.

## COMPARISON AND ENTITLEMENT –
## THE ROOTS OF MATERNAL ENVY

At the heart of envy lies social comparison – ironic,
considering that envy is such an anti-social emotion. Not all
negative social comparisons result in envy, however. We feel
envious chiefly of our peers, for reasons to do with notions of
justice. For instance, people do not necessarily envy the wealth
of celebrities, because the discrepancy in income does not
reflect badly on them. Envy only results when the discrepancy
between someone else's success and our failure serves to
demonstrate or call attention to our own shortcomings. Take

two mothers who are comparable in various respects – they are around the same age, have the same level of education, are both married and both first-time mothers – but one mother successfully breastfed while the other failed to do so. This discrepancy provides strong evidence to the failed mother that her inferiority, not other factors, was the source of her failure. Envy is ignited by her perception of her own inferiority more than by a perception of the other mother's superiority. The very closeness of the two mothers' traits (education, marital status and so on) exacerbates the tendency for the unsuccessful mother to equate the other's success with her own failure.

Anyone with a beating heart experiences envy as too painful to bear yet too shameful to reveal, and in mothers it is particularly insatiable. Mothers can be observed fleeing from unfavourable social comparisons everywhere they gather to chat; it's like a game – and a passionate one. Log onto any online parenting discussion forum and you will see formula-feeding mothers over-emphasising the differences between themselves and successful breastfeeders. They relish studies showing that socio-economic background predicts breastfeeding success, while downplaying studies that negate socio-economic differences. Their behaviour illustrates the ease with which envious mothers can create an imaginary world to justify their choices.

Alternatively, some mothers attempt to cope with envy by imagining that the breastfeeding mother didn't deserve her success. Remember Doris, the mother of nine from the previous chapter (see page 92)? She admits to using this strategy in the past:

'You see other mothers breastfeeding and you are simply green with envy. You justify it to yourself that they obviously had a much easier ride than you. Their baby could not possibly have been as hungry as yours. They do not have other children to take care of. Their skin is not as sensitive. Whatever the problem was or was perceived to be, you have a justification for having to give up.

And at the end of the day it's just milk, right? You love your baby just as much, you know your baby just as much. A happy mother = a happy baby! Formula is not poison; okay, breast milk is best, but formula is good enough....

Putting aside the obvious health issues here, you are deluding yourself. It does matter, and it matters a great deal – but you do not know that, because you have been robbed of your nursing relationship before it even started. And how could you know really? You simply do not know what you are missing, as you have not been able to experience it.'

Another way mothers convince themselves that other mums didn't deserve their breastfeeding success is to attribute their success to luck. Indignation flows from envy as readily as milk flows from an engorged breast. Psychologist Dr Joseph Berke has described the comforting allure of 'luck':

'Luck is the benign leveller. It removes the personal responsibility that contributes to feelings of inferiority and envy. With good luck or bad, whatever has happened appears to be outside human control.... Luck is a superbly efficient social-sanctioned device to rationalize inadequacy, incompetence, poor judgement, and, in general, dissimilar skills, traits, or resources. By giving the illusion of absolute equality, luck allows the envier to carry on without suffering a loss of status or becoming overwhelmed by hatred.'[444]

Thus, some envious mothers attempt to pacify themselves by framing breastfeeding as a matter of luck rather than a reflection of effort and so of character. This strategy has the potential to backfire spectacularly. For some it leads to feelings of anger and resentment at what the envious mother perceives to be the cards that 'fate' has dealt her – unsupportive husband, broken breasts et al. She experiences the gulf between the successfully breastfeeding mother and herself as a cruel turn of fate. Her own responsibility for – and thus control of – her breastfeeding outcome gets watered down or obscured altogether.

One reason women get so swept up in breastfeeding envy is that envy is most likely to be triggered when we make comparisons in areas *especially important* to how we define ourselves. When others surpass us in these domains, our 'self-evaluation' is threatened as the comparison process kicks in. There is arguably no domain more culturally and emotionally central to most women's self-image than motherhood. Because the act of mothering involves little direct feedback (particularly from babies, who freely issue complaints and demands but are largely mute on the good stuff), much of a mother's perception of her own competence comes from comparisons with other mothers. In the breastfeeding context, envy occurs when a mother notices the superior success (and thus personal qualities) of another mother and perceives them as reflecting badly upon herself: 'She is mothering "better" than me'. New mothers are particularly susceptible to this trail of thought. A new mother, lacking an internally secure sense of motherhood, builds a sense of herself as a competent mother based upon such outward achievements as breastfeeding.

Alongside comparison, entitlement is another prerequisite for envy. Only when a mother feels *entitled* to a successful breastfeeding experience will envy materialise. If she lacks this sense of entitlement, envy will not be detonated, because the mother perceives the gap between the unsuccessful mother and successful mothers as justified. In envy's place comes a sense of admiration, and perhaps even awe, accompanied by acceptance.[445]

A mother might feel entitled to a breastfeeding relationship but have a low estimation of her personal ability to achieve it – this creates a gap between successful breastfeeding mothers and herself, and from this gap spews forth envious begrudgement. Feeling incapacitated can emerge from a broad pool of 'self-perceived' physical, social or psychological causes. For instance, a mother may believe she does not have adequate support in the home to enable her to breastfeed, or she may need to return to work and regard employment as incompatible with breastfeeding. She may believe that she does not have strong-enough emotional capital – in the form of willpower or perseverance – to breastfeed. Or she may think her pain threshold is too low to endure breastfeeding because of past experience. Whatever the cause for her self-evaluated incapacity, a mother's sense of helplessness gives envy its harrowing edge. As the writer Joseph Epstein tactfully explained in his book *Envy: The Seven Deadly Sins*, 'Envy is an obsessive resentment over the good fortune or achievement of others...little more than the whining of those who lack the talent to succeed'.[446] The envious mother does not feel capable of equality with the breastfeeding mother, yet her sense of entitlement remains high. This creates tension and a feeling of victimhood. Sometimes she is not even aware that she is feeling envy and instead interprets the emotion as anger.[447] This translation of emotions is bolstered by her sense of entitlement.

So how does a feeling of entitlement to a breastfeeding relationship spring up? In communities where successful breastfeeding is seldom heard of, let alone seen, a feeling of entitlement may never materialise. Here, successful breastfeeding is conceptualised as something only elite 'others' do. Mothers in communities with little role-modelling of successful breastfeeding feel content, more often than not, to affirm their culture of formula feeding. They are aware that 'Breast is Best', but they believe formula is 'good enough'. However, in communities where some women successfully breastfeed, their visibility can invoke a sense of entitlement in other mothers. The number of successful breastfeeders need not be a majority; simply being visible is enough. Envy here is typically experienced as feelings of inferiority, longing or ill will towards these women.

Mother Nature – that incessant bringer of pain and torment to women – triggers another facet of breastfeeding envy. Since breastfeeding is intertwined with biological destiny, it is a relationship that women – and their bodies – expect to experience. So when breastfeeding fails, a feeling of loss arises, both psychological and physiological. Losing something (in this case a breastfeeding relationship) makes people twice as miserable as gaining the same thing makes them happy.[448] In more technical language, we are 'loss averse'. Seeing others enjoy what we have lost can arouse ugly feelings. By failing to breastfeed, a mother has not only lost the opportunity to give optimum nutrition to her baby, she has also lost the status and pride that comes with being a breastfeeding mother. It's painful to watch others succeed at breastfeeding while constantly telling yourself that you are doing the right thing by using formula. To understand this pain, think about the Three Types of Self we looked at in the Deception chapter. Envy occurs when we see aspects of our Desired Self reflected in someone else – a potent contrast to our Actual Self. Yet the Desired Self is never completely beyond our grasp, so when we see someone else living this self, her success seems tragically close to once being ours – so close we can literally feel the throb of longing in our breasts. In this sense, envy is accompanied by a bottomless sense of truth and pain. As the American satirical novelist Joseph Heller is said to have observed, 'There is no disappointment so numbing...as someone no better than you achieving more.'

Ironically, it's the mothers that hold breastfeeding in highest esteem who are likely to feel envy most painfully. In fact, it is possible to predict the strength of future breastfeeding envy by looking at a mother's intentions during pregnancy. Those mothers with the strongest intention to breastfeed and who fail to actualise this intention are likely to feel envy's wrath most mercilessly. In other words, the degree of envy experienced is largely tied to the degree to which mothers feel they are not measuring up to their Desired Self.

Another way to understand breastfeeding envy is to look at the intrinsic nature of breastfeeding. Unlike many objects of envy, successful breastfeeding is a non-transferable commodity, an unshareable asset – and all the more powerful for it. Psychology textbooks speak of men's 'breast envy',[449] defined as natural envy of the biological functions of women. Ironically, most women at some point in their lives contract a similar but even more crippling version of the disease: lactation envy. It's more crippling because, unlike men, women have the desired equipment but, for whatever reason, have failed to use it. The capacity to preserve life with one's own body is felt by many as the greatest of feminine gifts. The premature end of the breastfeeding relationship brings a change that evokes a crushing sense of inferiority. The target of breastfeeding envy is a non-transferable aspect of another woman: her ability to breastfeed, her skill, her talent. That is why envy of breastfeeding is particularly hopeless. The perpetual frustration that comes with wanting another person's traits arouses a chronic state of bitterness. Breastfeeding mothers remind formula-feeding mothers – merely by their presence – what the latter women *should* have, but do not have, and cannot feel.

## THE BABY GROUP – A BOILING POT OF ENVY

'We are ashamed to seem evasive in the presence of a straightforward man, cowardly in the presence of a brave one, and gross in the eyes of a refined one'.
Charles Cooley, 1902, *Human Nature and the Social Order*[450]

I'd like to use the quintessential 'baby group' environment as a backdrop to explain the dynamics of maternal envy, for envy is birthed and fed by social interaction. People attempt to gain clarity about their own social standing by seeking out others with whom to compare their standing. We're all motivated to maintain or increase our self-esteem, and much of the opportunity to obtain the feedback that allows us to do this originates in social interactions with similar people. For mothers, this means baby and toddler groups; however, feel free to replace the term 'baby group' with any maternal gathering in which the shared focus of attention is motherhood – the dynamics will be largely the same. In these environments the superior performances and attributes of peers are hard to ignore, and their prevalence is quite threatening to our self-esteem. These situations inevitably invoke comparisons, the first rung on the ladder to envy. It is easy to spot envious mothers in the baby group environment by observing their behaviour. The tension that often predominates in these female-dominated spaces has been captured eloquently by therapist Leyla Navaro in her essay 'On Being Envied: Heroes and Victims':[451]

'Untrained and unaccepted in overt expressions, most women use tactic codes and body language when feeling envious, jealous, or competitive. The use of eyes is a predominant nonverbal language: to use or withhold a glance, i.e. not to look at or address the envied person are tacit statements of invalidating the envied person's presence, that is, her very existence'.

Most women consciously or semi-consciously understand this characteristically female tacit language. This awareness brings with it discomfort but also an additional problem for breastfeeding mothers: they can never be sure whether such behavioural cues are a result of envy or our cultural unease with public displays of the female breast – or indeed both. In any cultural context where breastfeeding mothers are expected to negotiate an exceptionally complex minefield of 'tacit social codes' regarding privacy and publicity, the opaque, unpredictable and undefined nature of envy's non-verbal language makes its threat even more potent.

Although the breastfeeding mother cannot determine it for sure, the envious mother sees her as competition, and the positive pretense of the breastfeeder makes the envious mother feel as though she's losing that competition. In motherhood, the breast is a prestige symbol – it conveys honour, status and duty fulfilled. The bottle, on the other hand, is a stigma symbol – drawing attention to maternal discrepancy and thus raising questions as to the user's moral fabric. In this sense, envy reflects an eroding of a mother's social position (in her own eyes and the eyes of others), and the behaviour she engages in when envious controls this diminution of status. For example, the envious mother may try to prevent a breastfeeding mother's continued success (by giving poor advice); she may distort her own beliefs about the breastfeeding mother's success in a negative direction (by attributing the breastfeeding mother's success to mere luck); she may distort her beliefs about her own performance and attributes in a positive direction (by attributing her own lack of success to external forces); she may change her view of what is important or relevant in order to reject rather than compete with breastfeeding mothers (by rejecting the significance of breastfeeding); or she may reduce closeness with the breastfeeding mother (by avoiding environments where nursing mothers are likely to be present).[452] The latter example is common: avoidance that stems from envy is frequent and noticeable among mothers. Formula-feeding mothers suffering from envy tend to surround themselves with similar mothers while keeping breastfeeding mums at arms-length.

## FEAR OF ENVY – THE CURSE
## OF SUCCESSFUL BREASTFEEDING

In the world of breastfeeding, success is a double-edged sword, conferring dignity with one hand then taking it away with the other. For breastfeeding mothers in the presence of formula feeders, success can be downright uncomfortable. Because women derive so much of their identity and sense of well-being through attachment and relationships with others, the breastfeeding mother is acutely aware that nursing her baby may upset other women. Soon, a state of 'false responsibility' develops whereby she actually begins to feel guilt. It is deeply conflicting to feel success and accomplishment at one's own achievement, and at the same time empathy and sorrow for those who have failed. Such dissonance overshadows any boost to self-esteem that being envied could provide. Combine these factors with an underlying fear of retaliation, and many breastfeeding mothers nurse their babies almost apologetically: 'I breastfeed because I'm lazy, I couldn't do all the washing and sterilizing that comes with bottle feeding'.

Some women diminish or deny the joys of breastfeeding and exaggerate the burdens; some even belittle the meaning of the act altogether: 'As long as baby is fed, it doesn't really matter how'. Such exaggerated modesty is designed to reduce hostility. Unconsciously, the breastfeeding mother feels that if she makes breastfeeding less than it is – if she makes it less desirable, if she makes it appear less than it really means to her – it won't threaten or upset the other women. If the breastfeeding mother feels such self-deprecation is not sufficient to divert the envious eyes of other mothers, she may escalate her humility by excessively praising them, cooing in faux awe at their babies' arm folds and Buddha bellies. Essentially, after deflating herself, she inflates the other mothers. Such compliments are small gestures of goodwill given in the hope of soaking up envious resentment. A type of loser's compensation.

Playing oneself down, real or feigned modesty, shyness, self-effacement and resistance to acknowledging one's success are some of the inherently female dynamics adopted by breastfeeding mothers. They are covert means of attempting to change the relative balance of power – or at least its appearance – so formula-feeding mothers can have a sense of being better and more important than they are.[453] The breastfeeding mother finds it hard to distinguish between telling other mothers about some of the good aspects of breastfeeding, and the feeling that she is boasting. Consequently, she subdues her lights lest they blind other mothers. There is no way for a breastfeeding mother to share her pride without fearing she might stir up envy. So instead, she adopts the unconscious defence of 'de-selfing', that is, she publicly obscures the characteristics and attributes that made her successful.

Such is the stigma attached to women's pride, that both men and women recognise pride as a masculine emotion, one connected to power.[454] This gender stereotype is founded on the belief that men express powerful emotions, whereas women express powerless emotions. Powerless emotions have, at their core, a display of vulnerability, whereas powerful emotions imply dominance. When we look at maternal social exchange through this lens, we see that breastfeeding mothers are socially undermined and coerced to null their pride, whereas failed breastfeeders are encouraged to dwell expressively in their self-pity. The consequence of such social engineering? Only one half of the breastfeeding story is being told. The breastfeeding mother's strategy of deflating herself and inflating others also ironically serves to perpetuate the gender stereotype that makes women feel obliged to express emotions in a way that conveys modesty or vulnerability while bowing to the needs of others. What's more, these defence tactics are not even that effective. They reduce and delay hostility temporarily rather than eliminating it, and may actually aggravate the very envy mothers seek to avoid. By downplaying her success, the breastfeeding mother can lead others to believe she 'doesn't appreciate how lucky she is'. They may even end up thinking that her dished-out reassurances are a sign of the breastfeeding mother's superiority, a cruelty designed to belittle and humiliate. Basically, she can't win.

Not wanting to upset or arouse envy is a pervasive and overwhelming fear, particularly of women. Philosopher and wordsmith Joseph Berke[455] has described the fear of impending envy as akin to being in the gaze of a rattlesnake poised to strike. Another powerful metaphor for women's envy is the 'evil eye'. The curiously entitled book *Exploring the Dirty Side of Women's Health* features an interview transcript with an Asian mother describing the care a mum must take when breastfeeding to avoid anyone watching with an envious look, a look she referred to as 'the evil eye':

'Because we have this thing about the evil eye, Asian women will not breastfeed in front of other Asian women. They feel that the woman might cast an evil eye on their child and then you will stop producing milk. They are cautious about who they feed in front of, and will probably restrict it to just direct family. If there is someone else there, they will not come out and feed their child. It is not the shame of showing a boob; it is out of fear of casting the evil eye'.[456]

This recognition that successful breastfeeding triggers envy has existed for centuries in various geographical climates and religions.[457] In Anatolia, banning another lactating woman from entering the house of a new mum is believed to protect mother and baby from evil forces – the risk is that one of the lactating ladies may have a better breast milk supply than the other.[458] Even in our Western culture, a culture of consumerism, narcissistic self-preoccupation and competition, many breastfeeding mothers feel so uncomfortable at the prospect of arousing envy in their peers that they retreat to confinement. The performance of nursing acts as a strong, if unintended, signal to others that Mum belongs in Club Breastfeeder, with all the presumptive preoccupations that entails.

## DEGREES OF ENVY

When a mother fails at breastfeeding but one of her peers – be it a family member or friend – succeeds, instead of feeling proud of and positive about her peer's achievement, she feels inadequate, depressed and resentful. The other mother's success has brought her in contact with her own ambitions and longings. Tragically, she held herself back from fulfilling her breastfeeding dream when it was her turn, and now unconsciously feels driven to hold back another woman. Tarnished by her own unmet desires, she becomes frightened by her peer's capacity to fulfil hers. She admires her ability but cannot understand how her peer was able to successfully fulfil her breastfeeding goals when she herself felt unable to. When she sees her peer groping towards more and more success, she becomes threatened to the point that she tries to discourage her. If her peer's breastfeeding relationship then falls apart, the envious mother will experience *schadenfreude* – this cheeky German word means 'joy at another's misfortune'.[459]

One only has to observe mothers' interactions to see that envy is a dynamic emotion with varying degrees of potency. Some formula-feeding mothers look to their breastfeeding peers and experience a non-malicious envy – 'I wish I had what you have'. This can be experienced in a variety of ways: feeling inferior to the breastfeeder, longing for a breastfeeding relationship, despairing at ever having it, determining to improve oneself to enable successful breastfeeding next time, or admiring the breastfeeder. In this sense, envy is a sign that a mother hasn't given up her breastfeeding dreams; she still wants in. Envy holds within it an essence of hope, energy and motivation. See, it's not all bad.

Other formula feeders, however, experience a much more potent form of envy, termed 'malicious envy': 'I wish you did not have what you have'. When experiencing malicious envy, a mother may not necessarily desire what the breastfeeder has – only that it be taken away from her. Malicious envy is often the result of a mother's defensive reappraisal of circumstances, motivated by the desire to avoid feeling inferior.

When consumed with envy, a mother has several choices

for channelling her emotions: attempting to equalise herself with the target of her envy by successfully breastfeeding herself; avoiding breastfeeding mothers wherever possible and digging her head in the sand; or attempting to spoil and destroy the target of her envy by sabotage. Mothers inclined to choose the latter destructive option are not likely to identify their feelings as envy, and thus do not own them. They are more likely to have a low evaluation of their own capacity to breastfeed and a high evaluation of entitlement.[460]

A mother in the grips of such envy can be devastatingly masochistic. There is much truth in the German proverb 'Envy will eat nothing but its own heart'. Like excuse-making, malicious envy is a rusty sword. This emotion is remarkably self-destructive: while it is aimed at bringing other mothers down, it radically diminishes the envious mother's self-esteem. Robert Solomon, philosopher and previous president of the International Society for Research on Emotion, maintains that malicious envy, 'Like shame and guilt, involves a negative self-evaluation, but unlike those emotions, it lacks the dignity of a moral sense'.[461] Envious mothers do not get round to tackling the discontent in their own lives as long as they are busy focusing on other mothers. Their envy can sometimes involve the delusion that the breastfeeding mother is somehow the cause of their inferiority, and thus of their unhappiness. This may be experienced as anger or resentment over some alleged unfairness, and may become generalised, turning into an internal hatred of breastfeeding mothers or even the act of breastfeeding itself. Regardless of the validity of such beliefs, when we invoke comparisons, distinctions between cause and blame become lost. What is actually experienced is a sense of being wronged:

> 'Envy is a form of hatred. It is a belittling, or emptying out, of the value, meaning, and potential of another, because one feels that one cannot possess certain resources the other has'.[462]

Such mothers interpret the offending comparison as caused by the breastfeeding mother's agency ('She makes me look bad'). Indeed, the presence of the breastfeeding mother is 'the cause' of the formula feeder's inferiority, and this disparity creates uneasiness and tension. Although a breastfeeding mother cannot be faulted openly for her success, the envious discontent it evokes provokes a sense of injustice. Often, the envious mother knows that few people will sympathise with this brand of moral sentiment. Therefore, her hostility is the result of a necessarily *private* grievance. The hostile yet private aspect of envy is one of its most distinctive features. In feeling scorn for the object of her admiration – successful breastfeeders – the mother attacks their representation in her mind.

To reiterate, successful breastfeeding is envied by those who do not, or feel they do not, have the same choice. But envy involves more than just discontent with one's own possessions or attributes; it also includes hostility towards or resentment of those who have or appear to have advantages. The behaviour in which we engage when envious usually attempts to restore or maintain a positive view of the self when it is threatened by comparison to others. The formula-feeding mother is acutely aware that she lacks a breastfeeding relationship. Breastfeeding was something she aspired to, but for whatever reason couldn't achieve. Unable to examine her own envious feelings because she finds them disagreeable, she transforms them to something else: angry feelings for those who breastfeed. Does this anger flow both ways? Can breastfeeding mothers be equally vicious? All will be revealed in the next chapter – Contempt.

# 5

# CONTEMPT

'People who don't try to breastfeed are selfish and deluded if
they think that artificial milk is just as good'.

Breastfeeding mother[463]

While the bulk of this book explores the intentions of mothers
who fail to breastfeed (being, as they are, the bulk of women),
it is important to take a short pit stop at this juncture and pay
respect to those positive deviants of the world – successful
breastfeeding mothers. Certainly, the so-called 'Mummy
Wars'[464] of infant feeding could not exist without a counter-
camp. If you are a member of this elite minority camp, you
have probably enjoyed the book so far; however, you may find
the truths in this chapter hard to stomach, crawling as they do
over the tender scars of your success. This chapter will reveal
part of the breastfeeding mother's psyche; a condescending
and merciless place that hereto no one has dared explore. But
first, the easier to read, more respectable stuff....

I discussed what makes successful breastfeeders exceptional
in the Deception chapter, arguing that personality and the
related tendency to operate 'discriminative determination'
were key to success. Abraham Maslow, psychology professor
by profession, celebrity by reputation, recognised this positive
deviance but referred to such individuals as – it pains me to
say it – 'martyrs', although not in the derogatory sense of the
term. Rather, he believed such people to be extremely mentally
adjusted. His analysis pinpoints childhood experience as the

root of positive deviance:

> 'They will give up everything for the sake of a particular ideal or value. These people may be understood, at least in part, by reference to one basic concept (or hypothesis), which may be called increased frustration tolerance through early gratification. People who have been satisfied in their basic needs throughout their lives, particularly in their earlier years, seem to develop exceptional power to withstand present and future thwarting of these needs simply because they have strong, healthy character structure as a result of basic satisfaction.'[465]

This is essentially Maslow's psychobabbley way of revealing what we already suspect: quality parents create quality parents. His observations correlate with numerous data showing that mothers who were themselves breastfed as babies are more likely to breastfeed their own children, and for longer periods, than mothers who were not breastfed as babies.[466] Besides the positive influence of earlier parental role modelling, very little is known about what creates a successful breastfeeding mother. Studies of this rare breed have been few, due, in part, to their subjects' near-extinction; however what little research has been done exposes a handful of salient themes. It seems that, far from being martyrs in the pejorative sense, successful breastfeeding mothers take a reciprocal approach to breastfeeding. They tend to see it as 'mutually satisfying', with infant and maternal needs 'working in harmony'.[467] They speak of 'the joy of breastfeeding' with explicit reference to its meaningful, cooperative, intuitive and obvious nature, and the way it boosts pride and self-esteem. Even the quintessential maternal chip on the shoulder – tiredness – is reframed, with these mothers claiming that breastfeeding breeds a different kind of tiredness, a 'pleasant rest and a kind of sleepiness'.[468] Such mothers conceptualise breastfeeding not only as a way of channelling nutrition, but also as having a specific and distinct value: 'The emotional dimension of breastfeeding creates a feeling of having arrived in life',[469] one successful mum chirped.

Of course, it's not all butterflies and rainbows;

commitment is a biggy. For successful breastfeeding mothers, commitment begins antenatally, with the faith and conviction that breastfeeding is 'natural', interwoven with 'a sense of duty'.[470] Then, when the child is born, his needs are understood as paramount and their temporal nature recognised. Such sentiment helps these mothers to persevere in the face of physical, psychological or social difficulties.[471] They complement this commitment with an instinctive trust in the biological process of breastfeeding. Thus brews an empowering cocktail that, in turn, helps them reject contradictory and unhelpful advice. Instead of relying on the guidance of others, the mother trusts her child's needs and her 'feeling of what is right'.[472] In nursing successfully, the breastfeeding mother exhibits other priceless personality traits, including maturity, instinctiveness and an ability to accept the unpredictable nature of parenting – at least, according to a scholarly article in the *Journal of Obstetric Gynecologic, and Neonatal Nursing*. The same article claimed that, 'Mothers with contrasting qualities may experience difficulty or discomfort in the breastfeeding relationship'.[473]

Notice the conflict – even in peer-reviewed medical literature – between those mothers deemed to have desirable qualities and those deemed lacking. In most conflicts, there tends to be a winner and a loser, or at least one party holds a stronger position relative to the other. In the Mummy Wars this role is often, but certainly not always, appropriated by successful breastfeeders, marinating in the juices of their triumph. These specimens can often be found slapping each other on the back for being such prime cuts in the steak of motherhood. Successful breastfeeding endows these mothers with what sociologists like to call 'symbolic capital' – a form of power, prestige and respect.[474] Alongside this social kudos, breastfeeding mothers have science[475] on their side, and boy do they know it. Forget the old-school game 'Simon Says'. For a breastfeeding mum, it's fun to point up 'what science says' as a way of polishing their maternal halo,[476] the very same maternal halo they worked off their ta-tas to earn. Other mothers' failure affirms to the breastfeeding mother her default (and desired) relationship to success, and by extension, to elite mothering. Since breastfeeding is universally – and some may argue, dogmatically – recognised as the healthiest option, successful breastfeeders are more likely to see themselves as better mothers than their formula-feeding counterparts.[477] In enjoying such righteousness, breastfeeding mothers can easily become contemptuous of those who don't measure up. Because failed breastfeeders don't measure up, less warmth and affection is extended to them. The following narrative from a successful breastfeeding mother is a case in point:

'I met a woman who was changing her little one in a room with a few women breastfeeding. She was clearly feeling guilt about propping the bottle up into the face of her baby girl so she stated "I tried breastfeeding but I didn't make enough milk". I wanted to laugh because she had just told me her girl was only three weeks old. At that moment I realized that she simply didn't want to breastfeed. I thought about telling her all about how she could easily re-lactate at this point but I realized it would be falling on deaf ears'.[478]

Many breastfeeding mothers, perched upon the supercilious throne of success, turn against their unsuccessful counterparts with disdain. Most do it covertly with internal judgments or with subtle passive-aggressive digs – an approach adopted by this mother:

'When I got pregnant with my daughter I knew I would be breastfeeding, nothing was going to stop me! I felt that as a mother my body was made to provide this gift to my daughter and not giving her that gift would be selfish and uncaring of me.'[479]

Others mums are more expressive with their contempt; some even form a monolithic view of formula feeders as a group. For them, contempt is a reactive emotion, a mix of disgust and anger.[480] Indeed, the word 'contempt' takes its roots from the Latin word *contemnere*, meaning 'to scorn'. Of course, another person's failure to breastfeed does not necessarily elicit the same feeling of contempt at the same intensity in everyone.

Some people have dispositions or 'cognitive mechanisms' that predispose them to contempt, and these largely stem from personal breastfeeding experience. Let's take a look at the most common routes that lead a breastfeeding mother into the bitchy world of contempt.

## WHY CONTEMPT?

At first, it seems bizarre that some successful breastfeeding mothers feel such indignation towards mums who were unsuccessful. After all, in terms of social comparison, other mothers' lack of success poses no threat to the breastfeeding mother. To decipher this apparent psychosocial irregularity, we need to appreciate the way in which the human brain has evolved to understand its world. When humans have incomplete information, we are still able to make decisions, come to judgments and solve problems. How? By using mental shortcuts or 'cognitive biases'. I have referred to several of these in previous chapters to explain different mental quirks, such as mothers' tendency to give more weight to evidence that confirms their own beliefs (confirmation bias, see page 29), their tendency to view the availability of information as evidence of its probability and importance (availability bias, see page 71), and their presumption that the truth is being told at all times (truth bias, see page 141).

Cognitive biases are adaptive, a 'by-product' of our processing limitations. The human brain is awesome, but it is just that – human – and as such there are limits to its awesomeness. Often the human brain takes short-cuts in order to lighten its load (the cognitive biases). We all experience them to a certain degree; they are designed to enable more effective and speedier decision-making. However, because they are essentially time-saving short-cuts, their accuracy is imperfect. As we learned in the Excuses chapter, one such bias – extremely relevant for our present purposes – is mothers' tendency to attribute their successes to themselves, but blame their failures on chance or external factors.[481] Conversely – and here's where contempt manifests – when it comes to interpreting another mother's failure, they tend to attribute it to the mother herself.[482] So from the breastfeeding mother's perspective, she credits her success to herself and the failure of other mothers to their character. This feels damn good; it feels righteous. As American journalist and author Kathryn Schulz playfully pointed out:

'If it is sweet to be right, then – let's not deny it – it is downright savoury to point out that someone else is wrong. As any food scientist can tell you, this combination of savoury and sweet is the most addictive of flavours: we can never really get enough of revelling in other people's mistakes'.[483]

Contempt is porn for breastfeeding mothers. It's thrilling, rewarding and addictive. Their contemptuous analysis of other mothers is bolstered by another largely subconscious cognitive sleight-of-hand, what has been coined the 'just world hypothesis'. Essentially, we all have a belief in a 'just world', in which actions and conditions have predictable and appropriate consequences. In the infant-feeding context, the breastfeeding mother derogates the formula-feeding mother for being the victim of personal circumstances in an attempt to maintain the belief that such negative events will never affect the breastfeeder herself because we live in a 'just world'. She rationalises other mothers' misfortunes on the grounds that they deserve it.[484] This is not as illogical and unethical as it may at first seem. At the heart of the breastfeeding mum's ideology is the belief that hard work gets one ahead, and individuals are responsible for their life outcomes. Not an asocial idea, really, when you think about it.

When the successful breastfeeder made her decision to prioritise breastfeeding, she did so with an innate assumption that other mothers would – or should – have decided the same. This egotistical, albeit normal, mental mistake is another cognitive bias, known as the 'false consensus effect'.[485] It works like this: we see ourselves as largely rational and therefore consider our choices to be the default norm. Our own choices impact on how we expect others to behave in that situation. The successful breastfeeding mother cannot understand why anyone would not prioritise breastfeeding as she has done. Try as she might, she cannot identify with such people. As one breastfeeding mum confessed about formula-feeding mothers, 'I try to be understanding but ultimately I think they're selfish'.[486]

One way breastfeeding mothers demonstrate their 'non-identification' with formula feeders is to withdraw or distance themselves, sometimes physically, often psychologically.[487] This behaviour may be interpreted as 'cold and aloof' by those who observe it, and is typical of women, who tend to engage in more non-verbal forms of social aggression than men.[488] In this way, women's contempt is dismissive. It does not demand, nor even invite, response from its target. In distancing themselves, breastfeeding mothers remove the need to openly confront formula feeders – and to understand them.

However, human cognitive biases cannot wholly explain the depth of disdain some breastfeeders feel towards their unsuccessful counterparts. For those women, there are more oblique dynamics at play. It should come as little surprise that the breastfeeders who are apt to be the most unsympathetic also tend to be those who have overcome the most obstacles in order to breastfeed – 'It wasn't really working for me, but I stuck with it'.[489] There are two reasons why the waters of maternal emotion get muddier at this point. Firstly, the more hardship a breastfeeding mother endured to reach her goal, the higher she is likely to regard the virtues of breastfeeding. Why? Because why endure hardship if the result is of mediocre importance? In other words, the harder you work for something, the more you value it. To reassure herself that her plight was worthwhile, the breastfeeding mother feels driven to confirm the superiority of her decision.[490]

This behaviour is known in social psychology simply as 'effort-justification'. We all do it at various points in life to bolster our confidence in our choices. Learning that other mothers quit breastfeeding in circumstances similar to ones the successful breastfeeding mother overcame creates a type of cognitive dissonance in the latter – a conflict between the amount of effort she exerted into breastfeeding successfully and the implication that other mothers did not deem this effort to be worthwhile in their own experience. This riles the breastfeeding mother. To her, it almost feels as though other mothers are covertly suggesting that her hard work was disproportionate to her reward.

There is another, perhaps even more fascinating, reason why the tougher the challenges a breastfeeding mother overcomes, the more passionate her contempt towards those who fail. It concerns the way she reflects on her own struggles. In their book examining how we justify our choices, Carol Tavris and Elliot Aronson touched upon the mechanics at play:

> 'People who have been sorely tempted, battled temptation, and almost given in to it – but resisted at the eleventh hour – come to dislike, even despise, those who did not succeed in the same effort. It's the people who *almost* decide to live in glass houses who throw the first stones [their emphasis]'.[491]

To the successful breastfeeding mother, a failed breastfeeder represents a fragment of *herself* that she has great difficulty accepting. She recalls the times she thought she might bail under the pressure that comes with being a sole food source. Indeed, being a mobile 24-hour all-you-can-eat buffet pushes even the crunchiest of mothers to their limit. The failed mother reminds the breastfeeder of a part of her own past characterised by weakness, struggle and imperfection. Swiss psychiatrist Carl Jung aptly called this aspect of self – the part we like to judge, disown and reject – 'the shadow'.[492] The shadow is the 'sum of all personal and collective psychic elements which, because of their incompatibility with the chosen conscious attitude, are denied expression in life'.[493] The breastfeeding mother's former traits – inadequacy and imperfection provoked by challenges she later overcame – are incompatible with the elite self-view she enjoys at present. Yet, since it is impossible for her to completely erase these historical memories, her ego springs into action with a defence mechanism: it has her deny or repress the memories, and even project them onto other people. This instinct is a natural and universal part of being human. Freud recognised it decades ago and labelled it 'classical projection'. To use Freud's words, this cognitive technique enables the successful breastfeeder 'to fend off an idea that is incompatible with the ego by projecting its substance into the real world'.[494] Because the successful breastfeeding mother dipped her toe into the pool of failure but pulled it out at the last minute, she comes to resent those who, unlike her, did not withdraw their foot, but fell (or indeed, jumped) right in. Her own wishes for perfection, and her guilt and shame for not precisely meeting it, are projected onto other mothers.

So far, you would be forgiven for thinking that contempt has zero endearing value. After all, aside from a fleeting ego boost, what positive use can come from feeling superior to others as well as disconnected and dissimilar from them? Contempt is divisive. The behaviour that triggers it – breastfeeding failure – is regarded by the contemptuous mind not only as a negative choice (something that mothers can choose to do or not do) but also as morally wrong. Contempt is thus at its core a moral emotion. And this raises an intriguing question: in a so-called moral society, is contempt necessarily a bad thing? Here, our discussion turns from the personal to the political.

## THE CULTURAL REJECTION OF MATERNAL CONTEMPT

A breastfeeding mother's contempt is hierarchical – it presupposes a superior/inferior dichotomy between breastfeeding and formula feeding respectively. In this sense it is confirmed by scientific evidence: 'science says' breast is best (or more appropriately, biologically normal) and formula is sub-standard. Related to this dichotomy is a split between two ideologies: the individualistic and the collectivist. The distinction between individualistic and collectivist ways of thinking is important in deciphering the origins of maternal contempt. Whether a breastfeeding mum is collectivist or individualistic in her approach to achievement is a good indication of her likelihood of developing feelings of contempt.

An individualistic worldview holds that hard work gets one ahead and individuals are responsible for their outcome in life. If a breastfeeding mother has an individualistic world view, her contempt is more likely to be aroused towards those who do not adhere to her standards. People who hold a collectivist world view, on the other hand, are likely to blame breastfeeding failure upon external influences, like 'society'. The former mother regards success as a product of dedication, whereas the latter sees success as a product of 'luck' (if you succeed at breastfeeding, you do so 'despite' society). For those who wish to promulgate the latter view – and there are many, thanks to formula being the mainstream milk of choice – a major way they can attempt to strengthen the faux-link between success and luck is to raise concern about the morality of showing contempt. If breastfeeding success is simply down to good fortune in the form of societal privilege and working breasts, then, in theory, breastfeeding mothers should not feel contempt for those who are not lucky enough to enjoy these attributes, they argue.

This ideological war against maternal contempt can be exemplified by media pseudo-movements to 'End the Mummy Wars' exemplified by the whinge, 'Can't we all just support each other and stop judging?' Such collective missions are as old as our most primitive emotions and, on first glance, seem appealing. Almost a century ago, Freud referred to this phenomenon as part of the 'herd instinct'. Calls to end mother-on-mother conflict tend to build momentum because they allow negative feelings (formula feeders' envy; breastfeeders' fear of arousing envy) to be disguised but also acted upon. Borrowing rhetoric from social identity theory, these pseudo-movements emphasise the collective characteristics of mothers as a group while underplaying the distribution of differences between mothers. They appear to reverse hostility into positively toned ties of mutual support and solidarity. In a word, pleas to 'End the Mummy Wars' seem feminist. By participating in this group love-in, the shame and guilt produced by mothers' envy and fear of envy can be denied, while the participants bask in self-righteous identification with the common good.

Those fond of this stance are largely formula apologists, fighting for a stealthily self-serving utopia in which people – mothers in particular – are free to act without moral consequence. In other words, they believe that mothers do not have personal responsibility for the choices that they make; society does. One way they promulgate this view is by leaning heavily on collectivist rhetoric and denying individual self-determinism. They appeal to liberal ideology to shelter mothers from acknowledging the consequences of their choices. Facts regarding the risks of formula feeding are locked into this Pandora's Box and treated as hate speech. Woe betide mothers call each other out on their choices – that would cause hurt feelings, they argue. Indeed, formula apologists are heavily reliant on the rhetoric of emotion, demanding that we be mindful of mothers' subjective 'feelings', because logic and objective morality muddy the agenda they are seeking to advance. Essentially, they aim to replace a moral view of infant feeding with an emotional view.[495] The apologists deny that contempt has a positive role to play in a mother's moral life, they deem it an ugly, unfeminine and unfeminist emotion. Their argument is that contempt must be silenced since it has the power to rupture female solidarity; that when interacting with each other, mothers should demonstrate only positive emotions like empathy and acceptance. Yet this attitude is unduly paternalistic. It robs women of their individuality while ignoring the value of maternal contempt. So what is that value?

## IN DEFENCE OF MATERNAL CONTEMPT

Maternal contempt has a bad rep in mainstream consciousness, both academic and lay, largely because it involves downward-looking comparative evaluations between mothers, and thus poses a potential threat to dignity. The disapproval that many breastfeeding mothers feel toward their formula-feeding peers is referred to in derogatory terms: 'Breastfeeding Nazis' and the 'Brestapo' to cite Godwin's law. (This popular internet adage asserts that 'As an online discussion grows longer, the probability of a comparison involving Nazis or Hitler approaches'.[496]) I am about to argue that maternal contempt is not as unilaterally sinister as its reputation would suggest. In fact, I will go as far as to say that embracing contempt is *essential* if mothers are to partake fully in a moral society.

The backlash against maternal contempt is stiflingly conformist and does not allow for more challenging or counter-cultural attitudes. Our anti-contempt culture is overwhelmed by parenting permissiveness so pervasive that it is becoming socially and morally detrimental. We have a fear of judging, a fear of being seen as contemptuous. We try to do and say only those things that will be agreeable to other mothers. This disagreement deficit creates a culture in which we are seldom alerted to flaws in parental belief systems. Rather than being a sign of tolerance, shying away from contempt is a way to stay closed-minded. It is intellectually corrosive. Women are discouraged from forming opinions about the value of different choices, and this, in turn, dilutes their ability to have confident critical discussions. In the same vein, there are some lies that society accepts, and even encourages: motherhood is not political, formula is not harmful, parenting is not public, capitalism is not unjust and so on. Yet, as activists have quite rightly pointed out, the personal *is* political. What is and is not deemed sub-standard parenting is an issue of concern to us all. Unfortunately, because the issue is intimate, involves the ego and almost everyone has a personal stake in it, a blanket reluctance to discourse has emerged.

Should mothers be screened from judgement simply by virtue of being mothers? Is every choice to be revered because a mother made it? Mothers are not sacrosanct. Sometimes they make poor choices like everyone else and should be called out on them. Political correctness is designed to protect those who have no choice – on grounds such as disability, race and gender – but the vast bulk of formula feeders choose their group membership. At the heart of this issue lies a distinction between a quality like skin colour – which you cannot change – and a choice like infant feeding, which ought to be susceptible to debate and challenge.[497]

The general principle behind anti-contempt rhetoric seems to be that important life decisions are solely the concern of people who make them. There are several blinding flaws to this assumption. Firstly, by asserting that mothers should be free from accountability for their actions, formula apologists strengthen the myth that breastfeeding is merely a product of luck. When a breastfeeding mother criticises formula-feeding mothers she is conveying the message that they had sufficient ability to master the task of breastfeeding but didn't try hard enough. On the other hand, expressing pity or sympathy for the same poor performance communicates the belief that a mother's low ability was the reason for her failure. Sound familiar? It's the fuel for the Culture of Failure. In essence, by severing maternal accountability from breastfeeding outcome we feed the culture of failure and thus promulgate more failure.[498]

Secondly, by emphasising the individual nature of choice, formula apologists spit in the face of their cherished collectivist rhetoric. On the one hand, they argue that a mother's choice is her business and hers alone. Yet on the other, they contend that choices are mostly coordinated by 'society'. I argue that if a significant proportion of mothers are not breastfeeding for social or cultural reasons – as the latter point contends – then by supporting their decision without question, we are perpetuating the supposed social and cultural attitudes that supposedly got them there in the first place.

This links to the third major flaw: since choices are individual – as the apologist argument goes – they have no social consequences; thus women are relieved of the responsibility of considering the broader implications of their decisions. Aside from being far too sweeping, this assertion begs not one, but two questions: what about the baby's interests, which are not sufficiently taken into account? What about other people the infant-feeding decision affects? This last point requires some elaboration. Because our society has become increasingly interdependent, the proximity of a mother's failure to breastfeed can affect other members of society on a large scale. For example, if most mothers in the US breastfed for just six months, a colossal $13 billion in healthcare and other costs would be saved each year.[499] In many countries, including the UK, not breastfeeding costs the taxpayer dearly. The consequences of generations of formula feeding are so immense and far-reaching in terms of environmental damage, burdens on health care, and the denormalisation of breastfeeding[500] that one could argue that turning a moral blind eye is a grossly inadequate, ingenious and even dangerous response. In this sense, while the parent-child relationship is essentially a private relationship, it is a relationship bearing *public responsibility*.

Sadly, the debate has largely been muted by a self-pacifying, guilt-fuelled apologist agenda. Whether discussing stay-at-home motherhood, breastfeeding, vaccination or single parenthood, the politically correct fear of offence has slammed the door on dialogue. Such hypersensitive reactionism distorts reality by classifying certain groups of people (mothers) as victims in need of protection from criticism. Yet by discouraging judgement and debate on issues important to mothers, we not only infantilise women but prevent them from accessing information vital to informed choice. As journalist and passionate free speech advocate Anthony Browne has noted: 'Truth comes in two forms: the factually correct and the politically correct'.[501] In infant-feeding discourse, to point out the factual risks of formula is to sign a pact with political incorrectness. When women do this, they are seen by extension as turning against their gender. Ironically, this centrality of appeasement in popular perceptions of femininity has harmed women, dampening their expressiveness and causing an irrational fear of women's contempt.

In defence of contempt, I argue that mothers are not the passive wallflowers presupposed by apologists. They are adults. They are strong enough to deal with criticism. The breastfeeding mother, in showing contempt, is presupposing that the formula-feeding mother is capable of being held accountable for her actions, as any adult should be. When women judge each other's choices, they are doing exactly that – exploring each other's positions and claims. Judging is an excellent exercise in women's intellectual and observational skills and a route for personal development. It has an epistemic function, and in that sense, it *is* feminist.

Some people claim they never feel contempt. When they notice poor parenting, they try to slink into the background, hoping someone else will take the lead and call it out. When no one does, they simply downplay their reactions and convince themselves they had it wrong. This extremely common phenomenon is called 'pluralistic ignorance'. The people who do it are usually those who want to live their lives without thinking about anything verging on the political or discussing anything beyond the insulated walls of their own lives. The problem is that by not considering political issues (and infant-feeding is highly political[502]), they are supporting a system just as much as the lactivists who protest against formula company violations of the WHO code, or the 'intactivists' campaigning against non-essential circumcision. I argue that doing nothing – being apathetic towards parenting – is morally corrosive. It sends a simple and clear message to the community: parenting doesn't matter. Do what you like. Children are insignificant. Parenting is insignificant. As one mother passionately asserted:

> 'I think we are entitled to judge. I also judge people who I see taking overweight children to McDonalds and buying them pop. I judge people who smoke around children as well. It's not about me thinking I'm better. It has to do with being angry that these tiny innocent people are not getting the care they deserve. Maybe if people had to answer to their choices and if society wasn't required to passively accept them the world would be a better place'.[503]

In motherhood, as in any role with social consequences, confrontations with moral issues are inevitable. Clearly, contempt has a crucially important role to play as a way of provoking accountability. The injustice and harm caused by formula feeding, both on an individual level and on a macro-social level must be confronted. Given the manipulative moral stance of formula marketing ('Take it from us, you're doing great'[504]), the counter-stance – contempt – mitigates against corporate impairment of morality. Philosopher Macalester Bell[505] called its utility the 'ethic of contempt'. What I'm saying is that contempt is a morally valuable emotion. Without contempt, poor parenting in all its guises would go unchecked and poor parents would remain unaccountable. Contempt can be seen as an appropriate way to respond, attitudinally, to sub-par parenting choices. Contempt shines a spotlight on personal responsibility; it holds parents answerable for their behaviour. After all, the ultimate correction for the apologist tunnel vision afflicting poor parenting is not more darkness but more light. Contempt sparks debate and serves as a form of moral address.[506] We are all members of a moral community, and as philosopher Kurt Baier put it, matters of moral obligation are the moral community's 'business'.[507]

To sum up, I urge you to rethink your relationship to contempt, particularly maternal contempt. Triggered by a multifaceted blend of cognitive interactions, contempt is firstly innately human, and secondly has immense moral, political and intellectual utility. It promotes a searching, questioning and responsible attitude towards choice, an approach that forms the bedrock of a moral society. I argue that the risk of appearing contemptuous is preferable to the cowardice of not taking a position, or even worse, of reproducing a dominant false narrative ('formula is just as good as breast milk'). That some women feel safe and able to express contempt is a feminist achievement. I say 'some' women, because the process of judging one another – holding each other accountable for our decisions – is anything but easy. Many shy away from it. Being social creatures, mothers are naturally extremely sensitive to contempt, particularly if they perceive themselves as being on the receiving end. When they pick up the signals, their emotional systems flick to defensive mode. It is this reactionary recoil that we explore in the next chapter.

# 6

# DEFENSIVENESS

'Nature…has also given us pride to spare us the mortification of knowing our imperfections'.

François de La Rochefoucauld, 1678,
*Reflections; or Sentences and Moral Maxims*

Facing up to personal failure is tough for anyone, but it is particularly bothersome for mothers. Sometimes they are unable to do so because they are too exhausted, too angry, too sad or teetering on the brink of depression; acknowledging their own role in their failure would push them over the edge. Instead, they wax defensive.

In infant feeding, maternal defensiveness has a Siamese twin: resentment. When one is in view, you can be sure the other is hovering about. Robert Solomon, professor of philosophy,[508] placed resentment in the same emotional family as contempt, but emphasised an inverse relationship between the two: resentment is directed towards higher status individuals and contempt towards those of lower status. In the previous chapter, we examined the feelings of contempt that emanate from some breastfeeding mothers towards formula-feeding mothers. Because the target of this contempt is peers – fellow mothers – the threat to the latter is intensified.[509] What are formula-feeding mums to do with such hostility? Typically, their resentment of other mothers' contempt (real or perceived) and of the predicament of breastfeeding failure itself boils over into defensiveness. This state of mind is entertaining to spectate. It involves, as journalist Kathryn Schulz put it, mothers 'pulling up the drawbridge, manning the battlements, and skirting a confrontation with their fallibility'.[510]

## WHAT IS DEFENSIVENESS?

Before we marvel at the spectacle of defensive maternal behaviour, it helps to briefly explore the mental processes that lead to it. To understand how maternal defensiveness comes about, we need to revisit a phenomenon touched on in previous chapters, a popular and sexy psychological theory originating in the 1950s, known as 'cognitive dissonance' (see page 104). What is cognitive dissonance? In short, it describes the feeling of unease we experience when we have hypocritical thought patterns. In breastfeeding, the process typically begins with an initial thought (I will breastfeed) which then, for most women, is followed sometime later by a dissonant thought (I have failed to breastfeed). On failing, the mother becomes acutely aware that her attitudes, thoughts and beliefs (her cognitions) are inconsistent with her behaviour now she has given up breastfeeding. Mum knows she ought to have breastfed, that scientific evidence and government guidelines strongly point in this direction, yet she has not adhered to this standard. Such realisation brings with it an uncomfortable state of tension: cognitive dissonance. Mum experiences this as a state ranging from minor pangs to deep anguish. There's nothing quite like a dose of 'identity disconfirmation' to trigger zealous defensiveness. As philosopher Adam Phillips pointed out in his book, aptly titled *On Missing Out*, 'The only phobia is the phobia of self-knowledge'.[511]

There are three main reasons why cognitive dissonance is so powerful in the context of infant feeding. Firstly, mothers are acutely aware that their behaviour has important consequences for themselves and others. Their failure is, for the most part, irrevocable. Secondly, infant-feeding behaviour, largely because it overshadows the bulk of infancy, is central to a mother's sense of identity, self-worth and value. Thirdly, the availability of choice increases the strength of dissonance.

The latter point needs some elaboration. To quote that timeless beacon of paediatrics, Dr Benjamin Spock, 'Most women who choose to breastfeed can succeed if they give breastfeeding a fair trial'.[512] Since the number of women who physically cannot breastfeed is minuscule, whether a woman breastfeeds or formula feeds is commonly regarded as a choice. Very few women are literally 'forced' to formula feed, and the weaker the force compelling a woman to formula feed, the stronger the resulting dissonance when she does. Ouchers!

In laboratory studies using fancy technology – 'magnetic resonance imaging' if you must know – neuroscience boffins have found that the reasoning areas of the brain virtually shut down when a person is confronted with dissonant information. When consonance is restored, the brain's emotional circuits light up happily.[513] To restore a similar balance, a formula-feeding mother has two choices: she can either change her behaviour (relactate – i.e. get her breast milk flowing again) or she can change her attitude (rationalising the use of formula). Which option do you think is easiest? Well, to give an idea of the effort required to relactate, here's a brief, watered-down overview of the process: to get her now dry milk supply flowing again, not only does a mother have to feed her baby at the breast frequently – at least 12 times per 24 hours, including at least every three hours at night – she must hook herself up to a double electric breast pump every two hours. And because formula is still necessary at this point, she has to find a way to get it into her baby without said baby knowing. She can do this using a device from the *Alien* movies known as a 'Supplemental Nursing System'. And if she's *really* hardcore (find me a relactating mum who isn't!), she will also dowse her guts with lactation-friendly herbs and spices (fenugreek, marjoram, basil, anise, dill, caraway, ginger, turmeric) while bingeing on 'lactogenic foods' (brown rice, oatmeal, millet, coconut water, raw almonds, cashews, onions, macadamia nuts). If she is successful after all this, she will find she has not only emptied the contents of her local health food store, she now smells like a mobile curry house.[514]

Needless to say, folk tend to follow the path of least effort when attempting to restore their cognitive dissonance.[515]

Given a contradiction between an attitude and an item of behaviour, people have a tendency to change the attitude to make it consonant with the behaviour. It is far easier for a mother to ditch her lactivist leanings than to relactate. The Breast is Best message she once held so dear is no longer consonant with her current behaviour, and so she will suffer very little personal loss at having to relinquish it. Thus, rather than relactate, the vast majority of failed breastfeeders start a process of attitude change, of cognitive restructuring – a spring clean of the brain. This mental makeover is not spontaneous, like our old friends the cognitive biases. Rather, it is a strategically thought-out process,[516] the ease of which depends on how resistant to change the Breast is Best message is for the mother in question. Does the fact of breastfeeding's superiority fit with *her* reality?

'I was formula fed, and it didn't do me any harm'.

Obviously not if she trots out this sentence, or something similarly compelling. Often, a mother tangled in the net of cognitive dissonance, rationalises her behaviour by inventing a comfortable illusion. For example, she now perceives formula feeding to be less dangerous to her baby's health compared to her views when pregnant – thereby averting post-decisional regret through post-hoc rationalisation. In other words, the once pro-breastfeeding mother has made a stark about-turn. The cost of formula feeding is a price she has already paid, and as she is unable to get a refund, all she can do now is create an illusion that the cost was not so great or that the benefit of formula use is greater. It does wonders for her credibility to have an attitude consistent with her behaviour, at least in her now happily lit brain.

The new beliefs that result from this change ('Formula is just as good as breast milk' and 'My choice is as good as anyone else's') may be more internally consistent with one another, but they are not necessarily consistent with reality. Does Mum really think she can debunk Mother Nature? Does she sincerely believe the scientific links between formula and numerous health risks are so flimsy they can be ignored? Such wishful thinking can only stretch so far before bordering on irrational. Indeed, psychologist Robert Feldman once asserted, 'when the outside world conflicts with our thinking, sometimes we find ways to preserve the latter at the expense of how we perceive the former'.[517] Essentially, some mothers deny reality and then deny the denial. Consider the scenario of someone purchasing an item from a store and then losing the receipt. Studies have shown that people actually start to like items more when they cannot return them than when they can. After an irrevocable decision, the grass grows *less* green on the other side of the fence.[518] The same cognitive shift occurs when a mother abandons breastfeeding and switches to formula. She alters her thoughts, her beliefs and her attitudes at will. This kind of limitless cognitive refurbishment makes a paradox seem palatable: Mum is able to feel proud while she breastfeeds and then to question the value of breastfeeding once she has given up.

## PROVOCATION – A PREREQUISITE FOR MATERNAL DEFENSIVENESS?

Let's get back to our mate Freud. In his language, defensiveness occurs when the ego is called upon to justify a bad performance.[519] For infant feeding, this implies that defensiveness only occurs when mothers are explicitly or implicitly asked to justify their choices. However a Freudian analysis only tells part of the story. Now, I am going to argue that a mother doesn't need to be provoked into defensiveness, she can do it very well herself, thank you.

Mothers look at other mothers the way Jerry looks at Tom. They shore themselves up against the possibility of negative responses, long before circumstances call for such justification. Mums are literally primed to be defensive about their choices. Why? Because mothering, while originating in the private sphere, is to a large extent public property. Mother-work is under the media lens now more than ever. When we fail at a task privately, our chief loss is to our pride, but when we fail at a task publicly, the stakes of our mistake escalate to unsettling levels. Women – mothers in particular – are forever stalked by their choices. The explosion in recent years of reality television documentaries and 'Mummy Blogs' invites people to scrutinise each other's parenting technique in a way once reserved for the mother-in-law. And it's not just the media who are judging; in a recent study of more than 26,000 mothers, 84 percent admitted to judging other mothers.[520] A woman's self-image as a competent mother is thus periodically threatened. Given the new nakedness of what was once a private family life, the temptation felt by many mothers to defend their parenting rank is insatiable.

The plight of mothers is intensified by the fact that women are more 'field-dependent' than men: they are more receptive to the standards of others and tend to rely more heavily on external validation.[521] Consequently, mothers are more sensitive to the (real or imagined) disapproval of others. Because a woman's self-image is more vulnerable than a man's, the threat of external judgement has a more powerful influence over women than over men. A vicious circle is created: women, being more fearful of disapproval, are (as we saw in the previous chapter) more likely to use disapproval as a weapon of aggression or defence, and thus become more fearful of disapproval.

Being socially sensitive, a mother's image of herself always involves a sense of how others evaluate her behaviour. As with her experience of guilt and envy, even when a mother is not receiving explicit feedback from others, she can *imagine* how others perceive her. The mother's *perceptions* of other people's evaluations of her breastfeeding performance – rather than their actual evaluations – prompt her defensiveness. Most importantly, these perceptions are coloured by her personal take on breastfeeding. To illustrate, here's one mother's confession:

> 'It is not surprising that I felt that the other women in my [National Childbirth Trust] group would think of me as a failure. After all, this is how I had privately judged others who had failed in their attempt to breastfeed'.[522]

Here, we see how a breastfeeding mother can affect a formula feeder's self-image without even directing behaviour towards her. This behaviour is called 'self-reference ideation'[523] or as I like to call it, 'Stop breastfeeding AT me!' Shrinks and other mental-health professionals have long known about this defensive imaginary conflict. Essentially what happens is members of one group (in this case, failed breastfeeders) perceive the actions of another group (successful breastfeeders) to be aimed at and intended for them. So among the gaggle of voices at the baby group, hypersensitive mothers find their drama alarms triggered at the mere mention of breastfeeding – and before you know it, their ball of defensiveness is rolling.

## DEFENSIVENESS – THE MASK OF DENIAL

The more vociferously a mother defends her decision to formula feed, the more likely it is that she is defending it primarily against her own internal doubts. Remember that denial is a defence mechanism by which a mother represses certain emotions, for instance, humiliation, guilt, regret, betrayal and envy. These emotions are triggered when denial is challenged. A challenge can take many forms: a scientific study extolling the benefits of breastfeeding, a nursing mother who has overcome the challenges the formula-feeding mother could not, an ill-judged question and so on. In reaction to such a challenge, Mum switches to defensive-mode.

Most, if not all, mothers in this situation use the following strategy: they attribute their breastfeeding failure to specifics rather than 'global' reasons. What I mean is a mother frames her failure as evidence only of a minute maternal flaw – a temporary lapse of judgement – rather than a comprehensive reflection of her mothering as a whole.[524] We saw this type of behaviour in the Excuses chapter when we looked at the Mitigation Excuse (see page 121). Mum focuses on the circumstances that led to the failure, rather than on her own enduring characteristics.

Another, more indirect, defensive tactic relies on 'social comparison processes and projection'. What does that mean? Simply that mothers try to minimise the undesirability of formula feeding by comparing it with other things people do that are the same or worse. It is exemplified by statements such as, 'My generation was formula fed and we're okay'. The implication is that if most people do it, it must be reasonably normal or acceptable. A mother can then assert or imply that since most people formula feed, the criteria for labelling it 'bad' are in need of revision. We're teetering on the edge of the Redefining Standards excuse (see page 127). Indeed, some mothers supplement this defence by suggesting that because most people fail at breastfeeding, there must be something about breastfeeding that drives people to quit; that the guidelines are unrealistic, for instance. By doing this, mothers further deflect failure from their personal characteristics and position it on the external task. These projection tactics can be polished by adding a downwards comparison – 'There are worse things you can feed a child, like junk food'.[525] Or even the pearl-clutching, 'Formula is not poison'.

## HOSTILITY TO FACT

The drive of formula-feeding mothers to bolster their denial strongly affects their reaction to breastfeeding information. This scientific data has a persistent habit of going against the relativistic 'whatever feels right for you is therefore right' mindset. The very notion of formula feeding entailing a degree of risk is unsettling to formula feeders. It is dissonant with their understanding of themselves as good parents. When reminded of the inferiority of formula, the mood and self-esteem of those who use it plummet, depressing any positive illusions they have about their self-image as parents.[526] Two of the most common ways formula-feeding mothers are confronted with such data is via the media (newspaper reports and television documentaries) and the health service (NHS literature and meeting health professionals). Faced with such personal negative feedback (and that is precisely how formula-feeding mothers view this literature), mothers feel compelled to devalue the source of said feedback.[527] After all, if Mum can find a counterfactual way to criticise, distort or dismiss this disconfirming evidence, her self-esteem can recuperate. Mothers' defensiveness in this regard is not so much a response to scientific research and the facts it decrees. Rather, defensiveness is a response to the emotions those facts evoke.

Often these emotions (guilt and envy, to name a familiar duo) are painful and intolerable. To numb the discomfort, mothers are willing to manipulate or ignore triggering information.[528] Once they have made their choice to formula feed, they essentially put their heads in the sand to evade their regret. They are supremely unmotivated to educate themselves with facts that could rudely disrupt their sand-dwelling.

The behaviour of mothers illuminates the reality that facts don't exist in isolation; they are given meaning by the template each of us uses to view the world.[529] This template is formed thanks to our esteem-pandering urge to flatter ourselves[530] and it floats just under our consciousness. This thought-pattern is an obvious example: 'I formula feed and I'm a good mother, therefore studies detailing the risks of formula feeding are exaggerated'. By judiciously applying her template to 'describe' the facts, a mother can control the meanings the facts convey. Defensiveness overrides a mother's motivation to appraise information realistically. It can even produce the absurd result that the *absence* of evidence is taken as evidence for what Mum believes! For instance, studies have indicated that formula-fed babies are twice as likely to die from Sudden Infant Death Syndrome (SIDS) as their breastfed counterparts.[531] Yet because SIDS cannot be attributed to formula-feeding *alone*, Mum maintains that formula feeding has no part to play in SIDS. Logic is clearly being compromised in an effort to recoup lost esteem.

In this way, defensive mothers easily become overly insulated. Often they let their template manipulate the kind of information they are exposed to. In other words, they seek out or avoid certain types of 'truth', creating a mental filter that screens out any information that threatens to challenge their shaky self-image. Psychologists call this 'selective exposure'. We seek to minimise our exposure to information that contradicts our views, particularly our views about ourselves. For example, someone afraid of flying may seek out information detailing the horrors of airplane disasters, while avoiding factual information about safety records. Likewise, a formula feeder will seek out articles that extol the virtues of formula while simultaneously steering herself away from articles that point out its risks. New ideas are only mindfully absorbed if they are consistent with what already exists in the mind.[532] A good example is formula-feeding mothers' penchant for apologist media, particularly articles that blame 'society' for failing them or that omnipresent cliché 'inadequate support'. They spend time attending to such resources as a pacifying defence mechanism.[533]

Pro-formula propaganda is another self-medicative favourite. The claim that formula is a nutritionally valid substitute for breast milk is familiar, established and supported socially (if not factually). Soaking it up is both comfortable and efficient for a formula-feeding mother. This assimilation provides emotional advantages, namely comfort, pleasure and even a sense of kinship and security with the bulk of people doing the same thing as her. These psychological benefits are a powerful incentive for a mother to stay aligned with the pro-formula paradigm. Conversely, insight into the bodily mechanisms of breastfeeding, solutions to breastfeeding problems and information outlining sources of support all illuminate one pertinent fact: breastfeeding failure is seldom a result of uncontrollable factors. Essentially, many formula-feeding mothers have a fear of facts. Those who failed at breastfeeding want to believe that, as smart and rational individuals, their decision to formula feed was informed and ethical. Consequently they are not always happy with data that threatens to disprove this.

## THE LUCK SAFETY NET

'I'm not saying these [breastfeeding] problems are insurmountable, rather that however timeless and bountiful the activity is, there is a vast assortment of things, medieval and modern, that can go wrong with it, and generally speaking, they are not the mother's fault'.

Zoe Williams, 2012, *What Not to Expect When You're Expecting*[534]

The fool-proof defensive weapon of choice for many failed breastfeeders is to cite luck – as the reason they failed ('I was unlucky') and as an explanation for why some women succeed ('You got lucky'). Luck enables mothers to downplay their inadequacies while dimming the light of others' triumphs. If postnatal depression, mastitis, thrush, pushy health professionals, indifferent health professionals, insufficient milk, oversupply of milk, lethargic baby, ravenous baby, unsupportive husband, overzealous husband or simply the breasts's stubborn refusal to play ball aren't to blame for the outcome, there is always bad luck to fall back on. We saw that mothers are more prone to excuse-making if they say outside forces exert most control over their lives. The same mothers are also predisposed to leaning on the 'luck' explanation as their emotional crutch.[535] These are mothers who anxiously await life's inevitable negative feedback. They say they had no control over the breastfeeding process yet often, in reality, they remained active throughout.[536]

I spoke about luck in the Deception and Envy chapters. 'Oh not this again' you may be thinking. I hear you. But luck deserves – nigh demands – another mention here, not least because it is such a prolific rhetoric in breastfeeding discourse, and is insulting to many breastfeeding mothers. Luck, by its very nature, is beyond an individual's control. Winning the lottery is luck. Genes are luck. Being born into wealth is luck. Breastfeeding? Nuh-uh. Claiming that breastfeeding success is a product of luck is one of the weakest and most transparent of defensive tactics. Functioning breasts are no more 'lucky' than a functioning pair of legs, yet we don't incessantly dwell on the luck enjoyed by those of us who can walk. 'Luck' discounts the effort of breastfeeding mothers and – by extension – their success, explaining it as, for instance, simply the result of a higher quality support system or more generous maternity leave. Maternal agency is purposefully ignored.

Despite the deleterious effect of luck on the reputation of breastfeeding mothers, it is not a stretch to conclude that the true target of the luck rhetoric is not the breastfeeding mum, or even the world at large, but rather the failed breastfeeder. It is her self-esteem that is threatened by the success of others, her anxieties that demand some form of comfort. In this sense, whittling success down to 'luck' acts as a kind of self-administered sticking plaster that a mother can apply whenever her maternal esteem is in peril. Luck becomes the mechanism for softening a potentially unflattering spotlight. The tactic may not fool those listening, but it makes the mother feel better. And heck, if all else fails, she can always collapse into resignation and apathy and turn to transcendence, ('None of this will matter in a few years, anyway').

## HOOKED ON DEFENSIVENESS

So why do mothers twirl and toss the defensiveness baton, even at the risk of looking absurd? The irony is that however much mothers deny, distort or misconstrue the truth about breastfeeding, it continues to matter to them – enormously. In fact, they deny, distort and misconstrue breastfeeding *because* it matters to them. For mothers, defensiveness is crack cocaine. When practised often enough, it becomes habitual, a result of well trodden pathways and deeply established chemical dependencies. The mother becomes, in a sense, addicted to defensiveness, to the biochemical hit. She finds that it energises her. In this sense, defensiveness is not just a way of manipulating other people, but a pleasurable way of manipulating oneself. Some mothers end up enjoying their defensiveness not just because it invigorates them, but because it is capable of transforming the very way they see the world, and in particular, their parenting prowess.

Because mothers expect discussions on the topic of infant feeding to be judgemental, they often start off defensively or aggressively, thereby inviting an aggressive or defensive response. In doing so, they create a self-sustaining climate for breastfeeding dialogue. Their defensive framing of the topic both reflects and predicts the emotional orientation they experience. Paradoxically, like the contempt that often triggers it, defensiveness is by its nature a judgemental emotion. The offended mother turns the tables on the offender. Entering into the exchange feeling threatened, hurt and offended, the defensive Mum repositions herself as superior, even righteous. It is not hard to appreciate why this might feel energising. Then, after Mum has finished her defensive outburst, her painful emotions are repressed again and breastfeeding is not discussed unless it arises in the future. It becomes a taboo topic. Like the coyote cartoon character who runs off a cliff but doesn't fall until he glances down, defensiveness is the mother's way of not looking down.[537]

While defensiveness can start out as a smart face-saving strategy, it often ends up looking like a desperate emotional one. Mothers' failure all too easily becomes the soundtrack of their lives. Indeed, their lives become a protracted mourning for, or endless tantrum about, the breastfeeding relationship they were unable to have. They are haunted by, and forever running from, the myth of their maternal potential. Their discourse is defined by loss of what might have been. In the Guilt chapter, we discussed the powerful depth of grief many mothers feel on losing their breastfeeding relationship, a grief verging on mourning. To dispense with this pain, a mother must confront her loss, admit to it, grieve it, learn to live with it and work through the grief to find a renewed sense of meaning or purpose beyond the loss. Defensiveness prevents this healing process from taking place. Defensiveness is self-harm.

To sum up the essence of defensiveness, comparison with successful breastfeeding mothers inspires in formula feeders a sense of their own inadequacy. In order to numb this miserable feeling, mothers employ defensive tactics, insulating themselves against any social evaluation from others that differs from their ('competent but hard-lucked') view of themselves. A popular strategy is to actively solicit feedback that supports their self-image, and to regurgitate it on demand – that is, when their denial is challenged.

As we have seen, formula-feeding mothers are fearful and envious of their successful breastfeeding adversaries and also fearful and envious of the facts. While mentally corrosive and hard to handle, fear and envy are potent motivators. They house destructive potential. Sometimes, when fear and envy reach boiling point, a mother's frustration becomes so intolerable that the only solution seems to be the removal of the trigger – in other words, to sabotage the breastfeeding success of others. You're going to need a stiff drink for this next chapter.

# 7

# SABOTAGE

'We influence others' actions, and their
actions reflect, as a mirror, ourselves.'

Charles Horton Cooley, 1922,
*Human Nature and the Social Order*[538]

A dichotomy exists in our cultural consciousness, if not in
political correctness, between those mothers deemed successful
at breastfeeding and those deemed failures. Giving everyone
a fair share of failure by means of sabotage represents, for
many women, a tenaciously egalitarian answer to this painful
and discordant dichotomy. There are various methods of
sabotage that women (it is almost always women) tailor to the
breastfeeding scenario. In this chapter I am going to discuss
the most common techniques and examine their devastating
effectiveness. In keeping with the pro-individualism approach
of this book, I am not going to look at corporate undermining
of breastfeeding, largely because, while certainly relevant and
rife, it's been covered extensively elsewhere.[539] Instead, I am
going to focus entirely upon women-on-women sabotage, a
hugely neglected area. Neglected because since women are
socialised to fear being seen as aggressive or unaccommodating,
they tend to express their envious resentment in concealed,
more premeditated ways. In the breastfeeding domain, this
typically involves successful mothers being hurt in some way
without knowing by whom. This obscurity creates a veil,
making many sabotage missions hard to trace to their origins.
I hope by lifting the veil, this chapter can demystify sabotaging

forms of behaviour, draining them of much of their clout.

Let me begin by telling you a pertinent fact about sabotage: sabotage stems from admiration. This may sound like a bizarre assertion. After all, if you admire something, why seek to destroy it? The answer, of course, lies in that painful emotion – the one that conjures bilious anger and bitter vindictiveness – yes, I'm taking about the green-eyed bitch, envy. Envy has a lot to do with admiration, for it's the painful pangs of admiration that make a mother aware of her own shortcomings. Formula-feeding mothers envious of successful breastfeeding mothers feel this way precisely *because* they admire them. Sometimes this admiration motivates those mums to improve themselves. However, for many, the initial tendency towards idolisation cannot last too long because it arouses such intolerable inner torment. To escape these feelings of inferiority, a mother's immediate impulse is to reverse her admiration. She will come to denigrate breastfeeding, even wishing to annihilate it. At a time when she is feeling helpless, a sabotage mission offers an element of God-like control to an envious mother, and if the breastfeeding mother is similar in social status, it will feel natural and somehow fairer if their lots are equalised.

Being in the presence of a mother who is succeeding invariably damages the self-esteem of a failed mother, prompting an awkward and painful 'upwards comparison'. No woman likes to be reminded that there are other women out there who are more successful, more committed, more selfless, more dynamic – or indeed more womanly. Because envy is such a painful emotion, a mother feels compelled to remove it from within herself, and put it somewhere else. The Czech people have coined the word *litost* to describe the gnawing sense of inner torment one feels when faced by another's greater accomplishments, a feeling often swiftly followed by a desire for revenge. Indeed, neurological research has shown that envy is habitually followed by resentment, and that resentment is followed by *schadenfreude* – the pleasure derived from another's misfortune.[540] There is a flimsy border between *schadenfreude* and sabotage. As Mum blames what she envies – breastfeeding – for how she feels, her mission becomes to turn the object of her envy into something bad or non-existent.

Essentially, she tries to assuage her own discomfort by preventing or minimising the breastfeeding success of others.

## WITH FRIENDS LIKE THESE...

'Friends are like boobs. Some are big, some are small.
Some are real, and some are fake'.

Anon

Women are reported as showing greater need than men for affiliation with others.[541] Sensitivity to and protection of relationships are 'socially reinforced' as appropriate concerns for women. Consequently, women are acutely aware of the potential they have to arouse feelings of betrayal in their friends. A sense of implicit obligation constrains their choices. One study entitled 'Toward a situation-specific theory of breastfeeding' determined that a balancing of interests occurs between the mother-baby duo and her broader network of relationships.[542] Essentially, the study pinpointed the typical mother's choice: whether to do 'the right thing' by herself and her baby (breastfeeding), or adhere to social-normative values (formula feeding). Guess which is the route of least resistance? To give you a clue, the UK Infant Feeding Survey 2010 found that when most of their friends only formula fed their babies, mothers were more likely to stop breastfeeding within two weeks (26 percent) than mothers whose friends mostly breastfed (6 percent).

To understand the clout of peer pressure we need to appreciate that a huge part of the security a woman feels within her friendship network is based on commonality – a sameness. There is an unspoken pact between a woman and her friends, an ethos about staying together in the same place at the same rank. Difference is undesirable because it arouses feelings of abandonment. In most communities where breastfeeding is not the norm, a mother successfully breastfeeding signifies psychological differentiation: a break from the network, a change of rank. It implies 'better than, different than'. In this scenario, the nursing mother can feel as if she is doing something somehow forbidden, that she is betraying her network of friends and family. Breastfeeding success effectively threatens her relational ties.

It also can feel as if she is transitioning from one kind of self to another, a process that often invokes confusing feelings of 'depersonalisation' and loss. Choked by the tension between the urge for sameness to her peers and the urge to do better, a mother fears the implications of successful breastfeeding. The potential for her success to arouse envy in those close to her – and consequently lead to loss of support and solidarity – is a real threat to potential breastfeeding mothers. Combine this with women's oversensitivity to the opinions of others and we begin to understand why the fear of hostility and potential break of attachment paralyses many women. Indeed, psychoanalysis has taught us that women are more inclined to fear being the recipient of envy, and that this fear is intensified when that envy radiates from a female loved one.[543] On spying a glinting green eye, many mothers buckle and retire to the familiar ranks by bottle feeding. They trade individual success for communal fair play. Freud had a thing or two to say about this phenomenon, which he referred to as 'social conscious':

> 'Everyone must be the same and have the same. Social justice means that we deny ourselves many things so that others may have to do without them as well, or, what is the same thing, may not be able to ask for them'.[544]

In ancient Greece, the penalty for outstanding wealth or excellence was ostracism or death. While things have toned down a little since those days, successful breastfeeding mothers still have to field their fair share of indignation. Hassle from peers (sometimes subtle, sometimes less so) is the punishment for hard-won success. Often envy makes its presence felt in insidious ways, steadily infecting the atmosphere. Because women's capacities to display aggression, assertiveness and indeed envy are culturally limited, mothers have to express their competitive urges in more stifled, indirect and camouflaged ways. They are pigeonholed by patriarchal society into relying more on covert hostility and less on overt aggressiveness. This social straightjacket has resulted in a widespread phenomenon known as 'bitchiness'.

Take the following scenario: two close friends, Natalie and Sally, are having a play-date at Sally's house with their babies, both four months of age. Natalie is still breastfeeding her baby. Sally stopped breastfeeding when her baby was a few weeks old. Natalie is currently struggling and confides in Sally about a breastfeeding concern. Perhaps she has developed thrush or mastitis. While Natalie's guard is down (metaphorically as she confides in Sally, her armour is off – she is on her knees), Sally leaps at the opportunity to remind Natalie that she shouldn't expect more, that this is the way breastfeeding is. She then informs Natalie that formula feeding is much more convenient; since switching to formula she personally hasn't looked back.

What's going on here? For Sally, being the bearer of such an undermining response is an expression of her envy of Natalie's situation. She wants to pierce Natalie's breastfeeding relationship because she finds it painful to witness. The collapse of her own breastfeeding relationship seemed to confirm to her the futility of the entire endeavour. Spoiling, or attempting to spoil, Natalie's breastfeeding relationship is an attempt to deny what Natalie has, and, in doing so, suppress her own wanting. If she can somehow persuade Natalie to join her in formula feeding, she has perfect justification for her own decision to bottle feed. So she begins to proselytise.

This poisonous side of envy – the relentless ebb and flow between admiration and destructiveness – is subtle yet effective, and the consequent doubt it engenders is one of envy's hallmarks. Feminist sociologists Susie Orbach and Luise Eichenbaum[545] maintain that this is a common feminine phenomenon. They explain, 'The prohibitions against wanting are so strong in women, that it is very difficult to feel genuine joy about something a friend has which we ourselves desperately want'. Sabotage is a screen behind which an envious woman can hide from her longing. Focusing on sabotage diverts her energies away from exploring other feelings, feelings she finds even harder to cope with. A common tactic is to respond to a struggling mother's pleas for help with a suggestion to switch to formula because 'breastfeeding isn't the be all and end all'.

In this almost universal scenario, the mother has obviously chosen to breastfeed and so by suggesting a switch to formula, her 'friend' is not only undermining her choice, but rejecting it. This is akin to telling a vegetarian to eat meat. The fact is, for some women, breastfeeding IS the 'be all and end all', and for a friend to say it isn't just because it wasn't for *her* is a particularly insidious form of projecting. Consider if the circumstances were reversed and a bottle-feeding mother griped, 'I'm so tired of sterilising all these bottles'. Would her friends respond with 'Oh well, you should breastfeed, remember bottle-feeding isn't the be all and end all'? That's a rhetorical question obviously. My point is that when a mother's pleas for support are met with the bottle, she is being sent the condescending message that her struggles and sacrifices are worthless. The suggestion also promulgates the fallacy that bottle-feeding is void of inconvenience. Mothers who are unfortunate enough to be taken in by this ploy are left not only battling guilt, but also resentment, as they slouch exhausted over a sink full of bottles and teats. I argue that it is high time breastfeeding mothers exhibit the same public outrage as formula-feeding mothers do when someone suggests natural feeding is better for babies. If you mention to a formula-feeding mother that breast is best, many become offended and cite their rights. However, when a breastfeeding mother looks for help, it's socially acceptable to thrust a bottle in her face instead of supporting her.

Author, poet and freakishly insightful lady Maya Angelou has famously warned, 'Be careful when a naked person offers you a shirt'. No, she wasn't talking about men flashing in the street. Rather, she meant that it's unwise to take advice from someone who doesn't know what they are talking about. And she was certainly onto something. Studies have shown overwhelmingly that mothers, particularly during the early stages of their breastfeeding journey, and whether or not they are experiencing problems, want reassurance that they are 'doing it right'.[546] If a mother's entire social network comprises 'naked people' like Sally the Saboteur above, reassurance will be haphazard and insincere at best. The scenario reminds me of the fable 'The Fox Without a Tail'. Are you sitting comfortably?

Once upon a time, a fox fell into a trap. After a struggle he managed to get free, but without his beautiful bushy tail. He was so ashamed of his appearance that he thought life was not worth living unless he could persuade other foxes to part with their tails too, and thus divert attention from his own loss. So he called a meeting of the foxes, and advised them to cut off their tails: 'They're ugly things anyhow,' he said. 'Besides, they're heavy, and it's tiresome to be always carrying them about with you.'

Breastfeeding mothers should be wary of sly foxes. Numerous studies have found that friends are a prime source of breastfeeding negativity.[547] This finding is unlikely to win the Nobel Prize for the most earth-shattering discovery, considering that most women end up formula feeding and thus excuse-making. I touched on the efficiency of excuse-making as a tool of sabotage in the Excuses chapter, and I'm going to expand on it now, given that excuse-making is so epidemic in breastfeeding discourse.

As we saw in the aforementioned chapter, faulty anatomy – aka broken breasts – is a popular and grossly over-used claim of women giving up breastfeeding. It also happens to be an insurmountable fault independent of environmental factors or stamina – if a woman's breasts are broken, there's nothing she can do to prevent or correct it, a frightening message to send to any new mum. Such excuses can function as a tool of callous manipulation as well as a very personal shield to the user's self-esteem. Often, it's both. Who can say to what extent the friend suggesting that formula is just as good as breast milk is trying to influence the behaviour of the mother and to what extent she is comforting herself for her own choices?

Here, we begin to understand how far excuse-makers are saboteurs guised as victims. They lead other women down a treacherous thought path. Excuses have the effect of unfavourably colouring women's view of the feasibility of breastfeeding. The more women hear excuses, the more failure crystallises in their perception of breastfeeding and becomes a self-fulfilling prophecy. The conclusion drawn by those listening to excuses is that successful breastfeeding is bestowed by fate upon a few lucky mothers; that breastfeeding attempts are likely to end in failure. The assumption drawn from this subjective hearsay is of course inconsistent with the objective benchmark, also discussed in the Excuses chapter, that only a miniscule percentage of women cannot physically breastfeed.

Yet peer pressure wields a far more powerful influence over behaviour than scientific evidence. Particularly so the earlier it is wielded. For instance, mothers who are undermined during pregnancy – before they even attempt breastfeeding – are less likely to become successful breastfeeders than those sabotaged while breastfeeding. This effect, known as 'the primacy effect', means that early undermining has more influence than later undermining on a mother's perception of her breastfeeding 'competency'.[548] A mother's initial impressions are powerful in determining how she will select, retain and interpret subsequent information. Undermining a mother during pregnancy influences how she prepares for breastfeeding. It triggers the kind of selective attention to information described in the Deception chapter, whereby Mum discounts or withdraws her attention from new information. In short, antenatal sabotage, particularly by trusted peers, leads Mum to develop an unfavourable impression of her ability to breastfeed, an impression that, once planted, is hard to uproot.

Excuse-making creates a zeitgeist of pessimism. This is because widespread excuse-making alters our perception of breastfeeding's feasibility, turning functioning breasts from a biological fact to a fiction. We are primed to expect failure. We see all breasts as faulty by default. This erroneous expectancy not only drives the 'I'll try' fear-driven anticipatory excuses of pregnant women, but more concerning, alters the behaviour of every one of us. By expecting breastfeeding incompetence from the mothers in our life – family members, friends, colleagues et al – we inadvertently drive their behaviour towards failure. We can infer incompetence via subtle environmental and interpersonal cues. For instance, showering a mother with unsolicited advice and words of 'warning' ('Don't worry if you can't breastfeed'). Then, when faced with breastfeeding difficulties, the expectation of incompetence on the part of the mother (facilitated by similar expectations held by everyone around her) is often so perverse that other explanations for why breastfeeding does not appear to be going well are not even considered. When there is a ready explanation for an event – 'You can't breastfeed, your breasts are broken, like your friends' were' – one rarely feels compelled to search for other possible causes.

The negative effect of this mass lay-misdiagnosis is to rob a mother of the motivation to find more relevant cues that could help alleviate her difficulties. Here we see how, more often than not, a mother's community set-up means she is over-exposed to breastfeeding failure and under-exposed to sources that challenge formula feeding as a way of life. It is a painful fact that if a mother's social network only comprises inappropriate role models for breastfeeding, she is less likely to go on to successfully breastfeed. One reason for this phenomenon is that when she sees her peers' behaviour, a mother subconsciously internalises it so that she too has similar behaviour and attitudes. Psychologists call this process 'social learning theory':[549]

> 'Whether we spend so much time with these people because we agree with them, or agree with them because we spend so much time with them, the crucial point remains the same. We do not just hold a belief; we hold a membership in a community of believers'.[550]

But while we can choose our friends, our family is a non-negotiable contract....

## KEEPING IT IN THE FAMILY – FAMILY SABOTAGE

Families eh, who'd have them? A mother's family – immediate and extended – can provide a steady stream of breastfeeding encouragement, or a cannon of stress. We explored the marriage between familial ambivalence and breastfeeding failure in the Deception chapter when we looked at what a mother *believed* her family thought about her breastfeeding efforts. Now let's explore the actual behaviour of the family.

A woman's beliefs about breastfeeding are initially formed as a result of what she has already encountered. The more she encounters breastfeeding failure, for instance, the more she takes this as evidence of the inevitability of failure. Remember the black swans example discussed in the Deception chapter? Successful nursing mothers are black swans while failed nursing mothers are white swans. In our society, the black swans are lost in a sea of white swans, often to the point where the former become invisible. Probability theory tells us the more common something is, the earlier and more often we encounter it, the more driven we are to deem it probable. Combine this with the fact that looking for counter-evidence requires time, energy, resources, intellect, social capital and the confidence to question the current status quo in the face of those who bolster it, and we can see why many mothers are locked into formula-feeding from the very start.[551]

A study of nearly 1,400 US and Australian women found that breastfeeding help and encouragement from friends and family was more important than advice or support from health professionals.[552] It's hardly surprising. Thanks to their enduring prominence and omnipresence (indeed, they have a front row seat), family members are the most under-acknowledged architects of a mother's choices. Their behaviour exploits a mental shortcut in mothers that psychology nerds call 'the availability heuristic'. Let me explain this bad boy: we all have an inbuilt tendency to assess the likelihood of risks by how readily examples come to mind. Our brains are wired so that a risk that is familiar is seen as more serious than a less-familiar risk. A family member's story – that she failed at breastfeeding because of 'insufficient milk' for example – sticks in the mind. Indeed, Mum may even have spectated the failing performance of this family member first-hand. Consequently, she is likely to make her decisions influenced by this information rather than by more relevant but harder to obtain facts. Thus family members' biased presentation of breastfeeding creates a type of 'behavioural inheritance'.[553]

Unbeknown to most mothers, when they give birth they become a lot more powerful in the eyes of others. By giving birth, they have produced another human being, and in the pecking order of caring for that new human being, they reign supreme – particularly if they are breastfeeding. The powerful position of the breastfeeding mother as sole nutritional provider can frustrate other family members – and a family backdrop that is hostile or ambivalent towards breastfeeding is the match that lights the fuse of failure. Numerous studies have found that the higher the degree of social support received by a woman, the higher her feelings of 'self-efficiency', or breastfeeding confidence.[554] On the other hand, women whose family environment is characterised by anti-breastfeeding stories are more likely to abandon breastfeeding, and studies have suggested they do so to protect their physical and emotional well-being.[555]

Many mothers find themselves in this position, routinely encouraged to formula feed by family members.[556] Sometimes, a relative will urge the mother to switch to formula in order to give herself 'a break' or to salvage her mental health. Sometimes, family members provide the mother with skewed examples of evidence – the fable of the family friend who was breastfed yet has numerous allergies, or the formula-fed acquaintance who went on to become an Oxford professor. Anxious for some hands-on new-baby action, family members may even insinuate to the mother that breastfeeding is self-indulgent in so far as it places the baby in a situation of unparalleled dependence on its mother. Revered paediatrician Dr Benjamin Spock was attuned to such manipulation. He noted:

'A mother who is attempting to breastfeed may be subjected to a surprising amount of scepticism on the part of friends and relatives who are otherwise sympathetic. There are remarks like: "You aren't going to breastfeed are you?" "Your poor baby is hungry. Are you trying to starve the child to prove a point?" "Is he feeding again?" The milder remarks can be perhaps blamed on surprise; the meaner ones strongly suggest envy. Even later, if there is any question about continuing to nurse, you'll find several friends who'll urge you to stop'.[557]

Pressure from family members is particularly harmful not only because of its prominence but because it is strategically tailored to address the mother's specific circumstances, tapping into *her* concerns. For example, a mother's anxiety about her baby's crying can be exploited by an intimate relative who, aware of this anxiety, fabricates a link between the baby's crying and a suggestion that the mother has insufficient milk or that her milk is abnormal or inadequate in some way. The fact that such ideas are implanted into the mother by trusted kin makes them all the more potent and compelling. In his book on manipulation, professor of philosophy Thomas Carson described the harm caused:

> 'When we lie or attempt to deceive others, we do so in order to influence their attitudes or behaviour. Thus, generally, when we deceive others, we deceive them about matters of interest and concern to *them* and we try to influence them to do things (or have attitudes) that they would not do (or have) if they were not deceived, and ordinarily we *harm* them [his emphasis]'.[558]

It is far easier for family members to control a mother by employing manipulation and intimidation techniques than it is for the average Joe. Often, the closer we are to people, the harder it is to handle them when they are being cunning. We can't just walk away from the situation if we want to maintain our family relationship as well as our breastfeeding relationship. One of the two has to suffer. Being harmed by the manipulative tactics of others who claim to be acting in our best interests when they are not produces a unique sting for the mother – a feeling of intimate betrayal.

## GRANNY KNOWS BEST

'My parents advise me to stop every month or so.
My mother is envious that I still feed my son
when she "couldn't" breastfeed me'.
Breastfeeding mother[559]

Want to know a surprising fact? Many breastfeeding difficulties can be traced back to a mother's first relationship with a woman; the relationship in which she first felt affection and dependency, disappointment and rejection – the relationship to her own mother. Okay, okay, it's not that surprising. Not when you consider that women who were themselves entirely formula fed are significantly more likely to stop breastfeeding in the first two weeks (27 percent) than women who were only breastfed themselves (9 percent).[560] Indeed, countless studies have affirmed that grandmothers wield immeasurable clout over breastfeeding success.[561] One study even cited grandmothers as THE main source of breastfeeding discouragement.[562] It seems only right, therefore, that I devote a few pages to exploring Granny's shenanigans.

Typically, when a woman embarks on breastfeeding, particularly if she is from a family with little history of breastfeeding, there is some change of roles, norms and 'reference groups'. A reference group is a fancy sociological term meaning a group we use as a standard for evaluating our own qualities, attitudes, values and behaviour. One example is child discipline – does the family belong to an authoritarian reference group or a permissive reference group? Other reference group examples include religious ideals, work ethic, educational aspirations and so on. The changes that happen when a woman starts nursing push all the women of the family out of their comfort zones. None more so than Gran. Women who did not breastfeed their own children can find it particularly difficult to have their own daughters breastfeed successfully. A daughter's success has the potential to put the spotlight of doubt on Gran's own abilities to nurture. Envy is often an issue. Gran has built her identity around being an excellent nurturer, so there is always a touch of sadness and wistfulness when she sees her daughter breastfeed if she herself was unable to. In one study a grandmother confessed:

> 'I look at my daughter, and I look at what she has with her son, and I wish I had had that. And I mean my kids are great and they turned out great, but I wish... I envy what she has'.[563]

The daughter can easily begin to feel she is betraying or in some way deserting her mother by getting for herself something her mother never had. The scenario presupposes a win/lose situation in which she is the winner and her mother the loser. This competitive ambience is difficult to cope with in such an intimate relationship. She may experience the process of attempting to breastfeed as an aggressive, destructive act towards her mother. This discomfort with achievement makes any success less pleasurable and even guilt-inducing.

Often the grandmother interprets her daughter's breastfeeding as a beacon that her own maternal supremacy has been usurped; that can feel crippling. Her daughter's own mothering performance is a threat to the power Granny garners by having a monopoly on this role and the identity she has built around it. So by undermining her daughter's attempts at breastfeeding, Granny can somewhat weaken the foundations of this newly created hierarchical order. In their book *Baby-proofing Your Marriage*, the team of authors warned their readership that grandparents tend to feel a sense of 'ownership', a certain right of involvement that causes them to encroach on their children's parenting prerogative.[564] They blur the line between parenting and grandparenting. Is it any wonder that one of the most common complaints from new mothers is that their own mothers or mothers-in-law interfere?[565] Christine Crosby, founder of *GRAND* magazine, an American publication for grandparents, suspects that grandparents may act out because, well, baby boomers are used to getting their way. She says, 'Today's generation of grandparents were very empowered. They grew up in the 60s, and truly have had freedom that no previous generation ever had. Giving that control up doesn't come naturally.'[566]

At this point, you might want to re-evaluate having your mother over to stay next time you're postnatal: far from providing the bedrock of support it is often touted for, living with your own mother is in fact negatively correlated with breastfeeding outcome.[567] Heck, even having grandparents residing within the locality is predictive of shorter breastfeeding duration.[568] So what's going on here?

Well, the grandmother – particularly the maternal grandmother – has her own stake in relation to her daughter's infant-feeding journey. As elder, and thus more experienced, she naturally wants to be viewed as knowledgeable in such matters – at least more so than her fledgling daughter. For a grandmother, the birth of a grandchild represents both a blessing and a matriarchal crisis. Her daughter has entered the childbearing years as she is leaving hers behind. This milestone forces a grandmother to confront the ageing process and her dwindling competence while triggering vivid memories of her own experience of mothering. The daughter reawakens Granny's own historical breastfeeding struggles and reopens the psychological wounds. Her new motherhood challenges and disrupts whatever peace Granny had made with her breastfeeding past. Through her daughter, Granny relives her own discontent, her own shame at failing. She projects upon her daughter all the ambiguity of her relations with breastfeeding.

Therefore, the sense of satisfaction and achievement a grandmother feels with regard to her own parenting journey is of particular importance: if she lacks these sentiments, feelings of envy and competitiveness can surface and her capacity to appreciate and support her daughter's continuing maternal growth will be eroded. In other words, some grandmothers are unable to encourage ambition, conscientiousness and confidence in their daughters' breastfeeding because of their own underlying feelings of failure.

The acute realisation that her motherly status is coming to an end can be hard for Gran to cope with, particularly in a culture in which her nurturing qualities may have comprised much of her identity and sense of worth. Consequently, she may wish to keep her daughter in a subordinate position in order to maintain her own identity (which has hereto demanded respect and authority). In an attempt to pre-empt any shift in power or loss of control in the unforgiving arena of mothering, some grandmothers resort to manipulation techniques. This behaviour can begin at any time, but commonly starts in a subtle form prior to the birth of the baby, growing in strength from that point onwards. One study caught maternal grandmothers discouraging their daughters from attempting to breastfeed. The grannies in the study used genetic-related rhetoric to manipulate their daughters, telling them that they were 'biologically incapable of breastfeeding' and probably had 'an inherited inability to produce milk'.[569] And it's not just maternal grannies having a piece of the action. In another study[570] one mother explained how the paternal grandmother undermined her breastfeeding efforts:

> 'The baby cried all the time. My mother-in-law said it was because he was hungry and gave him a bottle of formula and he slept all night. That was all it took. I started pumping and I never got very much and it looked like water. My mother-in-law kept feeding the baby the bottle. I would lie down to have a rest and wake up to find her feeding him a bottle. Even after I had lots of milk, she took over the baby'.

Make no mistake, all interactions involve some degree of identity bargaining, and familial interactions are no exception. In trying to reassert her identity as the more skilled, if not principal, nurturer, Granny may exercise 360-degree criticism of her daughter's chosen parenting style. She might, for instance, find it inexplicable that her daughter chooses to sleep in the same room or bed as the baby. After all, as Granny proclaims, you all turned out fine without this breastfeeding nonsense, or co-sleeping nonsense or gradual weaning nonsense – so what are you worried about? When a mother is exhausted, overwhelmed and caked in breastmilk with a body resembling something from *National Geographic*, external criticism can break her will. To give you an idea of how low some grannies stoop, in a survey of 7,000 mothers, a sizable 45 percent said they got negative comments about their post-baby body from their parents.[571] Talk about hitting below the belt!

Criticism, in all its flavours, has two major effects. Firstly, Mum feels angry that someone else believes they know better than she does (this is normally her initial reaction). Secondly, Mum feels secretly worried that perhaps she's not doing the right thing (this subsequent reaction is normally more lingering). After all, few first-time mothers are entirely confident with their parenting skills. Stephanie Kutzen, an American social worker and author of *Grandparenting: Tales From The Crib — When Your Children Become Parents*[572] believes grandparents feel a 'dissonance' (to use the sexy buzzword) and some resentment that their children rely more on information gleaned from the internet or parenting classes than their hard-earned wisdom.[573] And what exactly does this hard-earned wisdom look like? A fascinating study from Brazil found that mothers' abandonment of breastfeeding in the first month was 'significantly associated' with maternal or paternal grandmothers advising them to give the baby water, tea or other milk.[574] Obviously what grandmothers say can have a huge effect on new mothers with little experience of babies, and indeed, this is the plan.

In controlling her own maternal identity, it is necessary for a grandmother to influence the identity of her daughter. Identities reflect relationships between people. If one person in a relationship wants to be seen as the dominant individual, the other person has to assume a more submissive role. Likewise, if one person wants to be regarded as knowledgeable, someone else must take the role of novice learner to whom knowledge can be imparted. To establish and protect her identity as matriarchal knowledge fount, a grandmother must strategically guide her daughter into believing she is lacking, and thus in need of her expertise. Psychologists call this shady behaviour 'altercasting': the use of social and emotional pressure to place another person in a particular identity.[575] In other words, people co-opt other people's behaviour in order to achieve their own purposes.

The grandmother wants to be viewed as the dominant matriarch, or at least as an irreplaceable utility, and so will try in a hundred ways to cause her daughter to assume a respectful posture: by pressuring her daughter, disparaging her ideas, refusing to follow her suggestions and so on. She will project feelings of inadequacy onto her daughter in order to justify perpetuating her own dominant stance. This hampers her daughter's capacities to experience herself as a competent parent. Perhaps Gran refuses to get on board with demand-feeding, forever asking 'Is he feeding *again*?' Their greater reliance on the judgement of others makes women particularly inclined both to being victims of altercasting and to being perpetrators of it.

Characteristic of altercasting is a competitive dimension that may comprise emotional blackmail, psychological manipulation and even emotional terrorism. Control of the infant-feeding process is stolen by a grandmother through exploitative manipulation. The mother is taken advantage of when she is arguably at her most vulnerable. Granny's technique may be subtle and passive – taking over care of the baby so her daughter has little choice but to become spectator – or more insensitive and heavy-handed – starting sentences with, 'If you were a good mother you would…'. Threats of withdrawing approval may additionally be sprinkled like salt on a wound. Then, if the altercasting is successful and Mum begins to behave submissively, Granny's own cherished identity is protected. By trying to appease and mollify a grandmother, the daughter simply encourages the cycle of control to continue. The process also undermines her own self-esteem as a mother because she begins to believe that she is indeed less competent than others.

'White-anting' is another strategy sometimes used by grandmothers in conjunction with altercasting. It refers to the process of undermining or eating away at something below the surface. Just as white ants eat away at the core of a tree without disturbing the surface, so too grandmothers and other intimate family members can eat away at the heart of a mother's confidence without their actions being noticed on the surface. As emotional manipulation strategies, altercasting and white-anting are most commonly used in intimate settings such as families, particularly when the user anticipates that their desires will be resisted or contested by the target. Yet because women are told to repress and disperse anger, as well as to be passive and show humility, a daughter faced with this kind of sabotage may have considerable difficulty in allowing herself to display the assertiveness necessary to defend herself. Assertiveness is culturally unfeminine, particularly when directed towards one's kin.

Of course, not all daughters will concede to their mother's attempts at altercasting and white-anting. Those who have carried out extensive independent research into breastfeeding, for whom it is of upmost importance and who are determined to carve out their own parenting style, are less likely to yield. The more central breastfeeding is to a mother's self-identity, the more likely she is to reject other people's altercasting attempts to threaten it.[576] A daughter who stands firm in the face of her mother's attempts to dim her light has crossed a threshold. She doesn't appear to need her mother in the same way any more. She has shown herself capable and confident – even better. Often in this scenario, mother and daughter do not know how to change and develop together or how to tolerate the differences emerging between them. They do not know how to talk about the emotional conflicts they are both experiencing. Some mother-daughter duos find it challenging to remain connected on this new basis.

Let's conclude this horror story of a chapter with a summary: sabotage enables the perpetrator (often a fellow mother) to restore her self-esteem through rearranging what she perceives to be the power imbalance caused by breastfeeding. Sabotage is a form of maternal social levelling that eases feelings of hurt, disappointment and vulnerability. Yet when women do this to each other, they gain nothing from their sabotage except, at best, temporary relief from their own anguish. The reason a sabotaging mother's relief is fleeting is because the actual source of her torment does not stem from what she envies (breastfeeding), but from herself (feelings of inferiority). In this sense, sabotage is inherently futile. The lovechild of guilt and envy, it springs up when we reject personal responsibility for our failings, and marinates within a private vat of seething bitterness. In the next chapter I venture to imagine what the world of infant feeding would look like if women took an altogether different path.

# In conclusion:
# a future for breastfeeding?

'At any given moment you have the power to say:
this is not how the story is going to end'.

Attributed to Christine Mason Miller

Mothers have fantasies, dreams and goals of successful breastfeeding that for a few pleasurably unfold into a triumphant performance. Everyone else's journey is tarnished by anxiety and dread, leaving them to deal nervously with their dishonour in the public eye. In this final chapter, I'll suggest how this woefully widespread and growing legacy can be halted – and indeed, inverted.

Mothers are tricksters, and breastfeeding is perhaps the biggest of confidence tricks. Living in a culture in which so many mothers stop breastfeeding as a result of difficulties has the inevitable consequence that women question whether or not they can sustain their own baby without artificial help. It does not have to be this way. In some parts of the world, babies are routinely swapped between mums, aunts, grandmas and neighbours. Women who have never given birth can breastfeed. Infertile women can breastfeed. Post-menopausal women can breastfeed. Transgendered women can breastfeed. In the same way various animals suckle other animals. [577] Even the World Health Organization has stressed:

'If a mother truly believes she can provide enough milk for her infant, she will encounter few problems with milk let-down, even in the stressful conditions and overwork experienced by most of the world's lactating women.... If on the other hand, a woman believes that modern life is incompatible with full breastfeeding, she may be more inclined to interpret any difficulties encountered – ironically, even those arising from producing too great a volume – as being due to too little milk. Women need basic information about the mechanics of breastfeeding, and the reliability of lactation'.[578]

Brought to their knees by lack of confidence, most mothers abandon the aspiration of breastfeeding in favour of the comfort of appearing in control. Their need to evolve artificial, strategic ways to experience a sense of control forces them to override their genuine feelings and wishes. These women soon find themselves overcome by guilt, despair, confusion and bitterness as a result of the tension between their original goals and these goals' seeming incompatibility with the drive for control. We need to help women cultivate this much-desired sense of control and incorporate it into their breastfeeding journey.

This task will not be met without resistance, not least from formula manufacturers, who promulgate untruths so they can, literally, capitalise on women's ignorance. The concept of women having control over breastfeeding is also threatening to the medical profession because the status of health professionals is reliant on mothers relinquishing control. One arsenal against such resistance is to follow the WHO's advice and educate women on matters of breast anatomy and the mechanics of lactation (see Epilogue). If a mother can understand the network of physiological processes involved in lactation, a sense of control will no longer seem so elusive. Understanding how the various breast tissues evolved to work in perfect sync with each other, and how a mother can manipulate the process by techniques such as hand-expression and positioning, can build in her a sense of empowerment and self-sufficiency.

But can mothers feel in control of breastfeeding to the same extent that they feel in control of formula feeding? Perhaps the answer to this conundrum is to take a reverse approach: mothers should be introduced to the notion that formula merely gives the *illusion* of control. Because of its inherent risks, formula is, in fact, far less controllable and reassuring than breastfeeding. When a mother nurses her child at her breast, she can be assured, to a relatively greater extent than if she chose other methods of feeding, that she and her child will be healthier. This knowledge, this confidence, is in itself a form of taking control – the mother is controlling her destiny and that of her child far more effectively than she ever could by formula feeding.

We can alert mothers to the fact that breastfeeding offers control on a practical level, too. A breastfeeding mother can offer her baby a quick drink now and then, enabling her to fit his needs around her other commitments. This level of flexible control isn't available for formula-feeding parents. A breastfeeding mother is not subservient to the bottle, the sterilizer – or the doctor for that matter. Breastfeeding enables her to avoid helplessness, dependence and victimhood. To give a real-world example of breastfeeding liberation, let's return to Doris, the mum of nine featured in the Guilt and Envy chapters. After formula feeding her first five babies, her story turns from tragedy to triumph. Doris is a born-again breastfeeder. She bags up her self-handicapping, excuse making and defensiveness, and dumps those fuckers in the trash:

'Fast forward a few babies. Quite a few babies in my case. You seek and find the right support while you are still pregnant. You listen, you learn, you surround yourself with other happily breastfeeding mothers and it is beginning to dawn on you that actually they did not have an easier ride than you. They had support when it mattered! So you grow quietly hopeful that maybe, just maybe, you will be able to feed this baby yourself.

And then your new baby girl is here, born at home surrounded by all your loved ones and she latches on beautifully; so far so good. There is no pain, as you both know what you are doing. You have the confidence to co-sleep from the start, making night feeds so much easier. You have your breastfeeding counsellor on speed dial (lol), but really you do not need her as it just works. And you fall hopelessly and utterly in love with this little bundle.

You treasure every moment you have with her at the breast. You love that drunken sailor look she gets all the time. You love the fact that she only wants you and all you have to do is lift your top and let her disappear under your jumper and she is happy.

You cannot stop sniffing her because she smells so good; so familiar and sweet and you get such a kick out of seeing her grow. Knowing that it is all your milk that has caused those chubby dimples. And then you get the first smile as she is coming off the boob, your milk dribbling down her chin. And then the first raspberry blow that has you both in fits of giggles. Chubby hands stroking your breasts, a little mouth contently glugging away and you just feel on top of the world.

Your older children imitating you by breastfeeding their dolls, suggesting baby needs feeding so they can get on with their play, and then your toddler comes up to you and asks to have some too. So you end up with both of them at the breast and of course your toddler does not know what to do, but you feel such a rush of love and it heals so many wounds, wounds you never even knew you had.

The conversations you have with your teenager, as to why she was not breastfed – did you not love her enough? Ouch! How do you answer that one?

And through it all those breastfeeding hormones are working their magic. Everyone around you is surprised at the change in you. The kids and your husband are commenting on how much calmer you are, "Mum you are a much nicer person you know!" From a friend, "What has happened to you, you have really changed!" (Incidentally that friend ended up breastfeeding her last baby for three years, having formula fed the first four!)

And what about you? You gain a new self-belief. You at long last feel comfortable in your own skin. You are WOMAN, hear me roar! Your milk has superpowers; it must have. Your baby grows into a toddler and tells you so! And you discover another thing about breastfeeding that you never knew. It is such a brilliant parenting tool when you have a toddler. How on earth did you ever manage without it before?

There are hardly any tantrums, you have the perfect tool right there, strapped to your chest – and you use it willingly and gladly. And there is such joy, such indescribable joy. You are finally doing what you were meant to be doing. It's natural and all of a sudden you are the one who other mums come up to and tell their breastfeeding story of pain and failure and justification and you see yourself and how you used to be.

Breastfeeding – it makes a difference it really does!'

Doris has the A B C of Breastfeeding Fidelity set out in the Deception chapter down to a T. Her story illustrates what can happen when we start to nurture women's confidence in their control of their own bodies's inherent abilities. Only then will excuses for not breastfeeding (both anticipatory and retrospective) be unnecessary – and our retrograde culture rejuvenate. At present, mothers adopt a dramaturgical approach to their interactions with each other and with the outside world. In a sense, they have become *performers*. For a gender famous for its intimacy, women are extraordinarily bad at being honest with each other. Their excuses popularise myths of broken breasts and insurmountable challenges, recycling a culture in which breastfeeding failure is the norm. This culture of failure robs mothers of a sense of having meaningful control over their bodies. Instead, mothers feel awash in an ebb and flow of situations beyond their influence, a scenario they understandably find profoundly distressing. It is no wonder excuses have become part of everyday maternal dialogue – mothers have lost faith in themselves.

The rationality of a woman listening to other women's excuses is skewed. When she tries to breastfeed, instead of feeling that she is doing the most natural thing in the world and assuming that she'll succeed, she feels that she's attempting to do the unusual, the difficult and the impossible. The A B C of Breastfeeding Fidelity framework is neither linear nor hierarchal; rather it is dynamic, with each factor interacting with the others. For instance, the Belief that most people formula feed affects a mother's perceived Control over her own breastfeeding ('If everyone else has failed, then so will I') while also affecting her Attitude about the perceived validity of the risks of formula feeding ('If everyone else formula feeds, it can't be that risky'). American journalist and author Kathryn Schulz once said, 'Few of us change the course of history when we make excuses for being wrong'.[579] Yet in a roundabout way, that is precisely what mothers have done and carry on doing: they have changed the course of history through excuse-making. Excuse-making impedes breastfeeding by denying the reliable heritage of lactation.

## FROM MICRO TO MACRO – THE POWER OF THE MOTHER AS INDIVIDUAL

While many of the factors discussed in this book are psychosocial in nature, the 'psycho' part – the part that looks at women's individualistic responses to breastfeeding – has been swept over in the real world by the broom of a collectivist agenda. As the preceding chapters have shown, it is not unfortunate cultural conditioning alone that 'causes' breastfeeding failure. A grassroots, more in-depth examination of women's experience reveals that particular emotional reactions set up the inclination to act in a certain way – and many of these courses of action are unfavourable towards breastfeeding. In the words of Australian professor of sociology, Jack Barbalet, 'Culture plays a role, certainly, in the details, but not the gross character of an actor's response to their circumstances'.[580]

If we take a micro-level analysis of breastfeeding (looking at the individual mother) rather than relying as we have always done on a macro-level analysis (looking at 'society'), we begin to understand – for perhaps the first time – the powerful agency of an individual mother. Breastfeeding behavior is shaped on a nationwide, and even global, scale through micro-level deception, guilt, envy and sabotage. Formula apologists like to parrot that, 'Society is to blame for poor breastfeeding rates' – as if society is something that exists externally to women. By looking at infant feeding through an individualistic micro-level lens, we see that, in reality, women participate in the erection and maintenance of the very breastfeeding hurdles they lament.

In this book I have held your hand as we encountered the most salient emotions felt by women during their infant-feeding journeys. We have explored the myriad ways mothers attempt to amplify some of these emotions while concealing others. For instance, we saw that envy and the sabotage are a mother's psychological shields against her fruitless longings. They allow her to project uncomfortable, often unpalatable, feelings onto someone else so they become less internally disruptive. Paradoxically, this tactic exacerbates her feelings of powerlessness. Envy keeps a mother in a constant state of emotional flux. It prevents her from exploring her desire to breastfeed and the difficulties that have impeded it. Her envy is an expression of her concealed feelings of entitlement. Left unchecked, it morphs into sabotage. This emotional current, which flows through significant life stages, has largely been overlooked by academics and policy-makers, but its importance cannot be overstated. For emotions cause or produce social processes; they are aggregated products of many individuals, which together act as a discrete force in society. Experts call this the 'macrosociology of emotions'.[881] The emotions we have explored in this book – guilt, envy, contempt and so on – are transformed everyday from personal events into social processes. As emotional behaviours, they double as defence mechanisms, working to displace responsibility and thereby fuel the macro-structures that maintain breastfeeding failure as a cultural norm. Evading personal responsibility for breastfeeding failure creates the illusion that the cause of failure is actually emanating from society itself.

I hope in the chapters of this book I have driven home the message that although emotions appear to be discrete, they are powerfully effectual, driving shockwaves through our culture. A continual flow of emotion exists between a mother and the culture of failure, a current that runs both ways. Sometimes the tide is strong enough to force mothers to feel what they don't feel. The sum of individual mothers' emotions has created a culture in which the worst sin is not envy, but exciting envy, a culture in which success is discouraged. Breastfeeding mothers find themselves at the mercy of a double-bind in which their achievement is likely to provoke admiration as much as it provokes envy and sabotage. The struggling breastfeeding mother told she has tried hard enough and should quit – 'Happy Mum, Happy Baby' – has to concede or risk offending and being labelled a neurotic, a perfectionist and a masochistic martyr.

The straightjacket enforced by emotional sensibilities has led to the stagnation of progress – a reluctance at best and inability at worst to discuss the issues most prevalent to breastfeeding failure, for fear of offending. Ironically, I believe the emotions we have explored in this book will be a pivotal mobilising force in the shift towards a breastfeeding counter-revolution. Both the personal and collective amalgamation of these emotions has the potential to create a 'moral shock' as mothers realise they have the control to turn things around. In fact, personal loss and vulnerability have been identified as the main incentives for active participation in activism.[582] In the breastfeeding context, guilt, regret, envy, defensiveness and sabotage speak of loss, rights and deserving. Instead of sinking into denial about their sense of entitlement to a breastfeeding relationship, mothers should be encouraged to harness it.

## TOWARDS A CULTURE OF TRUTH

'If we can't do the emotional work of fully accepting our mistakes, we can't do the conceptual work of figuring out where, how, and why we made them'.

Kathryn Schulz, 2010, *Being Wrong: Adventures in the Margin of Error*[583]

Women need sufficient contact with the facts if they are to make realistic and adaptive adjustments to their patterns of thinking and behaviour. If for instance, successful breastfeeders were encouraged to speak of their success instead of being shamed as 'smug', mothers everywhere would realise they share many of the same challenges. A new maternal zeitgeist – solidarity and success – would form. Only these black swans (breastfeeding mums) can tell us anything definitive about the nature of successful breastfeeding – and yet, other mothers persistently fail to seek them out because of 'confirmation bias', that is, they tend to give more weight to evidence that confirms their own beliefs than evidence that challenges them. Often other mothers censor breastfeeding mums because of painful feelings of personal conflict, otherwise known as, 'cognitive dissonance'. By sharing positive stories of breastfeeding success, mothers can accumulate 'embodied knowledge' – a type of knowledge gained through practical observation – and this has been proven to have a significant edge over theoretical knowledge at increasing mothers' confidence in breastfeeding.[584] Antenatal classes need to devote less resources to 'textbook' breastfeeding direction and more to providing opportunities for pregnant women to meet real breastfeeding mothers and see *successful* breastfeeding first hand.

Women routinely describe an incongruity between idealised expectations and early breastfeeding problems – which leads them to quit earlier than originally planned.[585] This is partly the result of a consumerist, convenience-driven mentality that expects every task to be convenient. If something requires a bit of effort, learning and *heaven forbid* discomfort, then it is seen as too inconvenient or 'not for me'. Breastfeeding advocates would be wise to provide accurate and realistic information on the realities of breastfeeding before mothers give birth – a type of 'feed-forward' preparation exercise. Aligning expectations and experience would provide valuable information that otherwise has to be learned by post-failure feedback.

The current behaviour of mothers conceals and distorts the physiological dependability of breastfeeding. If women are ever to have true sovereignty over their bodies, they need to be honest with each other and themselves. A radical change is called for. I recommend that women tell it like it is; tell the truth. Mums need to be transparent and lay their breastfeeding struggles on the table – their conflicting priorities, their discontent, their naivety, their fears, their tensions – both inwardly and out to others. By owning and indeed showcasing these painful, forbidden emotions, we separate the subjective from the objective. This would enable women to make choices based on the clear light of fact rather than the murky shadow of biased self-serving fictions. In short, truth is empowering. When a mother declares that others are to blame for her breastfeeding failure – her baby, her husband, health professionals et al – she is apt to stew in self-pity and smoulder with resentment. On the other hand, when a mother can blame *herself* and see her predicament as one for which *she* is largely responsible and which *she* can do something towards changing, she regains control. Indeed, studies have consistently found that when people are encouraged to attribute their failures to lack of effort, their future performance is significantly improved.[586] Taking personal responsibility – and indeed the blame – for failure helps a mother to understand what went wrong, and conveys the implication that she has the power to act to prevent such failure from recurring in the future.[587]

In just a few pages, I will be giving you a buffet of tips to facilitate this ownership process, but before that, I want to expand on why ownership of one's breastfeeding journey is so important. Remember the story of Natalie and Sally in the previous chapter? Their example illustrates the way in which deception – and its BFFs: guilt, envy and sabotage – sets up internal voices that constrain a mother from pursuing her breastfeeding ambitions, be they for relactation or for successful breastfeeding of future babies. After failing at breastfeeding herself, Sally sets out to undermine Natalie's breastfeeding efforts by infecting her with pessimism. Instead of facing her pain and the longing she has for a successful breastfeeding relationship, Sally wants to erase Natalie's breastfeeding relationship – and in doing so, erase the discomfort Sally feels at observing someone else with the very thing she wanted for herself. This strategy, while initially pacifying, is ultimately ineffective. Sabotaging Natalie won't actually do what Sally intends it to do. It will not remove Sally's feelings of entitlement. At best, it merely gives Sally temporary respite from her envy. On the other hand, by attributing her failure to herself and her own actions, Sally could restore a greater feeling of subjective control over future breastfeeding endeavours – by recognising that she can influence undesirable outcomes. Instead of feeling envy towards Natalie, she would feel inspired by her.

Mothers who are truthful about their responsibilities don't feel as though they are out of control or victims of circumstance. Accepting responsibility for their actions does not mean these mothers seldom make mistakes, rather it means that when they do, they can act to correct or at least improve upon them. Then breastfeeding failure becomes evidence not that a mother is broken, but that she can improve. While taking responsibility for one's mistakes doesn't do away with the pain, it does remove the focus of upset from guilt, envy and self-hatred, moving it into the realm of self-improvement. Conversely, running from responsibility merely exacerbates feelings of envy and deepens self-alienation.

The fogging of the causal chain between mothers' behaviour and breastfeeding outcomes – particularly the over-used anatomical excuse – has another detriment: it inhibits the ability of breastfeeding advocates to implement effective support strategies. Because the mother frames the cause of her failure as outside her volitional control, people wishing to support her find themselves, like bloodhounds, aimlessly sniffing red herrings, wasting their time and hers.

By giving accurate explanations of her behaviour, a mother equips health professionals and other breastfeeding advocates with more productive tools to help her. Honesty has the potential to improve the standard of support services by tailoring them to the actual (rather than 'theatrical') difficulties mothers face. In this new culture of truth, women will go into breastfeeding with open eyes, female solidarity will improve, and the inter-generational transmission of the art of breastfeeding will be invigorated again.

Openness would also strip malice of its power. When mothers are honest with themselves and each other, envy, guilt and contempt no longer seem too powerful to counter. When we start being honest, the enabling structure that makes formula feeding both more convenient and more desirable will collapse and take its belief system with it. Breastfeeding, freed from the shackles of censorship, would be taken more seriously as both a personal and political issue.

To put it bluntly, we need to admit our weaknesses, rather than haphazardly destroying each other with them. We need to be honest and acknowledge that breastfeeding is more likely to fail for behavioural reasons than for biological ones. Together, we can create a renegade social movement, a culture of confession, and lower the barriers of secrecy that have kept mothers in a flux of conflicting and often painful emotions.

# Epilogue: how to own your breastfeeding journey

'When you are writing the story of your life,
don't let anyone else hold the pen'.
Anonymous

So, how does one go about successfully breastfeeding in the face of so much emotional, social and cognitive adversity? What follows is a whistle-stop tour of what your successful breastfeeding journey could look like, and most importantly, how to own it. All aboard!

## BEFORE BREASTFEEDING

A note before we begin: do you remember the 'primacy effect' discussed in the Sabotage chapter? This explains that the earlier you set your emotional barometer for breastfeeding success or failure, the more likely you are to bring it about. Well, in tribute to that fact, this 'before' list centres on pro-active preparation. After all, there are nine months – or thereabouts – in which to prepare for breastfeeding blast off!

1.  First of all, remove the words 'I'll try' from your vocabulary. Instead, live by the words of Yoda in *Star Wars: The Empire Strikes Back*, 'Do or do not. There is no "try"'.
2.  Forget the benefits of breastfeeding. No, I didn't just commit a monumental typo. I want you to delete the

Breast is Best message from your brain's motherboard and instead install a new program: Understanding the Risks of Formula. Get yourself clued up on the cons of formula use, not just in relation to your baby but also in relation to yourself. I could list them here, but I'd run out of page space. Pubmed.com – a tardis of academic research papers – is your buddy. On the other hand, if you're time-strapped or not a nerd, then The Infant Feeding Action Coalition (INFACT) Canada have a nicely condensed online factsheet detailing the risks of formula: www.infactcanada.ca/RisksofFormulaFeeding.pdf

3. Write a list of all the reasons why breastfeeding is important to *you*. Leave no stone unturned – emotional, physical, financial, social, spiritual, intellectual – slam all those reasons down on paper. Make the list as thorough as you can, looking at both short-term and long-term motives. Now put the list somewhere safe.

4. I don't want to put a downer on you at this stage, but do read about the Burden of Breastfeeding (see page 35) and recap on why our culture frames breastfeeding as more of a hassle than it actually is. Psyche yourself up for the journey ahead – motherhood, which is the real 'hassle'!

5. Get clued up on your birthing options, and most importantly, your rights. Some medical interventions (for instance, pethidine pain relief, lack of skin-to-skin contact or separation of mum and baby after delivery) can interfere with your baby's nursing instinct. After you have conducted your research, use it to write your birth plan – aka your personal breastfeeding manifesto.[588]

6. If there is a UNICEF-accredited 'baby friendly' hospital in your area, aim to give birth there. These venues make it their business to be pro-breastfeeding (in theory at least).

7. While we're knee-deep in preparation,[589] it's time for Lactation 101. Recall in the Deception chapter we discussed mothers' Fear of Failure vs Hope of Success? Which camp do you want to kip in? Ignorance fuels fear; knowledge fuels success. I want you to educate yourself about the mechanics of lactation. Handy starting points include: establishing and maintaining breast milk supply,

feeding patterns of the breastfed baby, and potential problems. This epilogue cannot do justice to these broad and fascinating topics, so you'll need to do the legwork yourself. I recommend *Dr. Jack Newman's Guide to Breastfeeding*[590] as a go-to introduction.

8. Read about the Culture of Failure (see page 79). When you understand why everyone around you seems to have failed at breastfeeding and how this may impact on your own motivation and confidence, you are inadvertently robbing the culture of failure of much of its pessimistic brain-warping clout. Now come here and give me a fist-bump.

9. Anticipate visceral factors such as the effects of pain and lack of sleep on your motivation (see page 57) and plan for the time they kick in (they will, mark my words). Look into pain-relief options (at first breastfeeding can be a leeedle bit uncomfortable) and sleep strategies (the pros and cons of co-sleeping, for example). Remember, at this early preparation stage you are in a 'cold' state of visceral awareness – this is the perfect time to be making plans.

10. Using formula is detrimental to your long-term breastfeeding goals – put simply, formula consumption reduces your baby's inclination to nurse at your breast. I want none of this 'buying a tin just in case' business. That's not good prep, that's self-sabotage.

11. Increase the predictability of your social environment – aka round up your troops. I want you to write down at least three breastfeeding support telephone contacts. May I recommend La Leche League, NCT and your local peer supporter?[591]

12. Get nifty with positioning. Using a doll, a real baby or even one of those yappy little dogs, practise various breastfeeding holds: cradle, cross-cradle, football and the holy grail for nocturnal feeds, lying down. Want to watch how the pros do it? Google and YouTube are your besties.

13. Double Electric Breastpump – locate one. You may never have to use it, but I want you to know where you can access one if you need to at short notice. Your local breastfeeding counsellor may be able to lend you one for free.

14. Defuck your habitat. In the Sabotage chapter I mentioned that, more often than not, a mother's community set-up means she is over-exposed to breastfeeding failure and under-exposed to sources that challenge formula feeding as a way of life. Right, I want you to reverse this trend by sniffing out the veteran breastfeeders in your social circle and inviting them to discuss their success stories. Be sure to ask what challenges they faced and, most importantly, how they overcame them. Don't have any breastfeeding buddies? It's okay. Get yourself onto Google and type 'Alpha Parent Triumphant Tuesday' to find a massive collection of breastfeeding success stories you can dip in and out of. You are welcome.

## DURING BREASTFEEDING

1. You are now in a 'hot' state of visceral awareness (see page 59).[592] This is not the time to be making serious decisions. If you worked through the Before Breastfeeding list, you will have already made some stellar decisions anyway. So step away from the dummy. Avoid the formula aisle. Heck, fast-forward TV commercials. Stick to your plan and keep calm. You got this.
2. Remember, your ability to breastfeed is not 'fixed' but 'flexible' – that means it is open to adjustment, manipulation and change. Challenges are seldom insurmountable. Simply considering this fact on a regular basis will keep your mojo topped up.
3. Beware of 'sly foxes' (see page 213).
4. There's no such thing as 'the perfect latch', but some latches are better than others. Aim for your baby to take a good mouthful of breast: nipple, areola, the works! Your nipple should be in the upper part of your baby's mouth. That's because there needs to be enough room between the nipple and the lower lip for baby to compress the breast with his tongue, thus stimulating the ducts to release their coveted bounty.
5. Beware of nipple confusion. Now you've perfected your latch, let's not go sabotaging it. The synthetic teats on

bottles and dummies don't flex in the mouth the way your breast does. Allow your baby to master the art of suckling at your breast before you even THINK of introducing any of that shit. I'm talking six weeks MINIMUM, you got me?

6. Screw scheduled feeds. None of this 'every three hours' lark. Your baby knows her own appetite better than your living-room clock does. Watch for peckishness cues (gaping mouth, moving head from side to side, sucking fingers) and then open the milk bar. Alternatively, start up a 24-hour mobile milk buffet by wearing your baby in a sling against your chest.

7. Get to know the Timeline of a Breastfed Baby. Back in 2011, I created an online resource depicting (in minute day-by-day detail) the feeding, sleeping and behavioural patterns of the average breastfed baby. The resource gets, on average, 20,000 hits per day – and for good reason. The reassurance and comfort of knowing your baby is just fine can calm even the most visceral of factors. So log in when you're feeling anxious: www.thealphaparent. com/2011/12/timeline-of-breastfed-baby.html

8. You know those breastfeeding support numbers you wrote down? If you're feeling ropey, now is the time to ring them.

9. Ditto local breastfeeding support groups: La Leche League, NCT, ABM, BfN, NHS are great places to start. Google their contact numbers.

10. For goodness sake, EAT CAKE. Now is not the time to worry about your mummy tummy. As you're burning a good few extra calories per day by breastfeeding, you can afford to indulge. Replace the word 'cake' with any of your preferred food fetishes. We don't want 'visceral factors' like hunger and cravings bothering you right now.

11. At around three months you'll hit a minefield of boobie traps: your breasts will stop leaking, your baby will reduce the length of his feeds, weight gain will move at a slower pace, and your baby's bowel movements may go into hiding. Badass paediatrician and knower of all things breastfeeding Dr Carlos González called this turbulent time 'The Three-Month Crisis'. He was referring to the

way in which mothers get themselves all thong-wedgie misdiagnosing these happenings when, in reality, they are all perfectly normal bends on nature's breastfeeding path. La Leche League has called them simply 'false alarms'.[593] Keep calm and carry on.

12. Tempted to reach for the formula? One bottle won't hurt, right? Don't even go there, my friend. That's the boisterous toddler of your psyche speaking – 'the id', remember him (see page 60)? Instead, turn to page 57 and read Formula Feeding – the Control Paradox to remind yourself why formula is not the easy way out. Phew, that's better. The sensible parent of your psyche – the ego – just saved your bacon.

13. Are you Kate Middleton? If not, you have about as much chance of marrying a prince as of owning faulty breasts. Do bear this in mind when you're on the verge of freaking out. Your breasts work perfectly!

14. Recall that list of reasons why breastfeeding is important to you? Dig out that bad boy and stick it somewhere prominent (the location of your midnight nursing sessions would be ideal). Heck, photocopy it and stick versions all over your home – the fridge door, the bathroom mirror, the TV stand, your mother's face. Also, don't forget to slip a copy into your changing bag for out-and-about breastfeeding (this has the added benefit of enabling you to brandish it in the face of judgey naysayers – although at this stage, these people are largely fictional). What we're doing here is tapping into those 'gain goals' mentioned in the Deception chapter, the same goals prioritised by fellow positive deviants. Delayed gratification win!

15. While you're kicking ass and taking names, take a gander at your baby. Is he happy, active and looking healthy? Then, rest assured, all is well in the world. The lactivist mantra 'look at the baby, not at the scales' is sound advice.

16. Stimulation, stimulation, stimulation. No, this isn't a new political slogan; this is what you need to be doing with your breasts right now. Using your hands or a breast pump – but ideally a baby – ensure that your breasts are stimulated at least every three hours and especially

through the night. Sorry, I know it's a drag, but your body is more susceptible to milk-making hormones during the twilight hours; make re-runs on Dave your bedfellow for now.

## MAINTAINING BREASTFEEDING

1. High five! You're a bona fide positive deviant. Go you! Now, let's make sure you don't lose that title. Complacency is not your friend during this stage of breastfeeding,[594] so stay mindful.

2. Get some ear defenders (actual or metaphorical). You'll need them for the naysayers. If you've been feeding on demand, for instance, be prepared for cries of 'You'll spoil that child!' or 'Isn't he getting enough?' from frenemies and relatives. Give them the stink eye and ignore. If you wake up one day feeling particularly smart-arse, direct them to WHO or UNICEF guidelines.[595]

3. Has your baby hit the six-month mark? Is he raring to chew food? And do you think this is a good idea? Fair enough, just ensure that you offer the breast before giving solids to ensure baby receives all the milk he needs for optimum growth.

4. Remember positioning in the Before Breastfeeding list? Feel free to loosen the reigns on that now. Babies who have become veteran breastfeeders can nurse in almost any position. If she wants to go all *Cirque du Soleil* and you're fine with that, go for it!

5. Thinking about (or being forced to) return to work? It's time to dig out that breast pump I mentioned earlier and get tinkering. I find that a mixture of pumping and hand expression works best. Try expressing milk as often as you can – for 10–15 minutes each time, several times a day. Don't feel deflated (puntastic!) if nothing much comes out. This is normal at the start. And while I'm issuing warnings, don't try to habituate your baby to the bottle in advance (see Tip 5 on the During Breastfeeding list). When the time comes, your baby will feed from the bottle/cup/spoon if and when he is hungry.

6. Being hassled to give up breastfeeding by a jobsworth? Don't buckle under duress. Instead, plug those WHO/UNICEF guidelines again. If the offending busybody happens to be a health professional, consider submitting a complaint, citing said guidelines.

Congratulations! Preen those feathers – you're a Black Swan. My job here is done.

# Endnotes

1. Giles F. 2003. *Fresh Milk: The Secret Life of Breasts*. Simon & Schuster.
2. Marshall JL, Godfrey M, Renfrew MJ. Being a 'good mother': managing breastfeeding and merging identities. *Social Science & Medicine*. 2007. Nov 65(10):2147–59. Epub 2007 Aug 6.
3. Marshall JL, Godfrey M, Renfrew MJ. Being a 'good mother': managing breastfeeding and merging identities. *Social Science & Medicine*. 2007. Nov 65(10):2147–59. Epub 2007 Aug 6.
4. World Health Organization. Fact sheet N°342. Infant and young child feeding. Available at: www.who.int/mediacentre/factsheets/fs342/en/
5. Lupton D. 'A love/hate relationship': the ideals and experiences of first-time mothers. *Journal of Sociology*. 2000. 36(1):50–63.
6. Groleau D, Sibeko L. Breastfeeding in the Margins: Navigating Through the Conflicts of Moral and Social Order, p203, in Hall Smith P, Hausman BL, Labbok M (eds.). 2012. *Beyond Health, Beyond Choice. Breastfeeding Constraints and Realities*. New Brunswick, NJ: Rutgers University Press.
7. Wolf JB. 2010. *Is Breast Best?: Taking on the Breastfeeding Experts and the New High Stakes of Motherhood*. New York: NYU Press.
8. Kukla R. Ethics and Ideology in Breastfeeding Advocacy Campaigns. *Hypatia*. 21.2 2006. 157–18 p163.
9. McDowel MM, Wang C, Kennedy-Stephenson J. *Breastfeeding in United States, findings from the national health & nutrition examination survey*, 1999–2006. Number 5, 2008.
10. Perera PJ, Ranathunga N, Fernando MP, Sampath W, Samaranayake GB. Actual exclusive breastfeeding rates and determinants among a cohort of children living in Gampaha district Sri Lanka: A prospective observational study. *International Breastfeeding Journal*. 2012. Dec 22,7(1):21; Kaneko A, Kaneita Y, Yokoyama E, Miyake T, Harano S, Suzuki K, Ibuka E, Tsutsui T, Yamamoto Y, Ohida T. Factors associated with exclusive breast-feeding in Japan: for activities to support child-rearing with breast-feeding. *Journal of Epidemiology & Community Health*. 2006. 16(2):57–63; Otsuka K, Dennis CL, Tatsuoka H, Jimba M. The relationship between breastfeeding self-efficacy and perceived insufficient milk among Japanese mothers. *Journal of Obstetric, Gynecologic & Neonatal Nursing*. 2008. 37(5):546–555.
11. Betoko A, Charles MA, Hankard R, Forhan A, Bonet M, Saurel-Cubizolles MJ, Heude B, de Lauzon-Guillain B. EDEN mother-child cohort study group. Infant feeding patterns over the first year of life: influence of family characteristics. *European Journal of Clinical Nutrition*. 2013. Jun 67(6):631–7; Dashti M, Scott JA, Edwards CA, Al-Sughayer M. Predictors of breastfeeding duration among women in Kuwait: results of a prospective cohort study. *Nutrients*. 2014. Feb 20;6(2):711–28.
12. Al Juaid DA, Binns CW, Giglia RC. Breastfeeding in Saudi Arabia: a review. *International Breastfeeding Journal*. 2014. Jan 14;9(1):1; Perera PJ, Ranathunga N, Fernando MP, Sampath W, Samaranayake GB. Actual exclusive breastfeeding rates and determinants among a cohort of children

living in Gampaha district Sri Lanka: A prospective observational study. *International Breastfeeding Journal.* 2012. Dec 22;7(1):21; Skafida V. Change in breastfeeding patterns in Scotland between 2004 and 2011 and the role of health policy. *European Journal of Public Health.* 2014. Mar 17.

13. Thorisdottir AV, Gunnarsdottir I, Thorsdottir I. Revised infant dietary recommendations: the impact of maternal education and other parental factors on adherence rates in Iceland. *Acta Paediatrica.* 2013. Feb;102(2):143–8; Otsuka K, Dennis CL, Tatsuoka H, Jimba M: The relationship between breastfeeding self-efficacy and perceived insufficient milk among Japanese mothers. *Journal of Obstetric, Gynecologic & Neonatal Nursing.* 2008. 37(5):546–555.

14. Weitz.R 2013 The Sociology of Health, Illness, and Health Care: A Critical Approach. Boston: Wadsworth

15. Palmer G. 2009. *The Politics of Breastfeeding.* London: Pinter & Martin.

16. Akre J. 2006. *The Problem with Breastfeeding: A Personal Reflection.* Amarillo, Texas: Hale Publishing.

17. Loof-Johanson M, Foldevi M, Edvard Rudebeck C. 2013. Breastfeeding as a Specific Value in Women's Lives: The Experiences and Decisions of Breastfeeding Women. *Breastfeeding Medicine.* 8, 1. p39.

18. Donath SM, Amir LH, ALSPAC Study Team. Relationship between prenatal infant feeding intention and initiation and duration of breastfeeding: a cohort study. *Acta Paediatrica.* 2003. 92:352-356; also see: Forster DA, McLachlan HL, Lumley J. Factors associated with breastfeeding at six months postpartum in a group of Australian women. *International Breastfeeding Journal.* 2006. 1:18.

19. Burns E, Schmied V, Sheehan A et al. A metaethnographic synthesis of women's experience of breastfeeding. *Maternal & Child Nutrition.* 2010. 6:201–219.

20. Hauck Y, Reinbold J. Criteria for successful breastfeeding: Mothers' perceptions. *Australian College of Midwives Incorporated Journal.* 1996. Mar 9(1):21–7.

21. Iyengar S. 2010. *The Art of Choosing.* Twelve.

22. *For an example of this rhetoric, see*: Lemmon.G.T 2012 A Woman's Right to Choose (Not to Breastfeed). The Atlantic. JUL 31 2012. Available at: www.theatlantic.com/health/archive/2012/07/a-womans-right-to-choose-not-to-breastfeed/260530/.

23. NHS Infant Feeding Survey – UK, 2010.

24. *Indeed, one study revealed that even women who don't initiate breastfeeding are as aware of breastfeeding's benefits as their lactating counterparts:* Guttman N, Zimmerman DR. 2000. Low-income mothers' views on breastfeeding. *Social Science & Medicine.* 50: 1457–73.

25. Prochaska JO, Velicer WF. The transtheoretical model of health behavior change. *American Journal of Health Promotion.*1997. Sep-Oct 12(1):38–48.

26. *However, their model can be applied to various health-related domains. It is, for instance, the most commonly used in the health and fitness industry:* Coulson M, Bolitho S. 2012. *The Complete Guide to Pregnancy and Fitness.* London: Bloomsbury.

27. *Stay tuned – we'll explore this balance sheet very soon when we look at maternal*

*attitude.* Janis IL and Mann L. 1977. *Decision Making: a Psychological Analysis of Conflict, Choice and Commitment.* New York: Free Press.

28. Coulson M, Bolitho S. 2012. *The Complete Guide to Pregnancy and Fitness.* London: Bloomsbury.

29. Hoddinott P, Craig LC, Britten J, McInnes RM. A serial qualitative interview study of infant feeding experiences: idealism meets realism. *BMJ Open.* 2012. Mar 14;2(2).

30. *I refuse to use the word 'formula' in this context, lest the irony be lost.*

31. *If you're interested, I arrived at this framework by adapting the work of psychologist Icek Ajzen and his infamous Theory of Planned Behviour:* Ajzen I (1 December, 1991). 'The theory of planned behavior'. *Organizational Behavior and Human Decision Processes.* 50 (2): 179–211. To see its application to the breastfeeding context, read: Cabieses B, Waiblinger D, Santorelli G, McEachan RR. What factors explain pregnant women's feeding intentions in Bradford, England: a multi-methods, multi-ethnic study. *BMC Pregnancy and Childbirth.* 2014. Jan 28;14:50.

32. Andrew N, Harvey K. Infant feeding choices: experience, self-identity and lifestyle. *Maternal & Child Nutrition.* 2011. Jan;7(1):48–60; McCann MF, Baydar N, Williams RL. 2007. Breastfeeding attitudes and reported problems in a national sample of WIC participants. *Journal of Human Lactation.* 23, 314–324; Arafat I, Allen DE, Fox JE. Maternal practice and attitudes toward breastfeeding. *Journal of Obstetric, Gynecologic & Neonatal Nursing.* 1981. Mar-Apr 10(2):91–5; Kukla R. 'Ethics and Ideology in Breastfeeding Advocacy Campaigns'. *Hypatia.* 21.2 2006. 157–18.

33. Hannon PR, Willis SK, Bishop-Townsend V, Martinez IM, Scrimshaw SC. African-American and Latina adolescent mothers' infant feeding decisions and breastfeeding practices: a qualitative study. *Journal of Adolescent Health.* 2000. 26(6):399–407; Nelson AM. Adolescent attitudes, beliefs, and concerns regarding breastfeeding. *The American Journal of Maternal/Child Nursing.* 2009. 34(4):249–255; Wambach KA, Koehn M. Experiences of infant-feeding decision-making among urban economically disadvantaged pregnant adolescents. *Journal of Advanced Nursing.* 2004. 48(4):361–370.

34. Dungy C, Losch M, Russell D. 1994. Maternal attitudes as predictors of infant feeding decisions. *Journal of the Association for Academic Minority Physicians* 5 (4) 159–164; Scott JA, Landers M, Hughes R. 2001. Factors associated with breastfeeding at discharge and duration of breastfeeding amongst two populations of Australian women. *Journal of Paediatric and Child Health.* 37 254–261.

35. Perugini M, Bagozzi RP. 2001. The role of desires and anticipated emotions in goal-directed behaviours: broadening and deepening the theory of planned behaviour. *British Journal of Social Psychology.* 40 79–98.

36. Zajonc RB. Feeling and thinking: Preferences and no inferences. *American Psychologist.* 1980, 35, 151–175.

37. *Psychologist Erving Goffman referred to such behaviour as a 'strategic secret':* Goffman E. 1990. *The Presentation of Self in Everyday Life.* London:

Penguin Books, p141.

38. Forster DA, McLachlan HL, Lumley J. 2006. Factors associated with breastfeeding at six months postpartum in a group of Australian women. *International Breastfeeding Journal*. 1, 18–12; Lonstein JS. 2007. Regulation of anxiety during the postpartum period. *Frontiers in Neuroendocrinology*. 28, 115–141.

39. Clifford T, Campbell M, Speechley K, Gorodzinsky F. 2006. Factors influencing full breastfeeding in a southwestern Ontario community: Assessments at 1 week and at 6 months postpartum. *Journal of Human Lactation*. 22, 292–304; Lonstein JS. 2007. Regulation of anxiety during the postpartum period. *Frontiers in Neuroendocrinology*. 28, 115–141.

40. Belsky J. 1984. The Determinants of Parenting: A Process Model. *Child Development*. 55, 83-96. To find out more about some of the concepts applied to breastfeeding, see: Brown A. Maternal trait personality and breastfeeding duration. *Journal of Advanced Nursing*. 2014. Mar 70(3):587–98.

41. *A finding in a study of more than 400 women:* Scharfe E. 2012. Maternal attachment representations and initiation and duration of breastfeeding. *Journal of Human Lactation*. 28, 218–225. See also: Dix T. 1991. The affective organization of parenting: Adaptive and maladaptive processes. *Psychological Bulletin*. 110, 3–25; Leerkes E. 2010. Predictors of maternal sensitivity to infant distress. *Parenting: Science & Practice*. 10, 219–239.

42. Gratz KL, Roemer L. 2004. Multidimensional assessment of emotion regulation and dysregulation: Development, factor structure, and initial validation of the difficulties in emotion regulation scale. *Journal of Psychopathology and Behavioral Assessment*. 26, 41–54.

43. Dix T, Gershoff ET, Meunier LN, Miller PC. 2004. The affective structure of supportive parenting: depressive symptoms, immediate emotions, and child-oriented motivation. *Developmental Psychology*. 2004. Nov 40(6):1212–27; Mills-Koonce WR, Gariepy JL, Propper C, Sutton K, Calkins S, Moore G, Cox M. 2007. Infant and parent factors associated with early maternal sensitivity: A caregiver-attachment systems approach. *Infant Behavior & Development*. 30, 114–126.

44. Williams F. 2012. *Breasts: a Natural and Unnatural History*. New York: WW Norton and Company, p194. *On women's 'love-hate' relationship with breastfeeding, take a look at:* Forster DA, McLachlan HL. 2010. Women's views and experiences of breast feeding: positive, negative or just good for the baby? *Midwifery*. 26, 16–125; Andrew N, Harvey K. 2011. Infant feeding choices: experience, self-identity and lifestyle. *Maternal & Child Nutrition*. 7, 48–60.

45. Lawrence RA. 2009. Breastfeeding, in Benson JB, Haith MM (eds.). 2009. *Social and Emotional Development in Infancy and Early Childhood*. Academic Press, p59.

46. Leerkes E. 2010. Predictors of maternal sensitivity to infant distress. *Parenting: Science & Practice*. 10, 219–39; Dix T, Gershoff ET, Meunier LN, Miller PC. 2004. The affective structure of supportive parenting: depressive symptoms, immediate emotions, and child-oriented motivation. *Developmental Psychology*. 2004. Nov 40(6):1212–27.

47. Mathews E. 2013. Psychosocial Predictors of Breastfeeding Initiation and Duration. Human Development and Family Studies Thesis. Faculty of The Graduate School at The University of North Carolina at Greensboro; O'Brien ML, Buikstra E, Fallon T, Hegney, D. 2009. Strategies for success: A toolbox of coping strategies used by breastfeeding women. *Journal of Clinical Nursing*. 18, 1574–1582; Leerkes E. 2010. Predictors of maternal sensitivity to infant distress. *Parenting: Science & Practice*. 10, 219–239; Zeifman DM. 2003. Predicting adult responses to infant distress: Adult characteristics associated with perceptions, emotional reactions, and timing of intervention. *Infant Mental Health Journal*. 24, 597–612.

48. Mentro AM, Steward DK, Garvin BJ. 2002. Infant feeding responsiveness: a conceptual analysis. *Journal of Advanced Nursing*. 37, 208–216; Howard CR, Lanphear N, Lanphear BP, Eberly S, Lawrence RA. 2006. Parental responses to infant crying and colic: the effect on breastfeeding duration. *Breastfeeding Medicine*. 1, 146–155.

49. *This three step process is a watered down version of frameworks such as:* Kennerley.M and Mason.S 2008 The Use of Information in Decision Making, Literature Review for the Audit Commission. 15/02/2008

50. Andrew N, Harvey K. Infant feeding choices: experience, self-identity and lifestyle. *Maternal & Child Nutrition*. 2011. Jan 7(1):48-60. *On the topic of child-advice books, a massive 90 percent of US mothers are believed to have read at least one of them:* Ellison K. 2005. *The Mommy Brain*. New York: Basic Books. *When it comes to online research, 72 percent of internet users admit to using Dr Google for that all-important health information, with women being the most likely surfers: Health Online*. 2013. Pew Internet & American Life Project.

51. Payne JW, Bettman JR, Johnson EJ. 1993. *The Adaptive Decision Maker*. New York: Cambridge University Press.

52. Schrah GE, Dalal RS, Sniezek JA. 2006. No decision-maker is an island: integrating expert advice with information acquisition. *Journal of Behavioral Decision Making*. 19, 1, pp43–60.

53. Heath C, Tversky A. 1991. Preference and belief: Ambiguity and competence in choice under uncertainty. *Journal of Risk and Uncertainty*. 4, 5–28. *Of course, ignorance and uncertainty are often confounded, but if they can be teased apart people tend to show an aversion to ignorance rather than uncertainty per se. See:* Tversky A, Fox CR. 1995. Ambiguity aversion and comparative ignorance. *Quarterly Journal of Economics*. 100, 585–603; Tversky A, Fox CR. 1995. Weighing risk and uncertainty. *Psychological Review*. 102, 269–283. *This suggests that high quality antenatal education is of paramount importance in increasing the rate of breastfeeding.*

54. Mills J. 1965 The effect of certainty on exposure to information prior to commitment. *Journal of Experimental Social Psychology*. 1, 348–355.

55. Klayman J, Ha YW. 1987. Confirmation, disconfirmation, an information in hypothesis testing. *Psychological Review*. 94, 211–228; Wason PC. 1960. On the failure to eliminate hypothesis in a conceptual task. *Quarterly Journal of Experimental Psychology*. 12, 129–140; Mills J, Ross A. 1964. Effects of commitment and certainty in interest in supporting information.

*Journal of Abnormal and Social Psychology.* 68, 552–555.

56. Maslow AH. 1968. *Toward a Psychology of Being* (2nd edition). New York: Van Nostrad. p66.

57. Tracer DP. 2009. Breastfeeding structure as a test of parental investment theory in Papua New Guinea. *American Journal of Human Biology.* 21, 635–642; Lavender T, McFadden C, Baker L. 2006. Breastfeeding and family life. *Maternal & Child Nutrition.* 2, 145–155; Bentley G. 2007. Environmental effects on human reproduction. In: *Evolution and Medicine: How New Applications Advance Research and Practice* (Nesse R, ed.), London: Henry Stewart Talks Limited, The Biomedical & Life Sciences Collection. O'Campo P, Faden RR, Gielen AC, Wang MC. 1992. Prenatal factors associated with breastfeeding duration: Recommendations for prenatal intervention. *Birth.* 19(4), 195–201). *This study looked at women's beliefs about the consequences to themselves and their babies of breastfeeding and formula feeding and identified these as the most significant predictor of breastfeeding duration.*

58. *I say 'tenuous' because individuals tend to go about their daily lives in a practical, unreflective fashion. See:* Williams SJ. Theorising class, health and lifestyles: can Bourdieu help us? *Sociology of Health and Illness.* 1995. 17(5):577–604.

59. Blackburn ST. 2007. *Maternal, Fetal, and Neonatal Physiology: A Clinical Perspective* (3rd edition). St Louis: Saunders Elsevier.

60. Kinsella K, Williams K. Feeding Your Baby. NHS Foundation Trust. Available at: www.thh.nhs.uk/documents/_Patients/PatientLeaflets/breastfeeding/Feeding_Your_Baby_Folder.pdf Accessed January 24

61. Pearson RM, Lightman SL, Evans J. 2011. The impact of breastfeeding on mothers' attentional sensitivity towards infant distress. *Infant Behavior & Development.* 34, 200–205.

62. Tikotzky L, De Marcas G, Har-Toov J, Dollberg S, Bar-Haim Y, Sadeh A. 2010. Sleep and physical growth in infants during the first 6 months. *Journal of Sleep Research.* 19, 103–111.

63. Sadeh A, Mindell J, Rivera L. 2011. 'My child has a sleep problem': a cross-cultural comparison of parental definitions. *Sleep Medicine.*12, 478–482.

64. *To take a monetary example: the displeasure people feel when losing £100 is larger than the pleasure they feel from gaining £100. See*: Kahneman D, Tversky A. 1979. 'Prospect Theory: An Analysis of Decision under Risk', *Econometrica.* XLVII 1979, 263–291. *Think of the value mothers assign to the profits and costs of breastfeeding as a concave for profits and convex for losses, and as generally steeper for costs than it is for profits.*

65. *A new mother's psyche is vulnerable. She doesn't yet know what she's doing and doesn't yet have a fully developed maternal instinct (but has a nagging suspicion that she's supposed to). This vulnerability means that she is more susceptible to manipulation by people she perceives to have the coveted 'know-how'. Knowing this, formula company SMA ran a campaign aimed at mothers with the slogan 'We know', and one for health professionals with the slogan 'SMA know-how'. Such marketing techniques exploit personal fears about ignorance by downplaying the risks of formula whilst emphasising how formula use protects certain established values. In the aforementioned 'We know' campaign, a*

*common image was that of the father lovingly administering a bottle to his baby so that mother can enjoy her bodily autonomy and perceived marital equality. See*: Earle S. 2000. 'Why Some Women do not Breast Feed: Bottle Feeding and Fathers' Role.' *Midwifery*. 16(4): 323–30; Bailey C, Pain RH, Aarvold JE. A 'give it a go' breast-feeding culture and early cessation among low-income mothers. *Midwifery*. 2004. Sep 20(3):240–50; Schmidt J. 2008. 'Gendering in Infant Feeding Discourses: The Good Mother and the Absent Father'. *New Zealand Sociology*. 23(2): 61–74). *Of course, mothers aren't sponges, passively soaking up every marketing message. However, they consciously suspend disbelief because they want to – need to – believe what the formula company is claiming. Sociologist Colin Campbell describes such modern consumers as a self-deceiving 'dream artists', with 'the ability to create an illusion which is known to be false but felt to be true'.* (Campbell C. 1987. *The Romantic Ethic and the Spirit of Modern Consumerism*. Oxford: Basil-Blackwell. p78).

66. Kahneman D, Tversky A. 1979. Prospect Theory: An analysis of decision under risk. *Econometrica*. 47, 263–291.

67. Thaler RH, Sunstein CR. 2009. *Nudge: Improving Decisions about Health, Wealth and Happiness*. London: Penguin Books. p93.

68. 'To dodge the terrible feeling in the pits of our stomachs, we tend to act conservatively, so as not to deviate from the crowd too much'. Dobelli R. 2013. *The Art of Thinking Clearly*. London: Hodder and Stoughton. p251.

69. Salehnejad R. 2007. *Rationality, Bounded Rationality and Microfoundations: Foundations of Theoretical Economics*. New York: Palgrave MacMillan; Sloman J, Wride A. 2009. *Economics* (7th edition). Harlow: Pearson Education Limited.

70. *In this sense, breastfeeding is an 'investment': the costs are borne immediately, but the benefits are delayed. Whereas the mother gets relief from formula now and suffers the consequences later. The 'risks' associated with formula use are plentiful and well-publicised, however 'risk' by its very nature is temporal rather than immediate.*

71. Reiches MW, Ellison PT, Lipson SF, Sharrock KC, Gardiner E, Duncan LG. 2009. Pooled energy budget and human life history. *American Journal of Human Biology*. 21, 421–429p. 442.

72. Darwin C. 1871. *The Descent of Man and Selection in Relation to Sex*. New York: Appleton; Trivers RL. 1974. Parent-offspring conflict. *American Zoologist*.14, 249–264; Haig D. 1993. Genetic conflicts in human pregnancy. *Quarterly Review of Biology*. 68, 495–532; Vitzthum VJ. 2008. Evolutionary models of women's reproductive functioning. *Annual Review of Anthropology*. 37, 53–73.

73. *On choosing formula to enable a more equitable distribution of maternal time amongst offspring, see:* Andrew N, Harvey K. Infant feeding choices: experience, self-identity and lifestyle. *Maternal & Child Nutrition*. 2011. Jan 7(1):48–60.

74. Law J. The Politics of Breastfeeding: Assessing Risk, Diving Labor. Signs: *Journal of Women in Culture and Society*. 25, no.2 (2000): 407–50.

75. Tully KP, Ball HL. 2013. Trade-offs underlying maternal breastfeeding decisions: a conceptual model. *Maternal and Child Nutrition*. 9, pp90–98.

75b. *Dr Tully and Professor Ball argue that that this tipping point is different for every mum and baby (even consecutive babies for the same mum) because it can be influenced by many intrinsic and extrinsic factors that affect the costs and benefits and the mother's perception of these.*

76. *According to a survey of more than 7,000 mothers, only 1 in 10 reported 'problem-free' breastfeeding. That means 90 percent of breastfeeding mums have to overcome some sort of hurdle in order to continue breastfeeding* (Hoffman J. 2006. Today's Parent: *Nursing Confidential*).

77. Williams F. 2012. *Breasts: a Natural and Unnatural History*. New York: WW Norton and Company. p4.

78. Wall G. 2001. Moral constructions of motherhood in breastfeeding discourse. *Gender & Society*. 15(4): 590–608. p598.

79. ob cit, p598. *On breastfeeding 'tying mothers down' see also:* Zimmerman D R, 'Breast Is Best': Knowledge Among Low-Income Mothers Is Not Enough. *Journal of Human Lactation*. 2001. Feb Vol.17 no. 1 14–19.

80. *To see this tension played out in rant form, see:* Filipovic.J 2013 The choice to be child-free is admirable, not selfish. *The Guardian*. Friday 16 August 2013. Available at: www.theguardian.com/commentisfree/2013/aug/16/choice-child-free-admirable-not-selfish

81. *Google "Feeling suffocated" and "breastfeeding" and up pops the forum-laden rants of innumerous mums. For example:* Feeling suffocated- He won't take a bottle! (Babycentre) community.babycentre.co.uk/post/a17000945/feeling_suffocated-_he_wont_take_a_bottle

82. *For example,* Lee EJ. 2007. Infant feeding in risk society. *Health, Risk & Society*. 9:3, 295–309.

83. Andrew N, Harvey K. Infant feeding choices: experience, self-identity and lifestyle. *Maternal & Child Nutrition*. 2011. Jan 7(1):48–60, p56.

84. *There's a study to back this up, not that we needed a study to point out the bleedin' obvious:* Riordan CA. 1982. Intent, consequences, and locus of control: Some more efforts on judgements following harmdoing. Unpublished manuscript, University of Misouri-Rolla. See also: Rotenberg K. 1980. Children's use of intentionality in judgements of character and disposition. *Child Development*. 51, 282–284.

85. *This is a common reason why people make unsatisfactory decisions; they tend to regard their current preferences as much more stable and intrinsic than they actually are. See:* Loewenstein G, Angner E. 2003. Predicting and indulging changing preferences. In Loewenstein G, Read D, Baumeister R (eds.) *Time and Decision: Economic and Psychological Perspectives on Intertemporal Choice*. New York: Russell Sage Foundation. pp351–391.

86. Hoddinott P, Pill R. 1999. Qualitative study of decisions about infant feeding among women in East End of London. *British Medical Journal*. 318, 30–34.

87. *A type of self-imposed brain freeze called 'Motivated Selectivity'.*

88. Bäckström CA, Hertfelt Wahn EI, Ekström AC. Two sides of breastfeeding support: experiences of women and midwives. *International Breastfeeding Journal*. 2010. 5:20.

89. Zwedberg S, Naeslund L. 2011. Different attitudes during breastfeeding consultations when infant formula was given: a phenomenographic

approach. *International Breastfeeding Journal*. 2011. 6:1.

90. Bäckström CA, Hertfelt Wahn EI, Ekström AC. Two sides of breastfeeding support: experiences of women and midwives. *International Breastfeeding Journal*. 2010, 5:20.

91. González C. 2014. *Breastfeeding Made Easy*. London: Pinter & Martin.

92. Andrew N, Harvey K. Infant feeding choices: experience, self-identity and lifestyle. *Maternal & Child Nutrition*. 2011. Jan 7(1):48–60.

93. Nakamura M. Factors promoting breast feeding and nursing support [Article in Japanese]. *Ryukyu Medical Journal*. 2002. 21(2):9–17. See also: Nommsen-Rivers LA, Cohen RJ, Chantry CJ, Dewey KG. (2010b). The Infant Feeding Intentions scale demonstrates construct validity and comparability in quantifying maternal breastfeeding intentions across multiple ethnic groups. *Maternal & Child Nutrition*. 6, 220–227; Alexander A, Dowling D, Furman L. 2010. What do pregnant low-income women say about breastfeeding? *Breastfeeding Medicine*. 5, 17–23; MacGregor E, Hughes M. 2010. Breastfeeding experiences of mothers from disadvantaged groups: a review. *Community Practitioner*. 83, 30–33; Nommsen-Rivers LA, Chantry CJ, Cohen RJ, Dewey KG. (2010a). Comfort with the idea of formula feeding helps explain ethnic disparity in breastfeeding intentions among expectant first-time mothers. *Breastfeeding Medicine*. 5, 25–33; Bai Y, Middlestadt SE, Peng C-YJ, Fly AD. 2010. Predictors of continuation of exclusive breastfeeding for the first six months of life. *Journal of Human Lactation*. 26, 26–34; Swanson V, Power KG. Initiation and continuation of breastfeeding: theory of planned behaviour. *Journal of Advanced Nursing*. 2005. 50(3):272–282; Dennis CL. Breastfeeding initiation and duration: a 1990–2000 literature review. *Journal of Obstetric, Gynecologic & Neonatal Nursing*. 2002. 31(1):12–32; Rempel LA. Factors influencing the breastfeeding decisions of long-term breastfeeders. *Journal of Human Lactation*. 2004. 20(3):306–318; Lawson K, Tullock MI, Breastfeeding duration: prenatal intention and postnatal practices. *Journal of Advanced Nursing*. 1995. 22:841–849.

94. O'Campo, P, Faden RR, Gielen A C, Wang MC. 1992. Prenatal factors associated with breastfeeding duration: Recommendations for prenatal intervention. *Birth*. 19(4), 195–201.

95. Avery A, Zimmermann K, Underwood PW, Magnus JH. Confident commitment is a key factor for sustained breastfeeding. *Birth*. 2009. Jun 36(2):141–8.

96. Bottorff JL. Persistence in breastfeeding: a phenomenological investigation. *Journal of Advanced Nursing*, 1990. 15, 201–209. p203.

97. Mandel B. 1984. *Open Heart Therapy*. Berkley CA: Celestial Arts.

98. *The 'I'll try' noncommittal defence is common in other realms too:* Cialdini RB, Levy A, Herman CP, Evenbeck S. Attitudinal politics: The strategy of moderation. *Journal of Personality and Social Psychology*. 1973, 25, 100–108; Cialdini RB, Levy A, Herman CP, Kozlowski LT, Petty RE. Elastic shifts of opinion: Determinants of direction and durability. *Journal of Personality*. 1976, 34, 663-672; Hass RG, Mann EW. Anticipatory belief change: Persuasion or impression management? *Journal of Personality and Social Psychology*. 1976, 34, 105–111.

99. Murphy E. 2004. 'Anticipatory Accounts'. *Symbolic Interaction* 27(2): 129–154. pp24–25.

100. Ob cit.

101. *In contrast with just 25 percent of women who gave no anticipatory excuses.*

102. *A proven theory in motivational research, the origins of which are from:* Wright Mills C. 'Situated Actions and Vocabularies of Motive'. *American Sociological Review*, V (Dec):904–9 13, 1940.

103. Murphy E. 2004. 'Anticipatory Accounts'. *Symbolic Interaction* 27(2): 129–154. pp31–32.

104. Burger JM, Arkin RM. 1980. The role of prediction and control in learned helplessness. *Journal of Personality and Social Psychology.* 38, 482–91.

105. Dennis C-L. 1999. Theoretical underpinnings of breastfeeding confidence; a self-efficacy framework. *Journal of Human Lactation.* 15, 195–201; Dennis C-L, Faux S. 1999. Development and psychometric testing of the breastfeeding self-efficacy scale. *Research in Nursing and Health.* 22 399–409; Parkinson J et al. 2010. The Role of Mother-centred Factors Influencing the Complex Social Behaviour of Breastfeeding. ANZMAC Annual Conference 2010.

106. *Maternal confidence or breastfeeding self-efficacy has been shown to be positively associated with breastfeeding duration:* Dennis C-L, Faux S. 1999. Development and psychometric testing of the breastfeeding self-efficacy scale. *Research in Nursing and Health.* 22 399–409; Dick MJ, Evans ML, Arthurs JB, Barnes JK et al. 2002. Predicting early breastfeeding attrition. *Journal of Human Lactation.* 18 (1) 21–28; Martens PJ, Young TK. 1997. Determinants of breastfeeding in four Canadian Ojibwa communities: A decision-making model. *American Journal of Human Biology.* 9 (5) 579–593; Wambuch K. 1997. Breastfeeding Intention and Outcome: a test of the theory of planned behaviour. *Research in Nursing and Health.* 20 51–59.

107. *On the power and predictive nature of perceived self-efficiency, see:* Bandura A. 1997. *Self-Efficacy: The Exercise of Control.* New York: Freeman.

108. Heckhausen H. 1968. *The Anatomy of Achievement Motivation.* New York: Academic Press.

109. Haslam C, Lawrencea W, Haefeli K. 2003. Intention to breastfeed and other important health-related behaviour and beliefs during pregnancy. *Family Practice.* Vol. 20, No. 5.

110. Kelley DJ, Brush CG, Greene PG, Litovsky Y. 2013. *Global Entrepreneurship Monitor* (GEM). 2012. *Women's Report*, Global Entrepreneurship Research Association (GERA).

111. *Fear of failure has been proven to more frequently affect people who are relatively uncertain of their ability.* See: Conelley ES, Gerard HB, Kline T. 1978 Competitive behaviour: A manifestation of motivation for ability comparison. *Journal of Experimental Social Psychology.* 14, 123–131; Westin AF. 1970. *Privacy and Freedom.* New York: Atheneum. *This may in part explain why mothers who fail at breastfeeding their first child are less likely to even attempt to breastfeed their second or subsequent babies (UK National Infant Feeding Survey 2010, NHS).*

112. Wiessinger D, West D, Pitman T. 2010. *The Womanly Art of Breastfeeding*; London: Pinter & Martin.

113. *We're all a leeeedle bit egotistical, see:* Schlenker BR. 1980. *Impression Management: The Self-concept, Social Identity, and Interpersonal Relations.* Monterey, CA: Brooks/Cole.
114. James W. 1890. *Principles of Psychology.* Dover Publications.
115. Camus A. 1956. *The Fall.* New York: Vintage Books; Fingarette H. 1967. *Self-deception.* London: Routledge & Kegan Paul; Sartre JP. 1958. *Being and Nothingness: An Essay on Phenomenological Ontology* (translated H Barnes) London: Methuen.
116. Cooke K. 2009. *A Rough Guide to Babies and Toddlers.* Rough Guides. p73.
117. Smith E. 2012. *Luck: What It Means and Why It Matters.* London: Bloomsbury.
118. *If you wish to explore the socioeconomic arguments for breastfeeding failure, the bookstores are littered with offerings. May I recommend:* Palmer G. 2009. *The Politics of Breastfeeding.* London: Pinter & Martin; Baumslag N. 1995. *Milk, Money and Madness: The Culture and Politics of Breastfeeding.* Bergin & Garvey.
119. *To read assorted whinges on this tangent, see:* Wolf JB. 2010. *Is Breast Best?: Taking on the Breastfeeding Experts and the New High Stakes of Motherhood.* New York: NYU Press; Lee EJ. 2008. Living with risk in the age of 'intensive motherhood': Maternal identity and infant feeding. *Health Risk & Society.* 10 (5). pp467–477. ISSN 1369–8575; Barston S. 2012. *Bottled Up: How the Way We Feed Babies Has Come to Define Motherhood, and Why it Shouldn't.* CA: University of California Press.
120. *As one researcher of breastfeeding behaviour has noted, 'Social support has a significant indirect relationship with intentions, while subjective norms did not. This finding is interesting considering they both refer to social contact'.* Parkinson J et al. 2010. The Role of Mother-centred Factors Influencing the Complex Social Behaviour of Breastfeeding: Social Support and Self-efficacy. ANZMAC Annual Conference 2010.
121. *Really, someone actually commissioned a study to unearth this information.* See: Isabella PH, Isabella RA. 1994. Correlates of successful breastfeeding: a study of social and personal factors. *Journal of Human Lactation.* 10, 257–64.
122. Grassley J. and Eschiti V. 2008 Grandmother breastfeeding support: what do mothers need and want? *Birth.* Volume 35, Issue 4, pages 329–335, December 2008; Lavender T., McFadden C., Baker L. 2006 Breastfeeding and family life. *Maternal & Child Nutrition,* Volume 2, Issue 3, pages 145–155, July 2006; Cronin C. 2003 First-time mothers – identifying their needs, perceptions and experiences. *Journal of Clinical Nursing,* Volume 12, Issue 2, pages 260–267, March 2003.
123. Andrew N, Harvey K. Infant feeding choices: experience, self-identity and lifestyle. *Maternal & Child Nutrition.* 2011. Jan 7(1):48–60.
124. Bottorff JL. Persistence in breastfeeding: a phenomenological investigation. *Journal of Advanced Nursing.* 1990. 15, 201–209. p206.
125. *On the issue of the contagious nature of pessimism and optimism, see:* Hogg MA et al. 2007. Uncertainty, Entitativity, and Group Identification. *Journal of Experimental Social Psychology.* Vol. 43, No1: 135–142.
126. Tucker CM., Wilson EK., Samandari G. Infant feeding experiences

among teen mothers in North Carolina: Findings from a mixed-methods study. *International Breastfeeding Journal*. 2011. Sep 28;6:14.

127. *This is the way our brains are wired, a cognitive quirk known as the Availability Bias*: Schwarz N, Vaugn LA. 2002. The availability heuristic revisited: Ease of recall and content of recall as distinct sources of information. In Gilovich T, Griffin D, Kahneman D (eds.) 2002. *Heuristics and Biases*. Cambridge: Cambridge University Press. pp103–119.

128. *Qualitative interviews report that the Breast is Best message is reaching all mothers; the snag is that mothers are considering the message in light of their own experiences and those of their friends and family members, rather than considering it as fact. See:* Andrew N, Harvey K. Infant feeding choices: experience, self-identity and lifestyle. *Maternal & Child Nutrition*. 2011. Jan 7(1):48–60, and also see: Hoddinott P, Pill R. 1999. Qualitative study of decisions about infant feeding among women in east end of London. *British Medical Journal*. 318, 30–34.

129. Andrew N, Harvey K. 2011. Infant feeding choices: experience, self-identity and lifestyle. *Maternal & Child Nutrition*.7(1):48–60.

130. Fagerli RA, Wandel M. Gender differences in opinions and practices with regard to a 'healthy diet. *Appetite*. 1999. 32(2):171–190.

131. Thaler RH, Sunstein CR. 2009. *Nudge: Improving Decisions About Health, Wealth and Happiness*. London: Penguin Books.

132. Stern DN. 1998. *The Birth of a Mother: How Motherhood Experience Changes You Forever*. Basic Books.

133. Hughes T. April 15 2013. How having a baby boosts social life of new mothers. Available at: www.express.co.uk/news/uk/392003/How-having-a-baby-boosts-social-life-of-new-mothers Accessed May 14, 2013.

134. Infant Feeding Survey 2010: Early Results. The Information Centre, Government Statistical Service. 2011.

135. op cit.

136. Asch SE. 1951. Effects of group pressure on the modification and distortion of judgments. In Guetzkow H (ed.) *Groups, Leadership and Men* (pp177–190). Pittsburgh, PA: Carnegie Press; Asch SE. 1955. Opinions and social pressure. *Scientific American* 193, 35–35.

137. Kraft P, Rise J, Sutton S, Roysamb E. 2005. Perceived difficulty in the theory of planned behaviour: Perceived behavioural control or affective attitude. *British Journal of Social Psychology*. 44, 479–496.

138. Bandura A. 2004. Health promotion by social cognitive means. *Health Education & Behavior*. 2004. Apr 31(2):143–64. p144.

139. Ystrom E, Niegel S, Klepp KI, Vollrath ME. The impact of maternal negative affectivity and general self-efficacy on breastfeeding: the Norwegian Mother and Child Cohort Study. *Journal of Pediatrics*. 2008. Jan 152(1):68–72.

140. *Stress reduces perceptions of self-efficiency*: Budden JS, Sagarin B. 2008. Implementation intentions, occupational stress, and the exercise intention-behavior relationship. *Journal of Occupational Health Psychology*. 12, 391–401.

141. Andrew N, Harvey K. Infant feeding choices: experience, self-identity

and lifestyle. *Maternal & Child Nutrition*. 2011. Jan 7(1):48–60.

142. *Psychologists recognise our innate tendency to value certainty over mere probability and call it, funnily enough, the 'certainty effect'.*

143. Armitage C J, Conner M. 2001. Efficacy of the theory of planned behaviour: A meta-analytic review. *British Journal of Social Psychology.* 40, 471–499.

144. Indeed, mothers who feel that the process of breastfeeding is out of their control, may actually be predisposed to Postnatal Depression (Abramson LY, Seligman MEP, Teasdale JD. 1978. Learned helplessness in humans: Critique and reformation. *Journal of Abnormal Psychology.* 87, 49–74; Robins CJ. 1988. Attributions and depression: Why is the literature so inconsistent? *Journal of Personality and Social Psychology.* 54, 880–9; Sweeney PD, Anderson K, Bailey S. 1986. Attributional style in depression: A meta-analytic review. *Journal of Personality and Social Psychology.* 50, 974–91; Seligman MEP. 1975. *Helplessness: On Depression, Development and Death.* San Francisco: Freeman.

145. Dweck CS, Leggett EL. 1988. A social-cognitive approach to motivation and personality, *Psychological Review.* 95, 256–273; Dweck CS, Hong Y, Chiu C. 1993. Implicit theories: Individual differences in the likelihood and meaning of dispositional inferences. *Personality and Social Psychology Bulletin.* 19, 644–656.

146. Brewin CR. 1985. Depression and causal attributions: What is their relation? *Psychological Bulletin.* 98, 297–309.

147. Smith PH, Coley SL, Labbok MH, Cupito S, Nwokah E. Early breastfeeding experiences of adolescent mothers: a qualitative prospective study. *International Breastfeeding Journal.* 2012. Sep 29 7(1):13.

148. *For in-depth discussions of this, see*: Schmied V, Lupton D. 2001. Blurring the boundaries: breastfeeding and maternal subjectivity. *Sociology of Health and Illness.* 23, 234–250; Marshall JL, Godfrey M, Renfrew MJ. 2007. Being a 'good mother': Managing breastfeeding and merging identities. *Social Science & Medicine.* 65(10), 2147–2159.

149. Smith PH, Coley SL, Labbok MH, Cupito S, Nwokah E. Early breastfeeding experiences of adolescent mothers: a qualitative prospective study. *International Breastfeeding Journal.* 2012. Sep 29 7(1):13.

150. Otsuka K, Dennis CL, Tatsuoka H, Jimba M. The relationship between breastfeeding self-efficacy and perceived insufficient milk among Japanese mothers. *Journal of Obstetric, Gynecologic & Neonatal Nursing.* 2008. 37(5):546–555.

151. Barnes J, Stein A, Smith T, Pollock JI. Extreme attitudes to body shape, social and psychological factors and a reluctance to breast feed. ALSPAC Study Team. Avon Longitudinal Study of Pregnancy and Childhood. *Journal of the Royal Society of Medicine.* Oct 1997. 90(10): 551–559; Blum L. 1999. *At The Breast.* Boston: Beacon Press; Foster SF et al. 1996. Body image, maternal-fetal attachment, and breast-feeding. *Journal of Psychosomatic Research.* 41, no. 2: 181–84.

152. *Particularly for those women who identify themselves with roles they see as more important than motherhood*: Andrew N, Harvey K. Infant feeding choices: experience, self-identity and lifestyle. *Maternal & Child Nutrition.* 2011.

Jan 7(1):48–60; Lee E. 2007b. 'Infant Feeding in Risk Society.' *Health, Risk and Societ*. 9(3): 295–309.

153. Andrew N, Harvey K. Infant feeding choices: experience, self-identity and lifestyle. *Maternal & Child Nutrition*. 2011. Jan 7(1):48–60, p55.

154. *A popular technique whereby parents 'train' their babies to sleep by leaving them to cry for progressively longer periods of time. See*: Ferber R. 1986. *Solve Your Child's Sleep Problems*. Prentice Hall & IBD.

155. DiGirolamo AM, Grummer-Strawn LM, Fein SB. 2008. Effect of maternity-care practices on breastfeeding. *Pediatrics*. 2008. Oct 122 Suppl 2:S43-9; Merten S, Dratva J, Ackermann-Liebrich U. 2005. Do baby-friendly hospitals influence breastfeeding duration on a national level? *Pediatrics*. 116, 702–8.

156. McFadden A, Toole G. 2006. Exploring women's views of breastfeeding: a focus group study within an area with high levels of socio-economic deprivation. *Maternal and Child Nutrition*. 2, 156–168; Stewart-Knox B, Gardiner K, Wright M. What is the problem with breast-feeding? A qualitative analysis of infant feeding perceptions. *Journal of Human Nutrition and Dietetics*. 2003. Aug 16(4):265–73.

157. Andrew N, Harvey K. Infant feeding choices: experience, self-identity and lifestyle. *Maternal & Child Nutrition*. 2011. Jan 7(1):48–60.

158. Lee EJ. 2007. Infant feeding in risk society. *Health, Risk & Society*. 9:3, 295–309, p295.

159. Lee E. Health, morality, and infant feeding: British mothers' experiences of formula milk use in the early weeks. *Sociology of Health and Illness*. 2007. 29(7):1–16. p12.

160. Earle S. 2002. 'Factors Affecting the Initiation of Breastfeeding: Implications for Breastfeeding Promotion.' *Health Promotion International* 17(3): 205–21; Lee E. 2007. 'Infant Feeding in Risk Society.' *Health, Risk and Society* 9(3): 295–309.

161. NHS 'Making up infant formula'. Available at: www.nhs.uk/ Conditions/pregnancy-and-baby/pages/making-up-infant-formula. aspx#close Accessed April 4, 2014.

162. Lee EJ. 2007. Infant feeding in risk society. *Health, Risk & Society*. 9:3, 295–309, p301.

163. *Fact: pain, discomfort and tiredness, along with subsequent comfort with formula feeding, are among the most common 'reasons' mothers give for turning to formula. See*: Smith PH, Coley SL, Labbok MH, Cupito S, Nwokah E. Early breastfeeding experiences of adolescent mothers: a qualitative prospective study. *International Breastfeeding Journal*. 2012. Sep 29;7(1):13; Nommsen-Rivers LA, Chantry CJ, Cohen RJ, Dewey KG: Comfort with the idea of formula feeding helps explain ethnic disparity in breastfeeding intentions among expectant first-time mothers. *Breastfeeding Medicine*. 2010. Feb 5(1):25–33; Groleau D, Rodriguez C: Breastfeeding and poverty: negotiating cultural change and symbolic capital in Quebec, Canada. In 2009 Dykes F, Moran VH (eds.) *Infant and Young Child Feeding: Challenges to Implementing a Global Strategy*. Oxford: Blackwell Publishing; pp80–98; Bailey C, R Pain. 2001. 'Geographies of Infant Feeding and Access to Primary Health-Care'. *Health and Social*

*Care in the Community*. 9(5): 309–17; Lee E. 2007. 'Health, Morality, and Infant Feeding: British Mother's Experiences of Formula Milk Use in the Early Weeks'. *Sociology of Health and Illness*. 29(7): 1075–90; Lee E. 2007b. 'Infant Feeding in Risk Society'. *Health, Risk and Society*. 9(3): 295–309; Miller T, S Bonas, M. Dixon-Woods. 2007. 'Qualitative Research on Breastfeeding in the UK: A Narrative Review and Methodological Reaction'. *Evidence and Policy* 3(2): 197–230; Murphy E. 1999. 'Breast is Best': Infant Feeding Decisions and Maternal Deviance. *Sociology of Health and Illness*. 21(2): 187–208; Schmeid V, Deborah L. 2001. 'Blurring the Boundaries: Breastfeeding and Maternal Subjectivity'. *Sociology of Health and Illness*. 23(2): 234–50; Stapleton H, Fielder A, Kirkham M. 2008. 'Breast or Bottle? Eating Disordered Childbearing Women and Infant-Feeding Decisions'. *Maternal and Child Nutrition*. 4(2): 106–20.

164. Loewenstein G. Out of Control: Visceral Influences on Behaviour. *Organizational Behaviour and Human Decision Processes*. 65(3) March pp272–292, 1996.

165. Freud S. 1949. *The Ego and the Id*. London: The Hogarth Press Ltd.

166. Lee EJ. 2007. Infant feeding in risk society. *Health, Risk & Society*. 9:3, 295–309.

167. Loewenstein G. Out of Control: Visceral Influences on Behaviour. *Organizational Behaviour and Human Decision Processes*. 65(3) March pp272–292, 1996. *We will be more thoroughly exploring our Guilt, Excuses and Contempt in future chapters.*

168. Loewenstein G. Out of Control: Visceral Influences on Behaviour. *Organizational Behaviour and Human Decision Processes*. 65(3) March pp272–292, 1996, pp272–273.

169. Thaler RH, Sunstein CR. 2009. *Nudge: Improving Decisions About Health, Wealth and Happiness*. London: Penguin Books. p44.

170. *One study noted: 'Formula manufacturers focus on mothers' feelings and intuition rather than knowledge in making decisions'.* Hausman BL. Women's liberation and the rhetoric of 'choice' in infant feeding debates. *International Breastfeeding Journal*. 2008, 3:10.

171. *This emergence is not a sudden phenomenon but rather a gradual emergence by slow degrees. To learn more about how we prioritise our needs, see*: Maslow A. 1954. *Motivation and Personality*. New York: Harper; and also: Wahba MA, Bridwell LG. 1976. Maslow reconsidered: A review of research on the need hierarchy theory. *Organizational Behavior and Human Performance*. 15(2), 212–240.

172. *The drying-up process normally takes around seven to ten days.*

173. 166 Pettit P. 1991. Decision theory and folk psychology. In Bacharach M, Hurley S (eds.) *Foundations of Decision Theory*. Oxford: Blackwell.

174. Nisbett RE, Wilson DD. 1977. Telling more than we can know: Verbal reports on mental processes. *Psychological Review*. 84, 231–59; Ross M. 1989. Relation of impact theories to the construction of personal histories. *Psychological Review*. 96, 341–57.

175. Rottenstreich Y, Hsee CK. 2001. Money, kisses and electric shocks: On the affective psychology of risk. *Psychological Science*. 12, 185–190.

176. *If this statement amuses you, open up Mr Google and type "if formula was so*

*bad". Popcorn optional.*

177. Newell BR, Mitchell CJ, Hayes BK. 2005. Imagining low probability events: Contrasting exemplar cuing and frequency format accounts. In B Bara, L Barsalou, M Bucciarelli (eds.) *Proceedings of the 27ʰ Annual Conference of the Cognitive Science Society.* Mahwah NJ: Lawrence Earlbaum Associates Inc. pp1630–1635.

178. Awano M, Shimada K. Development and evaluation of a self-care program on breastfeeding in Japan: a quasi-experimental study. *International Breastfeeding Journal.* 2010. 5:9.

179. Seligman MEP. 1975. *Helplessness: On Depression, Development and Death.* San Fransisco: Freeman.

180. *In fact, much of the research in this area suggests that, even having an inaccurate perception of control over an impending task markedly reduces the averseness of that task*: Bowers K. Pain, anxiety and perceived control. *Journal of Consulting and Clinical Psychology.* 1968 32, 596–602; Glass D C, Singer JE. 1972. *Urban Stress: Experiments on Noise and Social Stressors.* New York: Academic; Kanfer FH, Seidner ML. Self-control: Factors enhancing tolerance of noxious stimulation. *Journal of Personality and Social Psychology.* 1973, 25, 381–389.

181. Lazarus RS, Alfert E. Short-circuiting of threat by experimentally altering cognitive appraisal. *Journal of Abnormal and Social Psychology.* 1964, 69, 195–205; Janis IL. 1958. *Psychological stress: Psychoanalytic and Behavioural Studies of Surgical Patients.* New York: John Wiley; Janis IL. 1971. *Stress and Frustration.* New York: Harcourt Brace Jovanovich. *Interestingly, the psychological and physiological consequences of control bear remarkable similarity. Lab experiments reveal that the galvanic skin response an individual experiences when stressed increases when she feels unable to predict or control a situation* (Staub E, Killet DS. Increasing pain tolerance by information about aversive stimuli. *Journal of Personality and Social Psychology.* 1972, 21, 198–203).

182. Kanfer FH, Goldfoot DA. Self-control and tolerance of noxious stimulation. *Psychological Reports.* 1966, 18, 79–85.

*183. Framework taken from*: Averill J. 1973 Personal control over adverse stimuli and its relationship to stress. *Psychological Bulletin.* 1973, 80, 286–303.

184. *See The Triumphant Tuesday Project for an archive of positive breastfeeding stories. Available at:* www.thealphaparent.com/search/label/Triumphant%20Tuesdays

185. Otsuka K, Dennis CL, Tatsuoka H, Jimba M: The relationship between breastfeeding self-efficacy and perceived insufficient milk among Japanese mothers. *Journal of Obstetric, Gynecologic & Neonatal Nursing.* 2008. 37(5):546–555.

186. Langer E. 1983. *The Psychology of Control.* Beverly Hills, CA: Sage Publications. p19.

187. Marshall, J. 2011. Motherhood, breastfeeding and identity. *Practising Midwife.* 14 (2). pp16–18. ISSN 1461–3123.

188. Orfali K, Gordon E. 2004. Autonomy gone awry: A cross-cultural study of parents' experiences in neonatal intensive care units. *Theoretical Medicine and Bioethics.* 2004. 25(4):329–65.

189. Ditto PH, Pizarro DA, Epstein EB, Jacobson JA, MacDonald TK. 2006. Visceral influences on risk-taking behaviour. *Journal of Behavioral Decision Making*. 19, 2, 99–113.

190. Walter M, Ebbesen EB, Raskoff Zeiss A. 1972. 'Cognitive and attentional mechanisms in delay of gratification'. *Journal of Personality and Social Psychology*. 21 (2): 204–218.

191. Thompson T and Richardson A. 2001 Self-handicapping status, claimed self-handicaps and reduced practice effort following success and failure feedback. *British Journal of Educational Psychology*. 2001 Mar;71(Pt 1):151-70

192. Andrew N, Harvey K. Infant feeding choices: experience, self-identity and lifestyle. *Maternal & Child Nutrition*. 2011. Jan 7(1):48–60.

193. *Maternal misinterpretation of infant fussiness have been noted in numerous studies, including*: Andrew N, Harvey K. Infant feeding choices: experience, self-identity and lifestyle. *Maternal & Child Nutrition*. 2011. Jan 7(1):48–60; Sacco LM, Caulfield LE, Gittelsohn J, Martinez H: The conceptualization of perceived insufficient milk among Mexican mothers. *Journal of Human Lactation*. 2006. 22:277–286; Osman H, El Zein L, Wick L. Cultural beliefs that may discourage breastfeeding among Lebanese women: a qualitative analysis. *International Breastfeeding Journal*. 2009. 4:12; Yamamoto H, Tanak M, Takano M: The perceptions of breastfeeding in mothers who believe that their breast milk is insufficient for their baby [Article in Japanese]. *Maternal Health*. 2009. 50(1):110–117.

194. Murphy, E. 2004. 'Anticipatory Accounts', *Symbolic Interaction*. 27(2): 129–154.

195. *For examples see*: Artiss K. 1959. *The Symptom as Communication in Schizophrenia*. New York: Grune and Stratton; Haley J. 1963. *Strategies of Psychotherapy*. New York: Anchor Books; Schlenker BR. 1980. *Impression Management: The Self Concept, Social Identity, and Interpersonal Relations*. Monterey, CA: Brooks/Cole.

196. *See, for example*: Gussler JD, Briesemeister LH. The insufficient milk syndrome: a biocultural explanation. *Medical Anthropology*. 1980. 4:145–174; and also: Rapley G, Murkett T. 2012. *Baby-Led Breastfeeding*. London: Vermilion.

197. Scheff TJ. 1971. *Being Mentally Ill: A Sociological Theory*. Chicago: Aldine.

198. *FYI, parading and exaggerating one's weaknesses is a behaviour called 'supplication'.*

199. Jones EE, Pittman T. 1982. Toward a general theory of strategic self-presentation. In Suls J (ed.) *Psychological Perspectives on the Self*. Vol. 1, 231–63. Hillside, NJ: Erlbaum.

200. Lewin K. 1936. *Principles of Topological Psychology*. New York: McGraw-Hill.

201. Stadlen N. 2004. *What Mothers Do*. London: Piatkus. p257.

202. Shaw ME. 1968. Attribution of responsibility by adolescents in two cultures. *Adolescence*. 3, 23–32; Shaw ME, Reitan HT. 1969. Attribution of responsibility as a basis for sanctioning behaviour. *British Journal of Social and Clinical Psychology*. 8, 217–226; Shaw ME, Sulzer JL. 1964. An

empirical test of Heider's levels in attribution of responsibility. *Journal of Abnormal and Social Psychology*. 69, 39–46; Sulzer JL, Burglass RK. 1968. Responsibility attribution, empathy and punitiveness. *Journal of Personality*. 36, 272–282.

203. Luginbuhl J, Palmer R. 1991. Impression management aspects of self-handicapping: Positive and negative effects. *Personality and Social Psychology Bulletin*. 17, 655–662.

204. Baumgardner AH, Lake EA, Arkin RM. 1985. Claiming mood as a self-handicap: The influence of spoiled and unspoiled social identities. *Personality and Social Psychology Bulletin*. 11, 349–358.

205. Humphreys AS, Thompson NJ, Miner KR: Intention to breastfeed in low-income pregnant women: the role of social support and previous experiences. *Birth*. 1998. 25:169–174; Persad MD, Mensinger JL. Maternal breastfeeding attitudes: association with breastfeeding intent and socio-demographics among urban primiparas. *Journal of Community Health*. 2008. 33:53–60; Shaker A, Scott JA, Reid M. Infant feeding attitudes of expectant parents: Breastfeeding and formula feeding. *Journal of Advanced Nursing*. 2004. 45:260–268; Andrew N, Harvey K. 2011. Infant feeding choices: experience, self-identity and lifestyle. *Maternal & Child Nutrition*. 7, 48–60.

206. Oleson KC, Poehlmann KM, Yost JH, Lynch ME, Arkin RM. 2000. Subjective overachievement: Individual differences in self-doubt and concern with performance. *Journal of Personality*. 68, 491–524.

207. Durkheim É. 1965. *The Elementary Forms of the Religious Life*. (1912, English translation by Joseph Swain, 1915). The Free Press.

208. Merton RK. 1948. The Self-fulfilling Prophecy. *Antioch Review*. 8, 193–210.

209. Snyder M. 1984. When belief creates reality. In Berkowitz L (ed.) *Advances in Experimental Social Psychology* (Vol. 18). New York: Academic Press. p293.

210. Hume D. 1910 [1748]. *An Enquiry Concerning Human Understanding*. PF Collier & Son.

211. *This phenomenon has been known for decades as the 'motive to avoid failure', or more recently as 'fear of failure'* . Birney RC, Burdick H, Teevan RC. 1969. *Fear of Failure*. New York: Van Nostrand Reinhold.

212. The Positive Deviance Initiative. Available at: www.positivedeviance. org/ Accessed August 4, 2013. See also: Sternin J, Choo R. 2000. *The Power of Positive Deviancy*. Harvard Business.

213. Lamontagne C, Hamelin A, St-Pierre M. The breastfeeding experience of women with major difficulties who use the services of a breastfeeding clinic: a descriptive study. *International Breastfeeding Journal*. 2008. 3:17.

214. Murphy E. 4a. 'Anticipatory Accounts', *Symbolic Interaction*. 27(2): 129–154.

215. Lindenberg S, Steg L. 2007. Normative, gain and hedonic goal frames guiding environmental behavior. *Journal of Social Issues*. 65, 117–137.

216. *Similar to the Belief dimension of my A B C analysis: Mum is highly influenced by those close to her.*

217. *Visceral factors spring to mind – the desire for sleep or to be free of breast*

*discomfort being pertinent examples in the breastfeeding context.*
218. McCaffery EJ, Baron J. 2006. 'Thinking about tax', *Psychology, Public Policy, and Law.* 12 (1): 106–35. p107.
219. Goleman D. 1995. *Emotional Intelligence.* New York: Bantam Books.
220. Hoddinott P, Craig LC, Britten J, McInnes RM. A serial qualitative interview study of infant feeding experiences: idealism meets realism. *BMJ Open.* 2012. Mar 14;2(2).
221. Lamontagne C, Hamelin A, St-Pierre M. The breastfeeding experience of women with major difficulties who use the services of a breastfeeding clinic: a descriptive study. *International Breastfeeding Journal.* 2008. 3:17.
222. Bottorff JL. Persistence in breastfeeding: a phenomenological investigation. *Journal of Advanced Nursing.* 1990.15, 201–209. p202.
223. Bottorff JL. Persistence in breastfeeding: a phenomenological investigation. *Journal of Advanced Nursing.* 1990.15, 201–209. p207.
224. Bottorff JL, Morse JM. 1990. Mother's perception of breast milk. *Journal of Obstetric, Gynecologic & Neonatal Nursing.* 19(6), 518–527. p520.
225. Bottorff JL. Persistence in breastfeeding: a phenomenological investigation. *Journal of Advanced Nursing.* 1990. 15, 201–209. p205.
226. Stern DN. 1995. *The Motherhood Constellation.* London: Basic Books. See also: Sills F. 2008. *Being and Becoming.* North Atlantic Books. p122.
227. Andrew N, Harvey K. Infant feeding choices: experience, self-identity and lifestyle. *Maternal & Child Nutrition.* 2011. Jan 7(1):48–60.
228. Parkinson J et al. 2010. The Role of Mother-centred Factors Influencing the Complex Social Behaviour of Breastfeeding: Social Support and Self-efficacy. ANZMAC Annual Conference 2010.
229. Marshall J. 2011. Motherhood, breastfeeding and identity. *Practising Midwife.* 14 (2). pp16–18. ISSN 1461–3123; Marshall JL, Godfrey M, Renfrew MJ: Being a 'good mother': Managing breastfeeding and merging identities. *Social Science & Medicine.* 2007. 65(10):2147–2159.
230. Maslow AH. 1970. *Motivation and Personality.* New York: Longman.
231. Maslow ob cit, p22.
232. Taylor E. 2007. *Choices and Illusions.* CA: Hay House.
233. Taylor 2007. ob cit, p18.
234. Lee EJ. 2007. Infant feeding in risk society. *Health, Risk & Society.* 9:3, 295–309.
235. Coulter J. 1986. Affect and social context: emotion definition as a social task. In Harre R (ed.) *The Social Construction of Emotions.* Oxford: Blackwell. pp120–134.
236. Thoits, P. A. (1990). Emotional deviance: research agendas. T. D. Kemper (Ed.), Research agendas in the sociology of emotions (pp. 180–203). Albany: State University of New York Press
237. Darwin C. 1965. The expression of the emotions in man and animals. Chicago: University of Chicago Press (Original work published 1872).
238. *This view is supported by:* Russell DW and McAuley E. 1986. Causal attributions, causal dimensions, and affective reactions to success or failure. *Journal of Personality and Social Psychology.* 50, 1174–85.
239. McFarland C, Ross M. 1982. The impact of causal attributions on affective reactions to success and failure. *Journal of Personality and Social*

*Psychology*. 43, 937-46.

240. Thibodeau. R & Aronson.E. 1992. Taking a closer look: Reasserting the role of the self-concept in dissonance theory. *Personality and Social Psychology Bulletin*. 18, 591–602.

241. Andrew N, Harvey K. Infant feeding choices: experience, self-identity and lifestyle. *Maternal & Child Nutrition*. 2011. Jan, 7(1):48–60.

242. Solomon RC. 2009. *True to Our Feelings: What Our Emotions Are Really Telling Us*. New York: Oxford University Press.

243. Lee EJ. 2007. Infant feeding in risk society. *Health, Risk & Society*. 9:3, 295–309; Murphy E. 1999. 'Breast is best': Infant feeding decisions and maternal deviance. *Sociology of Health and Illness*. 21, 187–208, Earle S. 2000. Why some women do not breast feed: Bottle feeding and fathers' role. *Midwifery*. 16, 323–330.

244. Freud S. 1924. *The Economic Problem of Masochism* (standard edition). 19:159–170, 1961.

245. Ystrom E. Breastfeeding cessation and symptoms of anxiety and depression: a longitudinal cohort study. *BMC Pregnancy Childbirth*. 2012. May 23;12:36.

246. Rudd MG, Viney LL, Preston CA. 1999. The Grief Experienced by Spousal Caregivers of Dementia Patients: The Role of Place of Care of Patient and Gender of Caregiver. *International Journal of Aging and Human Development*. 48: 217–240.

247. González C. 2014. *Breastfeeding Made Easy*. London: Pinter & Martin. p321.

248. *Does this behaviour sound familiar? Breastfeeding mothers often live on a leash too, for different reasons.*

249. Lee EJ. 2007. Infant feeding in risk society. *Health, Risk & Society*. 9:3, 295–309, p304.

250. *On formula feeders trying to hide from anticipated judgypants, see*: Andrew N, Harvey K. Infant feeding choices: experience, self-identity and lifestyle. *Maternal & Child Nutrition*. 2011. Jan 7(1):48–60.

251. Scheff TJ. 1988. Shame and Conformity: The Deference-Emotion System. *American Sociological Review*. 53: 395–406, Scheff TJ. 2000. Shame and the Social Bond. *Sociological Theory*. 18: 84–98; Shott S. 1979. Emotions and Social Life: A Symbolic Interactionist Analysis. *American Journal of Sociology*. 84: 1317–1334.

252. Cooley CH. 1902. *Human Nature and the Social Order* (revised edition). New York: Charles Scribner's Sons.

253. Fishbain DA. Secondary gain concept: Definition problems and its abuse in medical practice. *American Pain Society Journal*. Volume 3, Issue 4, Winter 1994, Pages 264–273

254. Mandler.G 1990 A constructivist theory of emotion, in Stein.N.L, Leventhal.B, and Trabasso.T (eds.) 1990 *Psychological and biological approaches to emotion*. New Jersey: Lawrence Erlbaum Associates, Inc.

255. Templar R. 2013. *The Rules to Break*. Harlow: Pearson. p158.

256. Nietzsche F. 1937. *The Philosophy of Nietzsche*. New York: Modern Library.

257. *On this pitiful process, see*: Lewis H, 1971. *Shame and Guilt in Neurosis*.

New York: International Universities Press.

258. Lynd HM. 1971. The Nature of Shame. In Morris H (ed.) *Guilt and Shame*. CA: Wadsworth Publishing Company.

259. Erikson EH. 1971. Autonomy v Shame and Doubt. In Morris H (ed:) *Guilt and Shame*. California: Wadsworth Publishing Company.

260. Trivers R. 2011. *Deceit and Self-Deception*. London: Penguin Books. p321.

261. Loewenstein G. Out of Control: Visceral Influences on Behaviour. *Organizational Behaviour and Human Decision Processes*. 65(3) March pp272–292, 1996. pp272–273.

262. *I have covered this in a blog post, available at*: www.thealphaparent. com/2011/10/why-way-you-feed-your-baby-is-my.html

263. *A comprehensive summary of the studies is available at:* www.thealphaparent. com/2011/07/virgin-gut-note-for-parents.html

264. Tangney.J.P 1994 The mixed legacy of the superego: Adaptive and maladaptive aspects of shame and guilt. In Masling.J.M and Bornstein.R.F (Eds) Empirical perspectives on object relations theory. , (pp. 1-28). Washington, DC, US: American Psychological Association 252 Nolen-Hoeksema S. 2004. *Women Who Think Too Much*. London: Piatkus.

265. Tavris C.1992. *The Mismeasure of Women*. New York: Simon & Schuster. *The bias is confounded by the rule of thumb that perpetrating physical harm to another person is generally seen as worse than harming oneself* (May R. 1984. Theory of excuses: positive images for others and self, in Snyder CR, Higgings RL, Stucky RJ. 1984. *Excuses Masquerades in Search of Grace*. Toronto: John Wiley & Sons; Murphy E. 2004. Risk, maternal ideologies, and infant feeding. In Germov J, Williams L (eds.) *A Sociology of Food and Nutrition*. Oxford: Oxford University Press). *In most other contexts, refusal to try or poor effort expenditure do not result in a transgression against another. Lack of action is often a victimless crime. However, the realm of parenting is a clear exception to this rule. Young children, in particular, are given elite victim status in this regard, due to their innocence and vulnerability* (Rozin P. 1997. *Morality*. In Brandt AM and Rozin P (eds.) *Morality and Health*. London and New York: Routledge; Jackson S, Scott, S. 1999. Risk, anxiety and the social construction of children. In Lupton D. (ed.) *Risk and Socio-cultural Theory: New Directions and Perspectives*. Cambridge: Cambridge University Press; Furedi F. 2001. *Paranoid Parenting*. London: Penguin Books). *In parenting, it is a moral duty to put forth effort. Achievement as a parent is intertwined with ideas about obligation. Responsibility is inherent even in the absence of intention.*

266. Tangney JP, Dearing RL. 2002. *Shame and Guilt*. New York: The Guilford Press; Baron-Cohen S. 2012. *The Essential Difference: Men, Women and the Extreme Male Brain*. Penguin Books; Brody LR. 1999. *Gender, Emotion and the Family*. Cambridge, MA: Harvard University Press.

267. Orbach S, Eichenbaum L. 1994. *Between Women*. London: Arrow Books.

268. UK Infant Feeding Survey 2010, NHS.

269. Robson, P. and Walter, T., 2012. Hierarchies of loss: a critique of disenfranchised grief. Omega: Journal of Death & Dying, 66 (2), pp. 97-119; Kenneth J. D 1989 Disenfranchised Grief: Recognizing Hidden

Sorrow. Lexington Books.

270. *No relation to the affordable high-street fashion retailer.*

271. Cooper J, Fazio RH. 1984. A new look at dissonance theory. In Berkowitz L (ed.) *Advances in Experimental Social Psychology* (Vol. 17, pp229–266). New York: Academic Press.

272. Higgins.R.L 2002  Reality Negotiation. In Higgins.R.L, Berglas.S 2002 Handbook of positive psychology. Oxford: Oxford University Press

273. Croghan R, Miell D. 1998. Strategies of resistance: 'bad' mothers dispute the evidence. *Feminism and Psychology*. 8: 445–465.

274. *But not incompatible with breastfeeding of course – provided dads know other ways to parent that don't involve a plastic teat.*

275. Earle S. 2000. 'Why Some Women do not Breast Feed: Bottle Feeding and Fathers' Role'. *Midwifery* 16(4): 323–30; Bailey C, Pain RH, Aarvold JE. A 'give it a go' breast-feeding culture and early cessation among low-income mothers. *Midwifery*. 2004. Sep 20(3):240–50; Schmidt J. 2008. 'Gendering in Infant Feeding Discourses: The Good Mother and the Absent Father.' *New Zealand Sociology*. 23(2): 61–74.

276. Janoff-Bulman R, Timko C. 1987. Coping with traumatic events: The role of denial in light of people's assumptive worlds. In Snyder CR, Ford CE (eds.) Coping with Negative Life Events. *Clinical and Social Psychological Perspectives*. pp135–59. New York: Plenum.

277. Galinsky A, Stone J, Cooper J. 1997. The reinstatement of dissonance and psychological discomfort following failed affirmations. Unpublished manuscript, Princeton NJ: Princeton University; Elliot A, Devine P. 1994. On the motivational nature of cognitive dissonance: Dissonance as psychological discomfort. *Journal of Personality and Social Psychology*. 67, 382–394.

278. Trivers R. 2011. *Deceit and Self-Deception*. London: Penguin Books.

279. *The study looked at the linear process of planning to breastfeed right through to sour grapes. In doing so, it identified seven distinct phases: planning, expecting, realising, questioning, getting on with it, defending and qualifying.* Sheehan A, Schmied V, Barclay L. 2010. Complex decisions: theorizing women's infant feeding decisions in the first 6 weeks after birth. *Journal of Advanced Nursing*. 66, 371–380.

280. Yates JF, Veinott ES, Patalano AL. 2003. Hard decisions, bad decisions: On decision quality and decision aiding. In Schneider SL, Shantaeu J (eds.) *Emerging Perspectives on Judgement and Decision Research*. New York: Cambridge University Press. pp13–63.

281. Freud A. 1936. *The Ego and the Mechanisms of Defence* (revised edition 1960). New York: International Universities Press.

282. NHS    www.nhs.uk/conditions/pregnancy-and-baby/pages/why-breastfeed.aspx#close

283. www.aap.org/en-us/about-the-aap/aap-press-room/Pages/AAP-Reaffirms-Breastfeeding-Guidelines.aspx

284. Schlenker BR. 1980. *Impression Management: The Self-Concept, Social Identity, and Interpersonal Relations*. Belmont, CA: Wadsworth.

285. The clearer the standard: Snyder M. 1985. The excuse: An amazing grace? In Schlenker BR (ed.) 1985. *The Self and Social Life*. New York: McGraw-

Hill. pp235–60; The more influential the source: Becker H. 1963. *Outsiders*. New York: Free Press.

286. *American entrepreneur, author and motivational speaker.*

287. Bailey C, Pain RH, Aarvold JE. 2004. A 'give it a go' breast-feeding culture and early cessation among low-income mothers 20:3, 240–250, September 2004.

288. Aronson E. 1999. Dissonance, hypocrisy, and the self-concept. In Harmon-Jones E, Mills J (eds.) *Cognitive Dissonance: Progress on a Pivotal Theory in Social Psychology*. Washington DC: American Psychological Association.

289. Ayers-Nachamkin B. 1982. Sex differences in self-serving biases: Success expectancies or role expectation? Unpublished doctoral dissertation, University of Kansas; Rosenfield D, Stephan WG. 1978. Sex differences in attributions for sex-typed tasks. *Journal of Personality*. 45, 244–259.

290. *Virtually (via my blog thealphaparent.com where I have interviewed mothers from around the world), professionally (via my previous work as a nursery nurse and now as a lab worker at Durham University's Baby Sleep Lab) and personally (as a fellow mother in my network of peers).*

291. Zuckerman M. 1979. Attribution of success and failure revisited, or: The motivational bias is alive and well in attribution theory. *Journal of Personality*. 47, 245–287.

292. *Oxford English Dictionary*. Oxford: OUP

293. Brock TC, Buss AH. 1962. Dissonance, aggression and evaluation of pain. *Journal of Abnormal and Social Psychology*. 65, 197–202; Harvey JH, Harris B, Barnes RD. 1975. Actor-observer differences in the perceptions of responsibility and freedom. *Journal and Personality and Social Psychology*. 32, 22–28.

294. Lamontagne C, Hamelin A, St-Pierre M. The breastfeeding experience of women with major difficulties who use the services of a breastfeeding clinic: a descriptive study. *International Breastfeeding Journal*. 2008. 3:17.

295. *If you take a look at the Belief section of the Deception chapter (see page 49), you'll see this more of this in action.*

296. Murphy E. 1999. 'Breast is best': Infant feeding decisions and maternal deviance. *Sociology of Health & Illness*. 21, 2, pp187–208 p194.

297. Darley JM, Zanna MP. 1982. Making moral judgements. *American Scientist*. 70, 515–21.

298. Austin W, Walster E, Utne MK. 1976. Enquiry into the law: The effect of a harmdoer's 'suffering in the act' on liking and assigned punishment. In Berkowitz L, Walster E (eds.) *Advances in Experimental Social Psychology* (Vol. 9). New York: Academic Press; Bramel D, Taub B, Blum B. 1968. An observer's reactions to the suffering of his enemy. *Journal of Personal and Social Psychology*. 8, 384–392.

299. Goffman E. 1990. *The Presentation of Self in Everyday Life*. London: Penguin Books; Hochschild AR. 1983. *The Managed Heart: The Communication of Human Feeling*. Berkley: University of California Press.

300. *Our sympathy reserves, or 'sympathy margins' as they are sometimes called, are serious business. Sociologist Candace Clark has written extensively about how we dish out sympathy in her paper:* Clark. C. Sympathy Biography and

Sympathy Margin. *American Journal of Sociology*. Vol. 93, No. 2, Sep., 1987. *If this topic tickles your fancy, you can read more about this mechanism in the books*: Swcheler. M 2008 *The Nature of Sympathy*. New Jersey: Transaction Publishers; Clark. C 1992 *Misery and Company: Sympathy in Everyday Life*. Chicago: University of Chicago Press.

301. Kahneman D, Tversky A. 1982. The simulation heuristic. In Kahneman D, Slovic P, Tversky A (eds.) *Judgement Under Uncertainty*, Cambridge: Cambridge University Press. pp201–8.

302. Gatti L. Maternal perceptions of insufficient milk supply in breastfeeding. *Journal of Nursing Scholarship*. 2008. 40(4):355–363; Yoshitome A, Gotoh Y, Tomiyasu T. Factors that negatively affected infant feeding methods within 3–4 months after birth [Article in Japanese]. *Perinatal Medicine*. 2003. 33(8):1040–1042; Li R, Fein SB, Chen J, Grummer-Strawn LM. Why mothers stop breastfeeding: mothers' self-reported reasons for stopping during the first year. *Pediatrics*. 2008. Oct, 122 Suppl 2:S69–76; Grossman LK, Harter C, Sachs L, Kay A. 1990. The effect of postpartum lactation counseling on the duration of breast-feeding in low-income women. *Journal of the American Dietetic Association*, 144, 471–474.

303. Smith TW, Snyder CR, Perkins SC. 1983. The self-serving function of hypochondriacal complaints: Physical symptoms as self-handicapping strategies. *Journal of Personality and Social Psychology*. 44, 787–797.

304. Feinberg J. 1970. Action and responsibility. In *Doing and Deserving*. Princeton NJ: Princeton University Press. pp119–51

305. *Time Magazine*, Is the Medical Community Failing Breastfeeding Moms? Available at: healthland.time.com/2013/01/02/is-the-medical-community-failing-breastfeeding-moms/ Accessed September 23, 2013. For more evidence for the 1–5 percent statistic see: Neifert MR. 1983. Infant problems in breastfeeding. In Neville MC, Neifert MR (eds.) *Lactation: Physiology, Nutrition, and Breastfeeding*. Plenum Press. See also: Akre J. 1989. Infant feeding: the physiological basis. Geneva: World Health Organisation. 108pp. *In one study, that looked at the clinical referrals to a breastfeeding-support service, only 1.3 percent of women were found to have a pathophysiology of milk production* (Woolridge MW. 1995. Breastfeeding: physiology into practice. In Davies DP (ed.) *Nutrition in Child Health*. Proceedings of conference jointly organised by the Royal College of Physicians of London and the British Paediatric Association. RCPL Press. *These statistics render the majority of breastfeeding success as so clearly effort-related that claims to the contrary ring hollow and lead to perceptions of dishonesty.*

306. González C. 2014. *Breastfeeding Made Easy*. London: Pinter & Martin.

307. *As there are only around a dozen princes on the planet, I would warn your mother to hold off buying that hat.*

308. Berglas S. The three faces of self-handicapping: Protective self-presentation, a strategy for self-esteem enhancement, and a character disorder. Zelen SL (ed.) *Self-representation: The second attribution-personality theory conference*, CSPP-LA. 1986, 1988. pp133–169.

309. Peterson C. et al Self-blame and depressive symptoms. *Journal of Personality and Social Psychology*, Vol 41(2), Aug 1981, 253-259; Janoff-

Bulman R. Esteem and control bases of blame: "Adaptive" strategies for victims versus observers. *Journal of Personality Volume* 50, Issue 2, pages 180–192, June 1982; Shaver, K.G. and Drown, D On causality, responsibility, and self-blame: A theoretical note. *Journal of Personality and Social Psychology*, Vol 50(4), Apr 1986, 697-702

310. Braginsky B, Braginsky D. 1967. Schizophrenic patients in the psychiatric interview: An experimental study of their effectiveness at manipulation. *Journal of Consulting and Clinical Psychology*. 1967. Dec 31(6):543–7; Braginsky BM, Gross M, Ring K. 1966. Controlling outcomes through impression-management: An experimental study of the manipulative tactics of mental patients. *Journal of Consulting Psychology*. 30, 295–300; Ludwig AM, Farrelly F. 1966. The code of chronicity. *Archives of General Psychiatry*. 15, 562—568.

311. Schlenker BR. 1980. *Impression Management: The Self-concept, Social identity, and Interpersonal Relations*. Monterey, CA: Brooks/Cole.

312. Murphy E. 2004. 'Anticipatory Accounts', *Symbolic Interaction* 27(2): 129–154. p14. *Most women are guilty of using one strain of the Happy Mum, Happy Baby rhetoric*. See: Blum L. 1993. Mothers, babies, and breast-feeding in late capitalist America – The shifting contexts of feminist theory. *Feminist Studies*. 19(2), 291–311. p297.

313. Dennis C. Breastfeeding Peer Support: Maternal and Volunteer Perceptions from a Randomized Controlled Trial. *Birth*. 29:3, 169–176, September 2002; Scott JA, Binns CW, Graham KI, Oddy WH. Temporal Changes in the Determinants of Breastfeeding Initiation. *Birth*. 33:1, 7–45, March 2006.

314. Zanardo V et al Elective cesarean delivery: does it have a negative effect on breastfeeding? Birth. 2010 Dec;37(4):275-9

315. *Recall in the Deception chapter we explored how mothers are selective in their research efforts.*

316. Loewenstein G. Out of Control: Visceral Influences on Behaviour. *Organizational Behaviour and Human Decision Processes*. 65(3) March pp272–292, 1996, pp272–273.

317. *Recall from the Deception chapter that mothers lacking a major sense of control over their lives are more excuse-prone. Numerous psychological studies also indicate a link between the degree of a mother's feelings of helplessness and the tendency to use the duress excuse. Unsurprisingly, this link is further strengthened by a lack of trust in interpersonal relationships* (Gregory WL, Steiner ID, Brennan G, Detrick A. 1978. A scale to measure benevolent versus malevolent perceptions of the environment. *Journal Supplement Abstract Service*. 8, No. 1679; Hochreich DJ. 1968. Refined analysis of internal-external control and behaviour in a laboratory situation. Unpublished doctoral dissertation. University of Connecticut; Rotter JB. 1967. A new scale for the measurement of interpersonal trust. *Journal of Personality*. 35, 651–665.

318. *And even if it did (resemble the true version of events), the experts – La Leche League – acknowledge that 'A mother's choices are not an accurate reflection of the quality of help she has received'.* Mohrbacher N, Stock J. 1997. *The Breastfeeding Answer Book* (revised edition). Illinois: La Leche League

International.

319. Bedard S. 1995. *Factors Associated with Breastfeeding Duration*. College of Nursing, University of Utah. p93. *Interestingly, the mother didn't see fit to correct her son's behaviour. Instead, she chose to wean the baby. Go figure!*

320. Kurtines WM. 1986. Moral behaviour as rule-governed behaviour: Person and situation effects on moral decision making. *Journal of Personality and Social Psychology*. 50, 784–91.

321. *A maternal interview from the study:* Earle S. Factors affecting the initiation of breastfeeding: implications for breastfeeding promotion. *Health Promotion International*. 2002. Vol. 77. No. 3.

322. *Yet interestingly, in some countries, Japan for instance, studies have found a positive association between returning to work and continued breastfeeding* (Kaneko A, Kaneita Y, Yokoyama E, Miyake T, Harano S, Suzuki K, Ibuka E, Tsutsui T, Yamamoto Y, Ohida T: Factors associated with exclusive breast-feeding in Japan: for activities to support child-rearing with breast-feeding. *Journal of Epidemiology & Community Health*. 2006. 16(2):57–63).

323. *The neon flaw in this facade is, of course, that a successfully breastfeeding mother can also be all of the aforementioned maternal reinventions.*

324. *For a textbook example of the redefining standards excuse in action, see*: Brody J E. The ideal and the real of breastfeeding. *New York Times*. July 23, 2012. Available at: well.blogs.nytimes.com/2012/07/23/the-ideal-and-the-real-of-breast-feeding/?_r=0 Accessed August 3, 2013.

325. *A form of 'reality negotiation' – a strategy we explored in the previous chapter – but this time rather than aiming her efforts at her internal audience, she aims them at an external one.*

326. *On the strategy of 'embedding', see*: Jellison JM. 1977. *I'm Sorry I Didn't Mean To, And Other Lies We Love to Tell*. New York: Chatham Square Press.

327. Frankfurt H. 2005. *On Bullshit*. Princeton NJ: Princeton University Press. p61.

328. Lamontagne C, Hamelin A, St-Pierre M. The breastfeeding experience of women with major difficulties who use the services of a breastfeeding clinic: a descriptive study. *International Breastfeeding Journal*. 2008. 3:17.

329. Smith PH, Coley SL, Labbok MH, Cupito S, Nwokah E. Early breastfeeding experiences of adolescent mothers: a qualitative prospective study. *International Breastfeeding Journal*. 2012. Sep 29;7(1):13; Kretchmar MD, Jacobvitz DB. Observing mother-child relationships across generations: boundary patterns, attachments, and the transmission of caregiving. *Family Process*. 2002. 41(3):351–374.

330. Andrew N, Harvey K. 2011. Infant feeding choices: experience, self-identity and lifestyle. *Maternal & Child Nutrition*. 7, 48–60.

331. Murphy E. 2004. 'Anticipatory Accounts'. *Symbolic Interaction* 27(2): 129–154.

332. Crockenberg S. 1986. Are temperamental differences in babies associated with predictable differences in caregiving? In Lerner JV, Lerner RM (eds.) New directions for child development: No. 31. *Temperament and Social Interaction in Infants and Children*. San Francisco, CA: Jossey-Bass.

pp53–73.

333. Hall CS. 1954. *A Primer of Freudian Psychology*. New York.

334. Hendrickson R. 2008. *The Facts on File Encyclopedia of Word and Phrase Origins*. Checkmark Books.

335. Knox RE, Inkster JA. 1968. Postdecision dissonance at post time. *Journal of Personality and Social Psychology*. 8, pp319–323.

336. *We'll look at this behaviour in more detail in the Sabotage chapter.*

337. Tavris C, Aronson E. 2007. *Mistakes Were Made (But Not By Me)*. London: Pinter & Martin. pp9–10.

338. Cody MJ, McLaughlin ML. 1985. Models for the sequential construction of accounting episodes: Situational and interactional constraints on message selection and interaction. In Street RL Jr, Cappella JN (eds.) *Sequence and Pattern in Communicative Behaviour*. London: Edward Arnold. pp50–69; McLaughlin ML, Cody MJ, O'Hair HD. 1983. The management of failure events: Some contextual determants of accounting behaviour. *Human Communication Research*. 9, 208–24; McLaughlin ML, Cody MJ, Rosenstein NE. 1983. Accounting sequences in conversations between strangers. *Communication Monographs*. 50, 102–25.

339. Shields NM. 1979. Accounts and other interpersonal strategies in credibility detracting context. *Pacific Sociological Review*. 22, 255–72.

340. From *As You Like It* 2:7.

341. Hughes T. April 15 2013. How having a baby boosts social life of new mothers. Available at: www.express.co.uk/news/uk/392003/How-having-a-baby-boosts-social-life-of-new-mothers Accessed May 14, 2013.

342. Durkheim É. 1995. *The Elementary Forms of Religious Life*. New York: Free Press. p217.

343. Douglas SJ, Michaels MW. 2005. *The Mommy Myth: The Idealization of Motherhood and How It Has Undermined All Women*. New York: Free Press. p6.

344. Swann WB Jr. 1987. Identity negotiation: Where two roads meet. *Journal of Personality and Social Psychology*. 53, 1038–1051.

345. Lee E. Health, morality, and infant feeding: British mothers' experiences of formula milk use in the early weeks. *Sociology of Health & Illness*. Vol. 29 No. 7 2007. ISSN 0141–9889, pp1075–1090, p1085.

346. Cozby PC. 1973. Self-disclosure: a literature review. *Psychological Bulletin*. 1973, 79, 73–91.

347. Goffman E. 1990. *The Presentation of Self in Everyday Life*. London: Penguin Books.

348. ob cit, pp161–162.

349. Stamper CL, Masterson SS. 2002. Insider or outsider? How employee perceptions of insider status affect their work behavior. *Journal of Organizational Behavior*. 23, 875–894.

350. Goffman 1959, ob cit, p169.

351. *To read more about how professionals have a chilling effect on excuse-making, see*: Arkin RM, Cooper H, Kolditz T. 1980. A statistical review of the literature concerning the self-serving attribution bias in interpersonal influence situations. *Journal of Personality*. 48, 435–48.

352. *Interestingly, some people say the word 'sincere' derives from the Latin words for 'without', sin, and 'wax', cere. They relate this back to ancient Rome when craftsmen covered cracks and defects in statues with wax. Conversely, when a mother is excuse-making, her tale of events can be said to contain 'cracks' or 'defects' that expose her pretence.*

353. *We delve into what breastfeeding mothers* really *think of formula feeders later, in the Contempt chapter.*

354. Petty RE, Cacioppo JT. 1986. The elaboration likelihood model of persuasion. In Berkowitz L (ed.) *Advances in Experimental Social Psychology* (Vol. 19) New York: Academic Press. pp123–205; Thomsen CJ, Borgida E, Lavine H. 1995. The causes and consequences of personal involvement. In Petty RE, Krosnick JA (eds.) *Attitude Strength: Antecedents and Consequences.* Mahwah, NJ: Erlbaum. pp191–214.

355. *The very act of offering excuses to the breastfeeding mother is itself as a sign of deference – a message that the formula feeder holds the breastfeeding mother in high regard. You may think this would be met favourably by the latter, being a boost to her self-esteem, however often, it is not, as I will explain in the next chapter – Envy.*

356. Weiner B. 1986. *Principles of Psychotherapy.* New York: Wiley.

357. Jones EE, Davis KE. 1965. From acts to dispositions: The attribution process in personal perception. In Berkowitz L (ed.) *Advances in Experimental Social Psychology* (Vol. 2). New York: Academic Press.

358. 'The Fundamental Attribution Error', see: Jones EE. 1979. The rocky road from acts to dispositions. *American Psychologist.* 34, 107–17.

359. Eiser JR. 1983. Attribution theory and social cognition. In Jaspars JMF, Fincham FD, Hewstone M (eds.) *Attribution Theory and Research: Conceptual, Developmental and Social Dimensions.* London: Academic Press.

360. Ross L, Amabile TM, Steinmetz JL. 1977. Social roles, social control and biases in social-perception processes. *Journal of Personality and Social Psychology.* 35, 485–94; Davies MF. 1985. Social roles and social-perception biases: the questioner superiority effect revisited. *British Journal of Social Psychology.* 24, 239–48. *However, excuse-makers can take some comfort from the fact that as the length of acquaintanceship with the other person increases, the tendency of the other person to neglect situational factors* decreases (Nisbett RE, Caputo C, Legant P, Maracek J. 1973. Behaviour as seen by the actor and as seen by the observer. *Journal of Personality and Social Psychology.* 27, 154–64.

361. *On failures judging other failures harshly, see*: Snyder M, Jones EE. 1974. Attitude attribution when behaviour is constrained. *Journal of Experimental Social Psychology.* 10, 585–600.

362. Gilbert DT, Malone PS. The correspondence bias. *Psychological Bulletin.* 1995. Jan 117(1):21–38.

363. Kawagoe T, Takizawa H. 'Why Lying Pays: Truth Bias in the Communication with Conflicting Interests'. Available at: www.rieti. go.jp/jp/publications/dp/05e018.pdf

364. May R. 1984. Theory of excuses: positive images for others and self, in Snyder CR, Higgings RL, Stucky RJ. 1984. *Excuses Masquerades in Search*

*of Grace.* Toronto: John Wiley & Sons. p24.

365. Kulik JA, Taylor SE. 1980. Premature consensus on consensus? Effects of sample-based versus self-based consensus information. *Journal of Personality and Social Psychology.* 38, 871–878; Major B. 1980. Information acquisition and attribution processes. *Journal of Personality and Social Psychology.* 39, 1010–1023; Orvis BR, Cunningham JD, Kelley HH. 1975. A closer examination of causal inference: The role of consensus, distinctiveness, and consistency information. *Journal of Personality and Social Psychology.* 32, 604-616; Wells GL, Harvey JH. 1977. Do people make consensus information in making causal attributions? *Journal of Personality and Social Psychology.* 35, 279–293; Kelley HH. 1972. Causal schemata and the attribution process. In Jones EE, Kanouse D, Kelley HH, Nisbett RE, Valins S, Weiner B (eds.) *Attribution: Perceiving the Causes of Behaviour.* Morristown, NJ: General Learning Press. *The mother can attempt to interfere with this process by offering the Embedded Excuse (see above), which directs the audience's attention to suggestions of her wider parenting prowess.*

366. Morris, M W. and Larrick, R P When one cause casts doubt on another: A normative analysis of discounting in causal attribution. Psychological Review, Vol 102(2), Apr 1995, 331-355; Ahn.W and Bailensonb.J Causal Attribution as a Search for Underlying Mechanisms: An Explanation of the Conjunction Fallacy and the Discounting Principle. Cognitive Psychology. Volume 31, Issue 1, August 1996, Pages 82–123 345 McArthur LZ, Post DL. 1977. Figural emphasis and person perception. *Journal of Experimental Social Psychology.* 13, 520–35.

366a.McArthur LZ, Post DL. 1977. Figural emphasis and person perception. *Journal of Experimental Social Psychology.* 13, 520–35.

367. *We are all overzealous in this way. The 'anchor and adjustment heuristic', as this behaviour has been called, can be found littered in psychological studies. For instance,* Tversky A, Kaheman D. 1974. Judgement under uncertainty: Heuristics and biases. *Science.* 185, 1124–1131; Jones EE. 1990. *Interpersonal Perception.* New York: Freeman and Company). *There's a cultural twist to anchoring. People in collectivist cultures, such as Asia, are more likely to make greater adjustments for circumstantial factors, whereas people in individualist cultures, such as North America and the UK, prefer solid dispositional attributions.*

368. Iyengar S. 2010. *The Art of Choosing.* Twelve.

369. *All thanks to that delightful human cognitive quirk 'false correspondence bias'.*

370. *Psychologists call this 'the need to believe in a just world' – we all experience it to certain degrees. We'll explore this sense of 'deservedness' later in the Contempt chapter, when we examine a thing called the Just World Hypothesis, so hold that thought!*

371. *The fact that excuses have consequences for both the excuse-maker and the listener is known as 'hedonic relevance'.*

372. *Psychologists call this 'bounded rationality'.*

373. *A pregnant mother takes the message about breastfeeding's challenging nature and projects it onto herself. Sadly, this projection is the first stage in the defensive pessimism that will motivate her subsequent decision-making* (Norem JK.

2001. Defensive pessimism, optimism, and pessimism. In Chang E (ed.) *Optimism & Pessimism: Implication for Theory, Research, and Practice.* Washington DC: American Psychological Association. pp77–100.

374. Burger JM. 1981. Motivational biases in the attribution of responsibility for an accident: A meta-analysis of the defensive-attribution hypothesis. *Psychological Bulletin.* 90, 496–512.

375. *According to a poll conducted by Today and Parenting.com, almost 90 percent of the 26,000 mothers surveyed admit they judge each other.* Available at: www.today.com/moms/mom-judging-olympics-competition-nobody-meant-enter-849454?f Accessed April 19, 2014.

376. Tesser A, Rosen S. 1975. The reluctance to transmit bad news. In Berkowitz L (ed.) *Advances in Experimental Social Psychology.* Vol. 8, pp193–232.

377. Buck RW, Savin VJ, Miller RE et al. 1972. Communication of affect through facial expression in humans. *Journal of Personality and Social Psychology.* 23, pp362–71; Wagner HL, Buck R, Winterbotham M. 1993. Communication of specific emotions: gender differences in sending accuracy and communication measures. *Journal of Nonverbal Behaviour.* 17, pp29–53; Hall JA. 1978. Gender effects in decoding nonverbal cues. *Psychological Bulletin.* 85, pp845–58; Hall J. 1984. *Nonverbal Sex Differences: Communication Accuracy and Expressive Style.* Baltimore: Johns Hopkins University Press; Rosenthal R, Hall JA, DiMatteo MR et al. 1979. *Sensitivity to Nonverbal Communication: The PONS Test.* Baltimore: Johns Hopkins University Press.

378. Brizendine L. 2008. *The Female Brain.* London: Random House.

379. Hoffman ML. 1977. Sex differences in empathy and related behaviours. *Psychological Bulletin.* 84, pp712–22; Zahn-Waxler C, Radke-Yarrow M, Wagner E, Chapman M. 1992. Development of concern for others. *Developmental Psychology.* 28, pp126–36; Maccoby EE. 1966. *The Development of Sex Differences.* Stanford University Press.

380. Hochschild AR. 1983. *The Managed Heart: The Commercialization of Human Feeling.* Berkeley: University of California Press.

381. Orbach S, Eichenbaum L. 1994. *Between Women.* London: Arrow Books. p44.

382. Maccoby EE. 1998. *The Two Sexes: Growing Apart, Coming Together.* Cambridge, MS: Harvard University Press; Campbell A. 1995. A few good men: evolutionary psychology and female adolescent aggression. *Ethology and Sociobiology.* 16, pp99–123.

383. Tetlock PE. 1981. The influence of self-presentation goals in attributional reports. *Social Psychology Quarterly.* 44, 300–11; Weiner B, Amirkan J, Folkes VS, Verette J. 1987. An atributional analysis of excuse giving: Studies of a naïve theory of emotion. *Journal of Personality and Social Psychology.* 52, 316–24.

384. Tesser A, Rosen S. 1975. ob cit.

385. *We tend to be highly receptive of self-esteem enhancing feedback*: Collins R, Dmitruk VM, Ranney JT. 1977. Personal validation: Some empirical and ethical considerations. *Journal of Consulting and Clinical Psychlogy*, 45, 70–77; Jones SC. 1973. Self and interpersonal evaluations: Esteem

theories vs. Consistency theories. *Psychological Bulletin*. 79, 185–199; Mosher DL. 1965. Approval motive and acceptance of 'fake' personality test interpretations which differ in favourability. *Psychological Reports*. 17, 395–402; Snyder CR. 1978. The 'illusion' of uniqueness, *Journal of Humanistic Psychology*. 18, 33–41; Snyder CR, Shenkel RJ. 1976. Effects of 'favourability', modality, and relevance upon acceptance of general personality interpretations prior to and after receiving diagnostic feedback. *Journal of Consulting and Clinical Psychology*. 44, 34–41; Snyder CR, Shenkel RJ, Lowery CR. 1977. Acceptance of personality interpretations: The 'Barnum effect' and beyond. *Journal of Consulting and Clinical Psychology*. 45, 104–114.

386. Jacobs L, Berscheid E, Walster E. 1971. Self-esteem and attraction. *Journal of Personality and Social Psychology*. 17, 84–91.

387. *On faking behaviour and the power of kinship endorsement, see*: McFarland LA, Ryan AM. 2006. Toward an integrated model of applicant faking behaviour. *Journal of Applied Social Psychology*. 36(4), 979–1016.

388. Leslie I. 2011. *Born Liars, Why We Can't Live Without Deceit*. Quercus.

389. Wahlroos S. 1981. *Excuses: How to Spot Them, Deal with Them, and Stop Using Them*. New York: Macmillan.

390. *Available at:* jezebel.com/5768349/not-breastfeeding-is-fine-but-what-about-her-reasoning

391. Goffman E. 1990. *The Presentation of Self in Everyday Life*. London: Penguin Books.

392. Bedard S. 1995. Factors Associated with Breastfeeding Duration. *College of Nursing*. University of Utah. p72.

393. Backman CW. 1985. Identity, self presentation, and the resolution of moral dilemmas: Towards a social psychological theory of moral behaviour. In Schlenker BR (ed.) *The Self and Social Life*. New York: McGraw-Hill. pp261–89.

394. Wahlroos S. 1981. *Excuses: How to Spot Them, Deal with Them, and Stop Using Them*. New York: Macmillan.

395. Elig TW, Frieze IH. 1979. Measuring causal attributions for success and failure. *Journal of Personality and Social Psychology*. Vol. 37(4), Apr 1979, 621–63.

396. McCrea SM, Hirt ER, Hendrix KL, Milner BJ, Steele NL. 2008. The worker scale: Developing a measure to explain gender differences in behavioral self- handicapping. *Journal of Research in Personality*. 42, 949–970.

397. McBride AB, Black KN. 1979. Sex differences in causal attributions of parenting. Paper presented at the Annual Meeting of the American Psychological Association (87th, New York, NY, September 1-5, 1979).

398. *A metaphor adapted from*: Kant I, *The Metaphysics of Morals*. 1785.

399. Forsyth DR, Berger RE, Mitchell T. 1981. The effects of self-serving vs. other-serving claims of responsibility on attraction and attribution in groups. *Social Psychology Quarterly*. 44, 59–64. *Of course, most mothers intuitively know this and so dilute their blame attempt by sandwiching it in a larger general context wherein blaming is not too salient. A common tactic is for a mother to blame someone else for her failure – 'the midwife pressured me' –*

*while simultaneously taking some responsibility – 'so reluctantly, I quit'.*

400. Schlenker BR. 1980. *Impression Management: The Self-concept, Social Identity, and Interpersonal Relations.* Monterey, CA: Brooks/Cole. p118. *Goffman calls such audience knowledge a 'dark secret':* Goffman E. 1990. *The Presentation of Self in Everyday Life.* London: Penguin Books. p141. *Just as it did with self-handicapping:*

401. Kelley HH. 1967. Attribution theory in social psychology. In Levine D (ed.) *Nebrasca Symposium on Motivation* (Vol. 15). Lincoln: University of Nebrasca Press.

402. Murphy E. 2004. 'Anticipatory Accounts'. *Symbolic Interaction.* 27(2): 129–154.

403. Murphy E. 2004. 'Anticipatory Accounts'. *Symbolic Interaction.* 27(2): 129–154.

404. Murphy was quoting Scott MB, Lyman S. 1963. Accounts. *American Sociological Review.* 33 (1):46–62 p52.

405. Kulik JA. 1983. Confirmatory attribution and the perpetuation of social beliefs. *Journal of Personality and Social Psychology.* 44, 1171–81.

406. *We all do this when we have a suspicion about someone. It's called 'Confirmatory Bias'.*

407. Bruner JS. 1957. Going beyond the information given. In Gruber HG, Terrell G, Wertheimer M (eds.) *Contemporary Approaches to Cognition.* Cambridge, MS: Harvard University Press.

408. Rhodewalt F, Sanbonmatsu DM, Tschanz B, Feick DL, Waller A. 1995. Self-handicapping and interpersonal trade-offs: The effects of claimed self-handicaps on observers' performance evaluations and feedback. *Personality and Social Psychology Bulletin.* 10, 1042–1050.

409. Schlenker BR, Pontari BA, Christopher AN, Excuses and Character: Personal and Social Implications of Excuses. Personality and Social Psychology Review. February 2001. Vol. 5 No. 1 15–32.

410. *The rule is known as the Norm of Internality, see:* Jellison JM, Green J. 1981. A self-presentation approach to the fundamental attribution error: The norm of internality. *Journal of Personality and Social Psychology.* 40, 643–9.

411. Holmes J. 1995. *Women, Men and Politeness.* Routledge; Hodgins HS, Liebeskind E, Schwartz W. 1996. Getting out of hot water: Facework in social predicaments. *Journal of Personality and Social Psychology.* 71, 300–314.

412. Goffman E. 1967. *Interaction Ritual: Essays on Face-to-face Behaviour.* Chicago: Aldine.

413. Brown P, Levinson SC. 1987. *Politeness: Some Universals in Language Usage.* Cambridge: Cambridge University Press. p61.

414. *On the anticipation of future interactions and its boost for face-saving, see:* Berscheid E, Graziano W, Monson T, Dermer M. 1976. Outcome dependency: Attention, attribution and attraction. *Journal of Personality and Social Psychology.* 34, 978–89; Miller DT, Norman SA, Wright E. 1978. Distortion in person perception as a consequence of the need for effective control. *Journal of Personality and Social Psychology.* 36, 598–607.

415. *Of course, just because something is socially acceptable it does not follow that it is morally or philosophically acceptable or that it does not have consequences.*

416. Leslie I. 2011. *Born Liars, Why We Can't Live Without Deceit.* Quercus.

417. O'Campo P, Faden RR, Gielen AC, Wang MC. Prenatal factors associated with breastfeeding duration: recommendations for prenatal interventions. *Birth.* 1992. Dec 19(4):195–201.

418. Buxton KE, Gielen AC, Faden RR, Brown CH, Paige DM, Chwalow AJ. Women intending to breastfeed: predictors of early infant feeding experiences. American Journal of Preventive Medicine. 1991. Mar-Apr;7(2):101–6.

419. Murphy E. 2004. 'Anticipatory Accounts', Symbolic Interaction 27(2): 129–154. p17.

420. Schlenker BR, Pontari BA, Chriostopher AN. 2001. Excuses and Character: Personal and Social Implications of Excuses. *Personality and Social Psychology Review.* 2001. Vol. 5, No. 1, 15–32.

421. *See the Guilt chapter to learn about reality negotiation.*

422. *Psychoanalysts have provided a wealth of field data on this behaviour, under the labels of 'repression' and 'dissociation'.*

423. McFarland C, Ross M. 1982. Impact of causal attributions on affective reactions to success and failure. *Journal of Personality and Social Psychology.* 43, 937–46.

424. *On reframing excuses as reasons, see:* Snyder CR. 1985. Collaborative companions: The relationship of self-deception and excuse-making. In Martin MW (ed.) *Self-Deception and Self-Understanding.* Lawrence KS: Regents Press. pp35–51.

425. Tavris C, Aronson E. 2007. *Mistakes Were Made (But Not By Me).* London: Pinter & Martin. p91.

426. *Karl Mannheim used the term 'self-distantiation' to describe this phenomenon*: Mannheim K. 1956. *Essays in the Sociology of Culture.* London: Routledge & Kegan Paul. p209.

427. Schulz K. 2011. Being Wrong – Adventures in the Margin of Error. Ecco. p218.

428. *For evidence of this behaviour, see*: Moore BS, Sherrod DR, Liu TJ, Underwood B. 1979. The dispositional shift in attribution over time. *Journal of Experimental Social Psychology.* 15, 553-69; Peterson C. 1980. Memory and the 'dispositional shift'. *Social Psychology Quarterly.* 43, 372–80.

429. *On excuse-making and memory-reconstruction, see*: Wells GL. 1982. Attribution and reconstructive memory. *Journal of Experimental Social Psychology.* 18, 447–63.

430. Ford CE, Berkman M. 1988. Women, dependency and depression. In Brehm SS (ed.) *Seeing Female: Social Roles and Personal Lives.* Westport, CT: Greenwood Press. pp91–100.

431. Allport, GW. 1943. *Becoming: Basic Considerations for a Psychology or Personality.* New Haven, CT: Yale University Press; Erikson EH. 1950. Childhood and Society. New York: Norton; Fromm E. 1955. *The Sane Society.* New York: Rinehart & Company; Rogers CR. 1959. A theory of therapy, personality, and interpersonal relationships, as developed in the client-centered framework. In Koch S (ed.) *Psychology: A Study of a Science, Vol. 3: Formulations of the Person and the Social Context.* New

York: McGraw-Hill. pp184–256); and Beck AT. 1976. *Cognitive Therapy and the Emotional Disorders*. International Universities Press.

432. Jahoda M. 1953. The meaning of psychological health. *Social Case Work*. October 349–354, p349.

433. DePaulo BM, Kashy DA. 1998. 'Everyday Lies in Close and Casual Relationships'. *Journal of Personality and Social Psychology*. 74: 63–79.

434. Lynd HM. 1971. The Nature of Shame. In Morris H (ed.) *Guilt and Shame*. California: Wadsworth Publishing Company.

435. Schlenker BR. 1980. *Impression Management: The Self-concept, Social identity, and Interpersonal Relations*. Monterey, CA: Brooks/Cole.

436. *Fact: lower future expectancies of success arise from lack of ability excuses. See*: Weiner B, Nierenberg R, Goldstein M. 1976. Social learning (locus of control) versus attributional (causal stability) interpretations of expectancy of success. *Journal of Personality*. 44, 52–68.

437. Goffman E. 1963. *Stigma: Notes on the Management of Spoiled Identity*. New Jersey: Penguin Books.

438. Tavris C, Aronson E. 2007. *Mistakes Were Made (But Not By Me)*. London: Pinter & Martin. pp9–10, p34.

439. Bulman RJ, Wortman CB. Attributions of blame and coping in the 'real world': severe accident victims react to their lot. Journal of Personality and Social Psychology. 1977, May 35(5):351–63.

440. Taylor SE. Adjustment to threatening events: A theory of cognitive adaptation. *American Psychologist*. Vol. 38(11), Nov 1983. 1161–1173.

441. And then spiral into Envy and Sabotage, as we will explore shortly.

442. Abramson LY, Seligman MEP, Teasdale JD. 1978. Learned helplessness in humans: Critique and reformation. *Journal of Abnormal Psychology*. 87, 49–74.

443. *As an extra bonus, taking responsibility is seen favourably by others: studies have shown that individuals are rated as more modest and honest when they attribute their failure to an internal rather than external source* (Carlston DE and Shovar N. 1983. Effects of performance attributions on others' perceptions of the attributor. *Journal of Personality and Social Psychology*. Vol. 44(3), Mar 1983. 515–525).

444. Berke JH. 1988. *The Tyranny of Malice*. New York: Summit Books.

445. *For more information on entitlement as a prerequisite for envy, see*: Berman A. 2007. Envy at the crossroad between destruction and self-actualization, and avoidance, in Navaro L, Schwartzberg SL. 2007. *Envy, Competition and Gender: Theory, Clinical Applications and Group Work*. London: Routledge.

446. *As cited by* Baumann P. 26 October, 2003. Joseph Epstein Assays Another Human Failing, *Chicago Tribune Books*. pp1–2.

447. *In fact, from an evolutionary perspective, people are biologically disposed to feel hostility when confronted with such experiences. The breastfeeding dyad has an evolutionary advantage over the non-breastfeeding dyad. Breastfed babies and their nursing mothers enjoy a wealth of physiological and psychological benefits; formula feeders are often painfully aware of this imbalance.*

448. Thaler RH, Sunstein CR. 2009. *Nudge: Improving Decisions about Health, Wealth and Happiness*. London: Penguin Books.

449. Warnes H, Hill G. 1974. 'Gender Identity and the Wish to be a Woman'. *Psychosomatics* 15 (1): 25–29.
450. Cooley CH. 1902. *Human Nature and the Social Order* (revised edition). New York: Charles Scribner's Sons. p184.
451. In Navaro L, Schwartzberg SL. 2007. *Envy, Competition and Gender: Theory, Clinical Applications and Group Work.* London: Routledge. p150.
452. We'll explore such strategic behaviour more thoroughly in the Sabotage chapter.
453. *Some Asian cultures take a slightly more unorthodox approach to fending off breastfeeding-related envy; they believe spitting on the suckling baby will help:* Dundes T. 1981. *The Evil Eye: A Folklore Casebook.* New York: Garland Publishing Inc.
454. Brody LR. 1997. Gender and emotion: Beyond stereotypes. *Journal of Social Issues.* 53: 369–394; Fabes RA, Martin CL. 1991. Gender and Age Stereotypes of Emotionality. *Personality and Social Psychology Bulletin.* 17: 532–540.
455. Berke JH. 1988. *The Tyranny of Malice.* New York: Summit Books.
456. Spiro A. 2005. Najar or bhut - evil eye or ghost affliction: Gujarati views about illness causation. *Anthropology and Medicine.* Routledge. p64.
457. Dundes T. 1981. *The Evil Eye: A Folklore Casebook.* New York: Garland Publishing Inc.
458. Geckil E, Sahin T, Ege E. Traditional postpartum practices of women and infants and the factors influencing such practices in South Eastern Turkey. *Midwifery.* 2009. 25:62–71.
459. Takahashi H et al. When Your Gain Is My Pain and Your Pain Is My Gain: Neural Correlates of Envy and Schadenfreude. *Science.* 13 February 2009: Vol. 323 no. 5916 pp937–939; Feather NT, Sherman R. Envy, Resentment, Schadenfreude, and Sympathy: Reactions to Deserved and Undeserved Achievement and Subsequent Failure. *Personality and Social Psychology Bulletin.* July 2002. Vol. 28 no.7 953–961; Van Dijk WW et al. When people fall from grace: Reconsidering the role of envy in schadenfreude. *Emotion.* Vol. 6(1), Feb 2006, 156–160; Shamay-Tsoory SG et al. The green-eyed monster and malicious joy: the neuroanatomical bases of envy and gloating (schadenfreude). *Brain.* 2007. 130 (6): 1663–1678.
460. Berman A. 2007. Envy at the crossroad between destruction and self-actualization, and avoidance, in Navaro L, Schwartzberg SL. 2007. *Envy, Competition and Gender: Theory, Clinical Applications and Group Work.* London: Routledge.
461. Solomon RC. 2009. *True to Our Feelings: What Our Emotions Are Really Telling Us.* New York: Oxford University Press. p103.
462. Young-Eisendrath P. 1997. *Gender and Desire.* Texas: A&M University Press. p40. *We see a form of hatred in those mothers who seek to avoid their breastfeeding peers. Webster's New World College Dictionary defines hate as 'to dislike or wish to avoid; shrink from'.*
463. Triumphant Tuesday: Cosleeping to Aid Breastfeeding. Tuesday, 3 September 2013. Available at: www.thealphaparent.com/2013/09/triumphant-tuesday-cosleeping-to-aid.html
464. *Guardian journalist Katha Pollitt summed up the general gist of the wars (well,*

*the media perception, at least):* 'Women are so eager to blame themselves and one another about, well, everything – weight, looks, clothes, sexual behaviour (you haven't lived till you've heard a seventh-grade girl refer to another as a "ho"), marriages and, of course, baybeez, every wrinkle of whose behaviour is directly attributable to their mothers' having made some small but fatal mistake'. See: Pollitt K. Attachment parenting: more guilt for mothers. *The Guardian.* Friday 18 May 2012. Available at: www. theguardian.com/commentisfree/2012/may/18/attachment-parenting-guilt-mothers

465. Maslow AH. 1970. *Motivation and Personality.* New York: Longman. p27.

466. Tarrant M, Fong DY, Wu KM, Lee IL, Wong EM, Sham A, Lam C, Dodgson JE. 2010 Breastfeeding and weaning practices among Hong Kong mothers: a prospective study. *BMC Pregnancy Childbirth.* May 29; 10–27; Horta BL, Victora IC, Gigante DP, Santos IJ, Barros FC. 2007. Breastfeeding duration in two generations. *Rev Saude Publica.* 41(1), 13–18; Battersby S. 2010. Understanding the social and cultural influences on breast-feeding today. *Journal of Family Health Care.* 20(4):128–31; Salt MJ, Law CM, Bull AR, Osmond C. 1994. Determinants of breastfeeding in Salisbury and Durham. *Journal of Public Health Medicine.* 16, 291–295; Riva E, Agostini C. 1999. Factors associated with initiation and duration of breastfeeding in Italy. *Acta Pediatrica.* 88, 411–415.

467. Leff EW, Gagne MP, Jefferis SC. Maternal perceptions of successful breastfeeding. *Journal of Human Lactation.* 1994. 10:99–104.

468. Loof-Johanson M, Foldevi M, Edvard Rudebeck C. 2013. Breastfeeding as a Specific Value in Women's Lives: The Experiences and Decisions of Breastfeeding Women. *Breastfeeding Medicine.* 8, 1, p41.

469. Loof-Johanson M, Foldevi M, Edvard Rudebeck C. 2013. Breastfeeding as a Specific Value in Women's Lives: The Experiences and Decisions of Breastfeeding Women. *Breastfeeding Medicine.* 8, 1. p41.

470. Loof-Johanson M, Foldevi M, Edvard Rudebeck C. 2013. Breastfeeding as a Specific Value in Women's Lives: The Experiences and Decisions of Breastfeeding Women. *Breastfeeding Medicine.* 8, 1. p39.

471. Manhire KM, Hagan AE, Floyd SA. A descriptive account of New Zealand mother's responses to open-ended questions on their breastfeeding experiences. *Midwifery.* 2007. 23:372–381.

472. Loof-Johanson M, Foldevi M, Edvard Rudebeck C. 2013. Breastfeeding as a Specific Value in Women's Lives: The Experiences and Decisions of Breastfeeding Women. *Breastfeeding Medicine.* 8, 1. p40.

473. Kearney MH. Identifying psychosocial obstacles to breastfeeding success. *Journal of Obstetric, Gynecologic & Neonatal Nursing.* 1988. Mar-Apr;17(2):98–105. See also: American Academy of Pediatrics. 2005. Breastfeeding and the use of human milk. *Pediatrics.* 115, 469–506 *in which mothers' willingness to share close proximity with a fussy infant is recognised as an 'essential skill for successful breastfeeding'.*

474. *When a mother quits breastfeeding prematurely (the definition of what constitutes 'premature cessation of breastfeeding' is, of course, highly culturally relative), she will lose at least some of this symbolic capital. The amount of capital lost is relative to the length of time she managed to breastfeed for. So,*

*for instance, a mother quitting after six months will be able to retain quite a significant amount of this symbolic kudos, whereas a mother who quit at the one-week mark will retain very little. Mothers who exclusively breastfeed for the 'gold standard' of six months earn the-mother-of-all-kudos. Interestingly, this cultural capital functions on a bell curve, with the amount mothers can earn ironically declining once the child reaches toddlerhood. And if the mother breastfeeds into the preschool years, she will have capital steadily deducted for being strange and culturally deviant. One study, for instance, found that mothers had 100 percent support in the first months of breastfeeding, silence/ noncommittal at six months, and open discouragement after 9–10 months. See:* Morse JM, Harrison MJ. 1987. Social coercion for weaning. *Journal of Nurse Midwifery.* 32(4), 205–209.

475. *By 'science', I'm using the term in its broadest sense, as illustrated by the UK Department for Innovation, Universities & Skills:* 'By science we mean all-encompassing knowledge based on scholarship and research undertaken in the physical, biological, engineering, medical, natural and social disciplines, including the arts and humanities, which is underpinned by methodologies that build up and test increased understanding about our world and beyond'. UK Department for Innovation, Universities & Skills. 2008. A Vision for Science and Society: A consultation on developing a new strategy for the UK. Available at: https://www.gov.uk/government/uploads/system/uploads/attachment_data/file/36747/49-08-S_b.pdf

476. Faircloth C. 2010b. '"If They Want to Risk the Health and Well-being of Their Child, That's Up to Them": Long-term Breastfeeding, Risk and Maternal Identity.' *Heath, Risk and Society.* 12(4): 357–67

477. Murphy E. 1999. 'Breast is best': infant feeding decisions and maternal deviance. *Sociology of Health and Illness.* 21, 187–208.

478. Triumphant Tuesday: Breastfeeding After Breast Trauma. Tuesday, 11 June 2013. Available at: www.thealphaparent.com/2013/06/triumphant-tuesday-breastfeeding-after.html

479. Triumphant Tuesday: Breastfeeding With Just One Breast. Tuesday, 23 July 2013. Available at: www.thealphaparent.com/2013/07/triumphant-tuesday-breastfeeding-with.html

480. *For more on this definition, see:* Tenhouten WD. 2007. *General Theory of Emotions and Social Life.* Routledge.

481. *So common is this behaviour, that it has attracted numerous labels, including 'Self Serving Attribution Bias', 'Beneffectance' and more crudely, 'Attributional Egotism'.*

482. Weiner B, Freize L, Kukla A, Reed L, Rest S, Rosenbaum R. Perceiving the causes of success and failure. In Jones EE, Kanouse DE, Nisbett RE, Valins S, Weiner B (eds.) *Attribution.* 1971. Morristown, NJ: General Learning Press; Streufert S, Streufert SC. The effects of conceptual structure, failure, and success on attributions of causality and interpersonal attitudes. *Journal of Personality and Social Psychology.* 1969, 18, 139–145; Wortman C, Costanzo PR, Witt TR. Effects of anticipated performance on the attributions of causality to self and others. *Journal of Personality and Social Psychology.* 1973, 27, 372–381.

483. Schulz K. 2010. *Being Wrong: Adventures in the Margin of Error*. London: Portobello Books.

484. *It is important not to poo-poo or underestimate this cognitive bias and its widespread application in all spheres of the 'Mummy Wars'. For more info on this bias, see*: Lerner MJ, Miller DT. 1978. 'Just World' research and the attribution process: Looking back and ahead. *Psychological Bulletin*, 85, 1030–51; Ryan W. 1971. *Blaming the Victim*. New York: Pantheon.

485. Ross L, Greene D, House P. 1977. The 'false consensus effect': An egocentric bias in social perception and attribution processes. *Journal of Experimental Social Psychology*. 13, 279–301.

486. Triumphant Tuesday: Breastfeeding a Baby with Facial Malformation. Tuesday, 8 January 2013, Available at: www.thealphaparent. com/2013/01/triumphant-tuesday-breastfeeding-baby.html

487. Bell M. 2005. 'A Woman's Scorn: Toward a Feminist Defense of Contempt as a Moral Emotion'. *Hypatia*. 20 (4): 80.

488. Underwood MK. 2004. 'Glares of Contempt, Eye Rolls of Disgust and Turning Away to Exclude: Non-Verbal Forms of Social Aggression among Girls'. *Feminism & Psychology*. 14 (3): 371.

489. Lamontagne C, Hamelin A, St-Pierre M. The breastfeeding experience of women with major difficulties who use the services of a breastfeeding clinic: a descriptive study. *International Breastfeeding Journal*. 2008. 3:17.

490. Aronson E, Mills J. 1959. The effect of severity of initiation on liking for a group. *Journal of Abnormal and Social Psychology*. 59, 177–181; Beauvois LJ, Joule RV. 1996. *A Radical Dissonance Theory*. London: Taylor & Francis.

491. Tavris C, Aronson E. 2007. *Mistakes Were Made (But Not By Me)*. London: Pinter & Martin, pp9–10, emphasis theirs.

492. Jung CG. 1996. *The Archetypes and the Collective Unconscious*. London: Routledge.

493. Jaffe A. 1984. *Jung's Last Years and Other Essays* (Jungian Classics Series). Spring Publications (revised sub. edition).

494. Freud S. 1895/1966. Extracts from the Fliess papers. In *The Complete Psychological Works of Freud* (Vol. 1). London: Hogarth Press. p270.

495. 'Is it ever OK to call someone a Nazi?'. BBC News. July 14, 2010. *To learn more about Godwin's Law and its anti-breastfeeding deployment, see my blog post* 'A Word About Nazis' available at: www.thealphaparent. com/2013/08/a-word-about-nazis.html

496. *A confusing state of affairs when you consider emotional relativism!*

497. *Consider also that moral and legal restraints on freedom of speech are designed to protect minorities. Yet formula-feeding mothers are far from a minority, and thus logically, should not especially vulnerable to the pain of being held in contempt.*

498. *Take as a metaphorical example, two teachers. One is authoritarian and the other permissive. The authoritarian teacher (pro-contempt) expects hard work and places responsibility for outcomes on the pupils themselves. In contrast, the permissive teacher (anti-contempt) offers reassurance to the pupils when things go wrong, regardless of the cause. Which of these teachers do you think would best cultivate the pupils's confidence in their own capabilities? Which*

approach do you think would best enhance breastfeeding rates: 1. 'With effort, you can breastfeed' or 2. 'Don't worry, it doesn't matter whether you succeed or not'. This analogy was adopted from psycho-analyst George Lakoff's dichotomy of conservative and liberal philosophies, which he respectively related to the metaphors of father as strict disciplinarian and mother as a source of unconditional love and comfort. See: Lakoff G. 2002. Moral Politics: How Liberals And Conservatives Think (2nd edition). University of Chicago Press.

499. Pediatrics. May, 2010.

500. A comprehensive run-down of how formula feeding affects each and every one of us is available at: www.thealphaparent.com/2011/10/why-way-you-feed-your-baby-is-my.html

501. Browne A. 2006. The Retreat of Reason: Political Correctness and the Corruption of Public Debate in Modern Britain. Civitas: Institute for the Study of Civil Society.

502. Palmer G. 2009. The Politics of Breastfeeding: When Breasts are Bad for Business. London: Pinter & Martin.

503. Kerri Norman, member of The Alpha Parent Facebook page. 2013.

504. ...said SMA formula in their 2013/14 television advertisement.

505. Bell M. 2013. Hard Feelings: The Moral Psychology of Contempt. Oxford: Oxford University Press.

506. Darwall S. 2009. The Second-Person Standpoint: Morality, Respect, and Accountability. Cambridge, MA: Harvard University Press.

507. Baier K. 1966. The Moral Point of View: A Rational Basis of Ethics. Cornell University Press. p223.

508. Solomon R. 2006. True to Our Feelings: What Our Emotions Are Really Telling Us. Oxford: OUP.

509. Bercheid E. 1966 Opinion change and communicator-comunicatee similarity and dissimilarity. Journal of Personality and Social Psychology. 4, 670–680; Bettinghous EP. 1968. Persuasive Communication. New York: Holt, Rinehart & Winston.

510. Schulz K. 2010. Being Wrong. London: Portobello Books. p200.

511. Phillips A. 2012. Missing Out: In Praise of the Unlived Life. Hamish Hamilton.

512. Spock B. 2004. Dr. Spock's Baby and Childcare. Simon & Schuster UK.

513. Westen D, Kilts C, Blagov P et al. 2006. The neural basis of motivated reasoning: an fMRI study of emotional constraints on political judgement during the U.S. presidential election of 2004. Journal of Cognitive Neuroscience. 18, pp1947–1958.

514. To read up on re-lactation, including the herbs, foods, pumping schedule and that alienesque supplemental nursing system, check out Hormann E. Breastfeeding an Adopted Baby and Relactation. La Leche League International.

515. Rosenberg MJ, Abelson RP. 1960. An analysis of cognitive balancing. In Rosenberg MJ, Hovland CI, McGuire WJ, Abelson RP, Brehm JW (eds.) Attitude Organization and Change. New Haven, CT: Yale University Press. pp112–163.

516. Goethals GR, Cooper J. 1975. When dissonance is reduced: The timing

of self-justificatory attitude change. *Journal of Personality and Social Psychology*. 32, 361–367.

517. Feldman R. 2009. *Liar: The Truth About Lying*. Virgin Books. p128.

518. Trivers R. 2011. *Deceit and Self-Deception: Fooling Yourself the Better to Fool Others*. Allen Lane.

519. Freud A. 1948. *The Ego and the Mechanics of Defence*. London: Hogarth Press.

520. Dube R. 2011. The Mom-Judging Olympics: A competition nobody meant to enter. Aug. 11, 2011, TODAY.com

521. Schenkel S. 1975. Relationship among ego identity status, field-independence, and traditional femininity. *Journal of Youth and Adolescence*. March 1975, Vol. 4, Issue 1, pp73–82.

522. Crossley ML. 2009. Breastfeeding as a moral imperative: An autoethnographic study. *Feminism and Psychology*. 19, 71–87, p82.

523. *Some have also labelled it 'vicarious personalism'* (Cooper J, Fazio RH. 1979. The formation and persistence of attitudes that support intergroup conflict. In Austin WG, Worchel S (eds.) *The Social Psychology of Intergroup Relations*. Monterey, CA: Brooks/Cole.

524. *On the utility to self-esteem of specific vs global attributions, see*: Greenberg J, Pyszczynski T. 1985. Compensatory self-inflation: A response to the threat to self-regard of public failure. *Journal of Personality and Social Psychology*. 49, 273–280.

525. *On the topic of downward comparisons, see*: Grunder CL. 1977. Choice of comparison persons in evaluating oneself. In Suls JM, Miller RL (eds.) *Social Comparison Processes: Theoretical and Empirical Perspectives*. Washington, DC: Hemisphere; and Wills TA. 1981. Downward comparison principles in social psychology. *Psychological Bulletin*. 90, 245–271.

526. Taylor SE, Gollwitzer PM. 1995. Effects of mindset on positive illusions. *Journal of Personality and Social Psychology*. 69, 213–226.

527. Clair MS, Snyder CR. 1979. Effects of instructor-delivered sequential evaluative feedings. *Journal of Educational Psychology*. 71, 50–57; Syder CR, Clair MS. 1976. Effects of expected and obtained grades on teacher evaluation and attribution of performance. *Journal of Educational Psychology*. 68, 75–82; Snyder CR, Shenkel RJ. 1976. Effects of 'favourability', modality, and relevance upon acceptance of general personality interpretations prior to and after receiving diagnostic feedback. *Journal of Consulting and Clinical Psychology*. 44, 34–41.

528. *We looked at this phenomenon, known as 'confirmation bias', in the Deception chapter when we examined how pregnant women attend to research.*

529. *This template is known as 'confirmation bias'. See*: Lord C, Ross L, Lepper M. 1979. Biased assimilation and attitude polarization: the effects of prior theories on subsequently considered evidence. *Journal of Personality and Social Psychology*. 37, pp2098–2109.

530. *Otherwise known as the Self-serving Bias.*

531. McVea KL, Turner PD, Peppler DK. 2000. The role of breastfeeding in sudden infant death syndrome. *Journal of Human Lactation*, 16: 13–20.

532. Mills J. 1965. Avoidance of dissonant information. *Journal of Personality*

*and Social Psychology.* 2, 589–593; Mills J. 1965. Effect of certainty about a decision on postdecision exposure to consonant and dissonant information. *Journal of Personality and Social Psychology.* 2, 749–752.

533. Monteith MJ. 1993. Self-regulation of prejudiced responses: Implications for progress in prejudice-reduction efforts. *Journal of Personality and Social Psychology.* 65, 469–485.

534. Williams Z. *What Not to Expect When You're Expecting.* Guardian Books. p90.

535. Lefcourt HM. 1976. *Locus of Control: Current Trends in Theory and Research.* Hillsdale, NJ: Lawrence Erlbaum Associates.

536. Phares EJ. 1973. *Locus of Control: A Personality Determinant of Behaviour.* Morristown, NJ: General Learning Press; Phares EJ. 1976. *Locus of Control in Personality.* Morristown, NJ: General Learning Press; Rotter JB. 1966. Generalized expectancies for internal versus external control of reinforcement. *Psychological Monographs.* 80 (Whole No. 609).

537. Analogy borrowed from Schulz K. 2010. *Being Wrong, Adventures in the Margin of Error.* London: Portobello Books.

538. Cooley CH. 1902. *Human Nature and the Social Order* (revised edition). New York: Charles Scribner's Sons.

539. Palmer G. *The Politics of Breastfeeding.* London: Pinter & Martin.

540. Conley C. 2013. *Emotional Equations.* London: Piatkus.

541. Maccoby EE. 1966. *The Development of Sex Differences.* Stanford: Stanford University Press.

542. Nelson AM. 2006. Toward a situation-specific theory of breastfeeding. *Research and Theory for Nursing Practice: An International Journal.* 20, 9–27.

543. Navaro L. 2007. Snow Whites, stepmothers, and hunters: gender dynamics in envy and competition in the family, in Navaro L, Schewartzbery SL. 2007. *Envy, Competition and Gender: Theory, Clinical Applications and Group Work.* London: Routledge.

544. Freud S. 1921. *Group Psychology and the Analysis of the Ego.* S.E. Vol.18.

545. Orbach S, Eichenbaum L. 1994. *Between Women.* London: Arrow Books. p93.

546. Marshall, J. 2011. Motherhood, breastfeeding and identity. *Practising Midwife.* 14 (2). pp16–18. ISSN 1461-3123.

547. For a typical example, see: Hall Smith P, Coley SL, Labbok MH, Cupito S, Nwokah E. 2012. Early breastfeeding experiences of adolescent mothers: a qualitative prospective study. *International Breastfeeding Journal.* 2012. 7:13.

548. Asch SE. 1946. Forming impressions of personality. *Journal of Abnormal and Social Psychology.* 41, 258–290.

549. Bandura A. 1977. *Social-learning Theory.* Englewood Cliffs, NJ: Prentice Hall.

550. Schulz K. 2010. *Being Wrong.* London: Portobello Books. p143.

551. Osman H, El Zein L, Wick L. Cultural beliefs that may discourage breastfeeding among Lebanese women: a qualitative analysis. *International Breastfeeding Journal.* 2009. 4:12.

552. Rochman B. Sep 20, 2010. In the Battle Over Breast or Bottle, Guilt

May Play a Role. *Time Magazine*. Available at: healthland.time.com/2010/09/20/in-the-battle-over-breast-or-bottle-guilt-may-play-a-role/

553. *A term used in* Hannon PA, Bowen DJ, Moinpour CM, McLerran DF. Correlations in perceived food use between the family food preparer and their spouses and children. *Appetite*. 2003. 40(1):77–83.

554. Parkinson J et al. 2010. The Role of Mother-centred Factors Influencing the Complex Social Behaviour of Breastfeeding: Social Support and Self-efficacy. ANZMAC Annual Conference 2010; Dennis C-L, 1999. Theoretical underpinnings of breastfeeding confidence; a self-efficacy framework. *Journal of Human Lactation*. 15, 195–201; Dennis C-L, Faux S. 1999. Development and psychometric testing of the breastfeeding self-efficacy scale. *Research in Nursing and Health*. 22 399–409.

555. Groleau D, Rodriguez C: Breastfeeding and poverty: negotiating cultural change and symbolic capital in Quebec, Canada. In Dykes F, Hall Moran V (eds.) *Infant and Young Child Feeding: Challenges to Implementing a Global Strategy*. Oxford: Blackwell Publishing; 2009. 80-98.

556. Brownell K, Hutton L, Hartman J, Dabraw S: Barriers to breastfeeding among African American adolescent mothers. *Clinical Pediatrics*. 2002. 41(9):669–673; Hannon PR, Willis SK, Bishop-Townsend V, Martinez IM, Scrimshaw SC. African-American and Latina adolescent mothers' infant feeding decisions and breastfeeding practices: a qualitative study. *Journal of Adolescent Health*. 2000. 26(6):399–407; Nelson AM. Adolescent attitudes, beliefs, and concerns regarding breastfeeding. *The MCM American Journal of Maternal/Child Nursing*. 2009. 34(4):249–255. Wambach KA, Koehn M. Experiences of infant-feeding decision-making among urban economically disadvantaged pregnant adolescents. *Journal of Advanced Nursing*. 2004. 48(4):361–370. Pierre N, Emans SJ, Odeidallah DA et al. Choice of feeding method of adolescent mothers: does ego development play a role? *Journal of Pediatric & Adolescent Gynecology*. 1999. 12:83–89. Black MM, Siegel EH, Abel Y, Bentley ME. Home and videotape intervention delays early complementary feeding among adolescent mothers. *Pediatrics*. 2001. 107(5):e67. Wiemann CM, DuBois JC, Berenson AB. Strategies to promote breastfeeding among adolescent mothers. *Archives of Pediatric & Adolescent Medicine*. 1998. 152(9):862–869. Moran VH, Edwards J, Dykes F, Downe S. A systematic review of the nature of support for breastfeeding adolescent mothers. *Midwifery*. 2007. 23(2):157–171. Lavender T, Thompson S, Wood L. Supporting teenage mothers with breastfeeding guardians. *British Journal of Midwifery*. 2005, 13(6):354–359; Dykes F, Moran VH, Burt S, Edwards J: Adolescent mothers and breastfeeding: experiences and support needs–an exploratory study. *Journal of Humam Lactation*. 2003. 19(4):391–401; Committee on Health Care for Underserved Women, Committee on Obstetric Practice: Breastfeeding: maternal and infant aspects. *ACOG Clinical Review*. 2007. 12:1S-16S; Martinez JC, Ashworth A, Kirkwood B. Breast-feeding among the urban poor in southern Brazil: reasons for termination in the first 6 months of life. *Bulletin of the World Health Organization*. 1989. 67:151–161.

557. Spock B. 2004. *Dr. Spock's Baby and Childcare*. Simon & Schuster UK.
558. Carson TL. 2010. *Lying and Deception, Theory and Practice*. Oxford: OUP.
559. Triumphant Tuesday: Breastfeeding with Large Nipples. Tuesday, 4 June 2013. Available at: www.thealphaparent.com/2013/06/triumphant-tuesday-breastfeeding-with.html
560. UK Infant Feeding Survey 2010.
561. *For example, see*: Kaneko A, Kaneita Y, Yokoyama E, Miyake T, Harano S, Suzuki K, Ibuka E, Tsutsui T, Yamamoto Y, Ohida T. Factors associated with exclusive breast-feeding in Japan: for activities to support child-rearing with breast-feeding. *Journal of Epidemiology & Community Health*. 2006. 16(2):57–63; Osman H, El Zein L, Wick L. Cultural beliefs that may discourage breastfeeding among Lebanese women: a qualitative analysis. *International Breastfeeding Journal*. 2009. 4:12; Grassley JS, Eschiti V. The value of listening to grandmothers' infant-feeding stories. *Journal of Perinatal Education*. 2011. Summer; 20(3):134–41; Liu P, Qiao L, Xu F, Zhang M, Wang Y, Binns CW. 2013. Factors associated with breastfeeding duration. *Journal of Human Lactation*. 2013. May, 29(2):253–9; Bedard S. 1995. *Factors Associated with Breastfeeding Duration*. College of Nursing, University of Utah. p71
562. Beske EJ, Garvis MS. Important factors in breast-feeding success. *MCN, American Journal of Maternal/Child Nursing*. 1982. 7:174–179.
563. Grassley JS, Eschiti V. The value of listening to grandmothers' infant-feeding stories. *Journal of Perinatal Education*. 2011. Summer; 20(3):134–41.
564. Cockrell S, O'Neill C, Stone J. 2007. *Baby-Proofing Your Marriage*. London: Collins.
565. Jolin L. 2009. *Coping with Birth Trauma and Postnatal Depression*. London: Sheldon Press.
566. 'Grandparents Behaving Badly'. NBC News. Available at: www.nbcnews.com/id/24842642/ns/health-childrens_health/t/grandparents-behaving-badly/#.U2f_7_ldVfg
567. *In one study, not living with their own mothers and fathers (grandparents of infants) was positively associated with mothers' breastfeeding status six months after birth, compared with those who lived with their parents* (Kaneko A, Kaneita Y, Yokoyama E, Miyake T, Harano S, Suzuki K, Ibuka E, Tsutsui T, Yamamoto Y, Ohida T. Factors associated with exclusive breast-feeding in Japan: for activities to support child-rearing with breast-feeding. *Journal of Epidemiology & Community Health*. 2006. 16(2):57–63).
568. Liu P, Qiao L, Xu F, Zhang M, Wang Y, Binns CW. 2013. Factors associated with breastfeeding duration. *Journal of Human Lactation*. 2013. May 29(2):253–9.
569. Osman H, El Zein L, Wick L. Cultural beliefs that may discourage breastfeeding among Lebanese women: a qualitative analysis. *International Breastfeeding Journal*. 2009. 4:12
570. Bedard S. 1995. *Factors Associated with Breastfeeding Duration*. College of Nursing, University of Utah. p71.
571. Baby Center 2010. Available at: www.babycenter.com/0_the-new-mom-

body-survey-7-000-women-tell-it-like-it-is_3653252.bc

572. Kutzen S, Brockman B, Shinkarev S. 2007. *Grandparenting: Tales From The Crib - When Your Children Become Parents*. Global Source Publishing.

573. 'Grandparents Behaving Badly'. NBC News. Available at: www.nbcnews. com/id/24842642/ns/health-childrens_health/t/grandparents-behaving-badly/#.U2f_7_ldVfg

574. Susin LR, Giugliani ER, Kummer SC. Influence of grandmothers on breastfeeding practices. *Revista de Saúde Publica*. 2005. Apr, 39(2):141–7.

575. Weinstein EA, Deutschberger P. 1963. 'Some dimensions of altercasting'. *Sociometry*. 26, 454–466.

576. Blumstein P. 1975. Identity bargaining and self-conception. *Social Forces*. 53, 476–485.

577. *To have a poke around the colourful world of lactation, see*: Giles F. 2003. *Fresh Milk: The Secret Life of Breasts*. Simon & Schuster.

578. WHO bulletin, OMS Supplement Vol. 87, 1989. p23. Available at: whqlibdoc. who.int/bulletin/1989/Vol67-Supp/bulletin_1989_67(supp)_2.pdf

579. Schulz K. 2010. *Being Wrong: Adventures in the Margin of Error*. London: Portobello Books. p213.

580. Barbalet JM. 1998. *Emotion, Social Theory and Social Structure: A Macrosoiological Approach*. Cambridge: Cambridge University Press. p27.

581. Barbalet.J.M. 1998 Macrosociology: Emotion, Social Theory and Social Structure. Cambridge: Cambridge University Press

582. Maxwell JC. 1995. Coping with Bereavement through Activism: Real Grief, Imagined Death, and Pseudo-Mourning. Douglas W. 2003. *Bad News, Good News: Controversial Order in Everyday Talk and Clinical Settings*. Chicago: University of Chicago Press; Milligan MJ. 2005. Ambivalent Passion and Passionate Ambivalence: Emotions and the Historic Preservation Movement. Presented at the annual meeting of the American Sociological Association, Philadelphia, PA.

583. Schulz K. 2010. *Being Wrong: Adventures in the Margin of Error*. London: Portobello Books. p207.

584. Hoddinott P, Pill R. 1999. Qualitative study of decisions about infant feeding among women in East End of London. *British Medical Journal*. 318, 30–34.

585. Mozingo JN, Davis MW, Droppleman PG, Merideth A. 'It wasn't working.' Women's experiences with short-term breastfeeding. *MCN, American Journal of Maternal/Child Nursing*. 2000. May–Jun, 25(3):120–6.

586. Andrews GR, Debus RL. 1978. Persistence and the causal perception of failure: Modifying cognitive attributions. *Journal of Educational Psychology*. 70, 154–66; Dweck CS. 1975. The role of expectations and attributions in the alleviation of learned helplessness. *Journal of Personality and Social Psychology*. 31, 674–85; Anderson CA. 1983. Motivational and performance deficits in interpersonal settings: The effect of attributional style. *Journal of Personality and Social Psychology*. 45, 1136–47.

587. *On the virtues of self-blame, see*: Bains G. 1983. Explanations and the need for control. In Hewstone M (ed.) *Attribution Theory: Social and Functional Extensions*. Oxford: Basil Blackwell; Langer EJ. 1975. The illusion of

control. *Journal of Personality and Social Psychology*. 32, 311–28; Wortman C. 1976. Causal attributions and personal control. In Harvey JH, Ickles WJ, Kidd RF (eds.) *New Directions in Attribution Research* (Vol. 1). Hillsdale NJ: Erlbaum.

588. *While you're researching, be mindful of the cognitive biases we discussed in the Deception chapter. Glance over the section entitled Learning to Choose, Choosing to Learn.*

589. *Recall the fancy Transtheoretical Model of Behaviour Change in the deception chapter? You're currently in stage 3 – the preparation stage. By virtue of reading this book, you already passed through stages 1 and 3 – precontemplation and contemplation – so most of your 'attitude-work' is already done!*

590. Newman J. 2014. *Dr. Jack Newman's Guide to Breastfeeding* (updated edition). London: Pinter & Martin.

591. *Peer supporters possess the practical acumen that certificate-laden health 'professionals' often lack. See my blog post*: Why Some Lactation Consultants Fail Breastfeeding Mothers available at: www.thealphaparent. com/2014/08/why-some-lactation-consultants-fail.html;   also   see: Battersby S, Aziz M, Bennett K, Sabin K. 2004. The cost-effectiveness of breastfeeding peer support. *British Journal of Midwifery*. 12 (4) 201-205.

592. *This is Stage 4 of the Transtheoretical Model of Behaviour Change – the action stage. Beware: while residing in this stage, you are most susceptible to quitting.*

593. Mohrbacher N, Stock J. 1997. *The Breastfeeding Answer Book* (revised edition). Illinois: La Leche League International. p28.

594. *This is stage 5 – the Maintenance stage – of the Transtheoretical Model of Behaviour Change.*

595. Available at: www.who.int/nutrition/topics/exclusive_breastfeeding/ en/ and www.unicef.org.uk/Documents/Baby_Friendly/Guidance/ Implementation%20Guidance/Step_8_Implementation.pdf

# Bibliography

Akre J. 2006. *The Problem with Breastfeeding: A Personal Reflection.* Amarillo, Texas: Hale Publishing

Allport, GW. 1943. *Becoming: Basic Considerations for a Psychology or Personality.* New Haven, CT: Yale University Press

Artiss K. 1959. *The Symptom as Communication in Schizophrenia.* New York: Grune and Stratton

Baier K. 1966. *The Moral Point of View: A Rational Basis of Ethics.* Cornell University Press

Bandura A. 1997. *Self-Efficacy: The Exercise of Control.* New York: Freeman

Bandura A. 1977. *Social-learning Theory.* Englewood Cliffs, NJ: Prentice Hall

Barbalet JM. 1998. *Emotion, Social Theory and Social Structure: A Macrosoiological Approach.* Cambridge: Cambridge University Press

Baron-Cohen S. 2012. *The Essential Difference: Men, Women and the Extreme Male Brain.* Penguin Books

Barston S. 2012. *Bottled Up: How the Way We Feed Babies Has Come to Define Motherhood, and Why it Shouldn't.* CA: University of California Press

Baumslag N. 1995. *Milk, Money and Madness: The Culture and Politics of Breastfeeding.* Bergin & Garvey

Beauvois LJ, Joule RV. 1996. *A Radical Dissonance Theory.* London: Taylor & Francis

Beck AT. 1976. *Cognitive Therapy and the Emotional Disorders.* International Universities Press

Becker H. 1963. *Outsiders.* New York: Free Press

Bedard S. 1995. *Factors Associated with Breastfeeding Duration.* College of Nursing, University of Utah

Bell M. 2013. *Hard Feelings: The Moral Psychology of Contempt.* Oxford: Oxford University Press

Berke JH. 1988. *The Tyranny of Malice.* New York: Summit Books

Berkowitz L (ed.) *Advances in Experimental Social Psychology* (Vol. 2). New York: Academic Press

Bettinghous EP. 1968. *Persuasive Communication*. New York: Holt, Rinehart & Winston

Birney RC, Burdick H, Teevan RC. 1969. *Fear of Failure*. New York: Van Nostrand Reinhold

Blackburn ST. 2007. *Maternal, Fetal, and Neonatal Physiology: A Clinical Perspective* (3rd edition). St Louis: Saunders Elsevier

Blum L. 1999. *At The Breast*. Boston: Beacon Press

Brandt AM and Rozin P (eds.) *Morality and Health*. London and New York: Routledge

Brehm SS (ed.) *Seeing Female: Social Roles and Personal Lives*. Westport, CT: Greenwood Press

Brizendine L. 2008. *The Female Brain*. London: Random House

Brody LR. 1999. *Gender, Emotion and the Family*. Cambridge, MA: Harvard University Press

Brown P, Levinson SC. 1987. *Politeness: Some Universals in Language Usage*. Cambridge: Cambridge University Press

Campbell C. 1987. *The Romantic Ethic and the Spirit of Modern Consumerism*. Oxford: Basil-Blackwell

Camus A. 1956. *The Fall*. New York: Vintage Books

Chang E (ed.) *Optimism & Pessimism: Implication for Theory, Research, and Practice*. Washington DC: American Psychological Association

Cockrell S, O'Neill C, Stone J. 2007. *Baby-Proofing Your Marriage*. London: Collins

Conley C. 2013. *Emotional Equations*. London: Piatkus

Cooke K. 2009. *A Rough Guide to Babies and Toddlers*. Rough Guides

Cooley CH. 1902. *Human Nature and the Social Order* (revised edition). New York: Charles Scribner's Sons

Coulson M, Bolitho S. 2012. *The Complete Guide to Pregnancy and Fitness*. London: Bloomsbury

Darwall S. 2009. *The Second-Person Standpoint: Morality, Respect, and Accountability*. Cambridge, MA: Harvard University Press

Darwin C. 1871. *The Descent of Man and Selection in Relation to Sex*. New York: Appleton

Dobelli R. 2013. *The Art of Thinking Clearly*. London: Hodder and Stoughton

Douglas SJ, Michaels MW. 2005. *The Mommy Myth: The Idealization of Motherhood and How It Has Undermined All Women*. New York: Free Press

Douglas W. 2003. *Bad News, Good News: Controversial Order in Everyday Talk and Clinical Settings*. Chicago: University of Chicago Press

Dundes T. 1981. *The Evil Eye: A Folklore Casebook*. New York: Garland Publishing Inc

Durkheim É. 1995. *The Elementary Forms of Religious Life*. New York: Free Press Dykes F, Moran VH (eds.) *Infant and Young Child Feeding: Challenges to Implementing a Global Strategy*. Oxford: Blackwell Publishing

Ellison K. 2005. *The Mommy Brain*. New York: Basic Books

Erikson EH. 1950. Childhood and Society. New York: Norton

Feldman R. 2009. *Liar: The Truth About Lying*. Virgin Books

Feinberg J. 1970. *Doing and Deserving*. Princeton NJ: Princeton University Press

Ferber R. 1986. *Solve Your Child's Sleep Problems*. Prentice Hall & IBD

Fingarette H. 1967. *Self-deception*. London: Routledge & Kegan Paul

Frankfurt H. 2005. *On Bullshit*. Princeton NJ: Princeton University Press

Freud A. 1936. *The Ego and the Mechanisms of Defence* (revised edition 1960). New York: International Universities Press

Freud S. 1949. *The Ego and the Id*. London: The Hogarth Press Ltd

Freud S. 1895/1966. *The Complete Psychological Works of Freud* (Vol. 1). London: Hogarth Press

Freud S. 1921. *Group Psychology and the Analysis of the Ego*. S.E. Vol.18

Fromm E. 1955. *The Sane Society*. New York: Rinehart & Company

Furedi F. 2001. *Paranoid Parenting*. London: Penguin Books

Germov J, Williams L (eds.) *A Sociology of Food and Nutrition*. Oxford: Oxford University Press

Giles F. 2003. *Fresh Milk: The Secret Life of Breasts*. Simon & Schuster

Gilovich T, Griffin D, Kahneman D (eds.) 2002. *Heuristics and*

*Biases*. Cambridge: Cambridge University Press

Goffman E. 1967. *Interaction Ritual: Essays on Face-to-face Behaviour*. Chicago: Aldine

Goffman E. 1963. *Stigma: Notes on the Management of Spoiled Identity*. New Jersey: Penguin Books

Goffman E. 1990. *The Presentation of Self in Everyday Life*. London: Penguin Books

Goleman D. 1995. *Emotional Intelligence*. New York: Bantam Books

González C. 2014. *Breastfeeding Made Easy*. London: Pinter & Martin

Gruber HG, Terrell G, Wertheimer M (eds.) *Contemporary Approaches to Cognition*. Cambridge, MS: Harvard University Press

Haley J. 1963. *Strategies of Psychotherapy*. New York: Anchor Books

Hall J. 1984. *Nonverbal Sex Differences: Communication Accuracy and Expressive Style*. Baltimore: Johns Hopkins University Press

Hall CS. 1954. *A Primer of Freudian Psychology*. New York

Harmon-Jones E, Mills J (eds.) *Cognitive Dissonance: Progress on a Pivotal Theory in Social Psychology*. Washington DC: American Psychological Association

Harvey JH, Ickles WJ, Kidd RF (eds.) *New Directions in Attribution Research* (Vol. 1). Hillsdale NJ: Erlbaum

Heckhausen H. 1968. *The Anatomy of Achievement Motivation*. New York: Academic Press

Hendrickson R. 2008. *The Facts on File Encyclopedia of Word and Phrase Origins*. Checkmark Books

Hewstone M (ed.) *Attribution Theory: Social and Functional Extensions*. Oxford: Basil Blackwell

Hochschild AR. 1983. *The Managed Heart: The Communication of Human Feeling*. Berkley: University of California Press

Holmes J. 1995. *Women, Men and Politeness*. Routledge

Hume D. 1910 [1748]. *An Enquiry Concerning Human Understanding*. PF Collier & Son

Iyengar S. 2010. *The Art of Choosing*. Twelve

James W. 1890. *Principles of Psychology*. Dover Publications

Janis IL. 1971. *Stress and Frustration*. New York: Harcourt Brace

Jovanovic

Jaspars JMF, Fincham FD, Hewstone M (eds.) *Attribution Theory and Research: Conceptual, Developmental and Social Dimensions.* London: Academic Press

Jellison JM. 1977. *I'm Sorry I Didn't Mean To, And Other Lies We Love to Tell.* New York: Chatham Square Press

Jolin L. 2009. *Coping with Birth Trauma and Postnatal Depression.* London: Sheldon Press

Jones EE, Kanouse D, Kelley HH, Nisbett RE, Valins S, Weiner B (eds.) *Attribution: Perceiving the Causes of Behaviour.* Morristown, NJ: General Learning Press

Jones EE. 1990. *Interpersonal Perception.* New York: Freeman and Company

Kahneman D, Slovic P, Tversky A (eds.) *Judgement Under Uncertainty,* Cambridge: Cambridge University Press

Kutzen S, Brockman B, Shinkarev S. 2007. *Grandparenting: Tales From The Crib - When Your Children Become Parents.* Global Source Publishing

Jung CG. 1996. *The Archetypes and the Collective Unconscious.* London: Routledge

Lakoff G. 2002. *Moral Politics: How Liberals And Conservatives Think* (2nd edition). University of Chicago Press

Langer E. 1983. *The Psychology of Control.* Beverly Hills, CA: Sage Publications

Lefcourt HM. 1976. *Locus of Control: Current Trends in Theory and Research.* Hillsdale, NJ: Lawrence Erlbaum Associates

Leslie I. 2011. *Born Liars, Why We Can't Live Without Deceit.* Quercus

Lewin K. 1936. *Principles of Topological Psychology.* New York: McGraw-Hill

Lewis H, 1971. *Shame and Guilt in Neurosis.* New York: International Universities Press

Loewenstein G, Read D, Baumeister R (eds.) *Time and Decision: Economic and Psychological Perspectives on Intertemporal Choice.* New York: Russell Sage Foundation

Lupton D. (ed.) *Risk and Socio-cultural Theory: New Directions and Perspectives* Cambridge: Cambridge University Press

Maccoby EE. 1966. *The Development of Sex Differences*. Stanford University Press

Maccoby EE. 1998. *The Two Sexes: Growing Apart, Coming Together*. Cambridge, MS: Harvard University Press

Mandel B. 1984. *Open Heart Therapy*. Berkley CA: Celestial Arts

Mannheim K. 1956. *Essays in the Sociology of Culture*. London: Routledge & Kegan Paul

Maslow A. 1954. *Motivation and Personality*. New York: Harper

Maslow AH. 1968. *Toward a Psychology of Being* (2nd edition). New York: Van Nostrad

Mohrbacher N, Stock J. 1997. *The Breastfeeding Answer Book* (revised edition). Illinois: La Leche League International

Morris H (ed.) *Guilt and Shame*. CA: Wadsworth Publishing Company

Navaro L, Schwartzberg SL. 2007. *Envy, Competition and Gender: Theory, Clinical Applications and Group Work*. London: Routledge

Neville MC, Neifert MR (eds.) *Lactation: Physiology, Nutrition, and Breastfeeding*. Plenum Press

Newman J. 2014. *Dr. Jack Newman's Guide to Breastfeeding* (updated edition). London: Pinter & Martin

Nietzsche F. 1937. *The Philosophy of Nietzsche*. New York: Modern Library

Nolen-Hoeksema S. 2004. *Women Who Think Too Much*. London: Piatkus

Orbach S, Eichenbaum L. 1994. *Between Women*. London: Arrow Books

Palmer G. 2009. *The Politics of Breastfeeding*. London: Pinter & Martin

Payne JW, Bettman JR, Johnson EJ. 1993. *The Adaptive Decision Maker*. New York: Cambridge University Press

Petty RE, Krosnick JA (eds.) *Attitude Strength: Antecedents and Consequences*. Mahwah, NJ: Erlbaum

Phares EJ. 1973. *Locus of Control: A Personality Determinant of Behaviour*. Morristown, NJ: General Learning Press

Phares EJ. 1976. *Locus of Control in Personality*. Morristown, NJ:

General Learning Press

Phillips A. 2012. *Missing Out: In Praise of the Unlived Life*. Hamish Hamilton

Rapley G, Murkett T. 2012. *Baby-Led Breastfeeding*. London: Vermilion

Salehnejad R. 2007. *Rationality, Bounded Rationality and Microfoundations: Foundations of Theoretical Economics*. New York: Palgrave MacMillan

Rosenthal R, Hall JA, DiMatteo MR et al. 1979. *Sensitivity to Nonverbal Communication: The PONS Test*. Baltimore: Johns Hopkins University Press

Ryan W. 1971. *Blaming the Victim*. New York: Pantheon

Sartre JP. 1958. *Being and Nothingness: An Essay on Phenomenological Ontology* (translated H Barnes) London: Methuen

Scheff TJ. 1971. *Being Mentally Ill: A Sociological Theory*. Chicago: Aldine

Schlenker BR. 1980. *Impression Management: The Self-concept, Social Identity, and Interpersonal Relations*. Monterey, CA: Brooks/ Cole

Schlenker BR (ed.) 1985. *The Self and Social Life*. New York: McGraw-Hill

Seligman MEP. 1975. *Helplessness: On Depression, Development and Death*. San Francisco: Freeman

Schulz K. 2011. Being Wrong - Adventures in the Margin of Error. Ecco

Sills F. 2008. *Being and Becoming*. North Atlantic Books

Singer JE. 1972. *Urban Stress: Experiments on Noise and Social Stressors*. New York: Academic

Sloman J, Wride A. 2009. *Economics* (7th edition). Harlow: Pearson Education Limited

Smith E. 2012. *Luck: What It Means and Why It Matters*. London: Bloomsbury

Snyder CR, Higgings RL, Stucky RJ. 1984. *Excuses Masquerades in Search of Grace*. Toronto: John Wiley & Sons

Solomon RC. 2009. *True to Our Feelings: What Our Emotions Are Really Telling Us*. New York: Oxford University Press

Spock B. 2004. *Dr. Spock's Baby and Childcare*. Simon & Schuster UK

Stadlen N. 2004. *What Mothers Do*. London: Piatkus

Stern DN. 1998. *The Birth of a Mother: How Motherhood Experience Changes You Forever*. Basic Books

Stern DN. 1995. *The Motherhood Constellation*. London: Basic Books

Sternin J, Choo R. 2000. *The Power of Positive Deviancy*. Harvard Business

Tangney JP, Dearing RL. 2002. *Shame and Guilt*. New York: The Guilford Press

Tavris C.1992. *The Mismeasure of Women*. New York: Simon & Schuster

Tavris C, Aronson E. 2007. *Mistakes Were Made (But Not By Me)*. London: Pinter & Martin

Taylor E. 2007. *Choices and Illusions*. CA: Hay House

Templar R. 2013. *The Rules to Break*. Harlow: Pearson

Tenhouten WD. 2007. *General Theory of Emotions and Social Life*. Routledge

Thaler RH, Sunstein CR. 2009. *Nudge: Improving Decisions about Health, Wealth and Happiness*. London: Penguin Books

Trivers R. 2011. *Deceit and Self-Deception*. London: Penguin Books

Wahlroos S. 1981. *Excuses: How to Spot Them, Deal with Them, and Stop Using Them*. New York: Macmillan

Weiner B. 1986. *Principles of Psychotherapy*. New York: Wiley

Wiessinger D, West D, Pitman T. 2010. *The Womanly Art of Breastfeeding*; London: Pinter & Martin

Williams F. 2012. *Breasts: a Natural and Unnatural History*. New York: WW Norton and Company

Williams Z. *What Not to Expect When You're Expecting*. Guardian Books

Wolf JB. 2010. *Is Breast Best?: Taking on the Breastfeeding Experts and the New High Stakes of Motherhood*. New York: NYU Press

Young-Eisendrath P. 1997. *Gender and Desire*. Texas: A&M University Press

# Glossary of terms

*Altercasting*: using social and emotional pressure to place another person in a particular identity.

*Cognitive*: mental activity related to how we process knowledge.

*Cognitive bias*: a deviation in judgment, whereby existing knowledge is applied to a novel situation in an illogical fashion.

*Cognitive dissonance*: the painful feeling of holding two simultaneous beliefs that are incompatible with each other.

*Collectivism*: a social ideology that fixates on the interdependence of every human.

*Confirmation bias*: the human tendency to give more weight to evidence that confirms our beliefs than to evidence challenging them.

*Constructivist theory*: the belief that emotions should be interpreted in terms of the social functions they serve.

*Culture of failure*: a widespread lack of confidence in breastfeeding at societal level.

*Dyad*: two humans meshed as one by virtue of their interdependency.

*Effort-justification*: the subjective tendency to attribute a greater value to an outcome when effort was put into achieving it.

*Individualism*: a social ideology that fixates on the moral worth of the individual.

*Internalisation*: the process of coming to believe one's own attitudes and values are truth.

*Ingratiation*: a manipulation technique in which an individual attempts to become more likeable to their target.

*Malingering*: fabricating or exaggerating the symptoms of mental or physical disorders in order to receive some anticipated benefit.

*Positive deviance*: the behaviour of certain individuals that enables them to find better solutions to problems than their peers, despite sharing the same circumstances and resources.

*Rationalisation*: a largely subconscious process whereby an individual explains his or her actions in a way that is not threatening.

*Reality negotiation*: a process of cognitive restructuring whereby reality is denied and then replaced by a new reality.

*Schadenfreude*: the feeling of pleasure derived from another person's misfortune.

*Self-deception*: a type of emotional defence-mechanism whereby threatening emotions are buried in the subconscious.

*Self-efficacy*: a strong belief in the ability to succeed.

*Self-handicapping*: a strategy in which one withdraws effort from a task with the aim of keeping potential failure from harming self-esteem.

*Visceral factors*: rewarding or punishing sensations – for example the urgent desire to escape pain – that alter the attractiveness of certain activities.

*White-anting*: the process of undermining or eating away at something below the surface.

# Index

ABC of breastfeeding fidelity 24–57, 230–1
ability to breastfeed
    anatomical excuses for inability 118–21, 160, 213, 236
    'broken breasts' excuses for quitting 48, 74–5, 118–21, 153, 213, 215, 243
    and claimed self-handicapping 74–5
    as flexible rather than fixed 56, 241
    grandmothers claim inheritable inability 221–2
    mother's poor self-perception of 45, 166–7
    psychological 54–6
ABM (Association of Breastfeeding Mothers) 242
accountability *see* personal responsibility
Actual Self 88–9, 149, 156, 168
addiction, to guilt 99
admiration, as source of sabotage 208, 211
advice-seeking *see also* information-seeking
    be wary of who you seek from 212
    compassion-seeking disguised as advice-seeking 78
    listening to the one person advising you to quit 38, 71
    seeking advice and then not following 77
    unwise to ask new formula-feeders for advice 130
    'yes, but...' responses to advice 77
advocacy, breastfeeding
    the breastfeeding counter-revolution 226–37
    empowerment of women 67–70, 227–45
    needs to raise mother's self-expectations 155, 234
    self-advocacy (owning your journey) 238–45

and the self-handicapping mother 77
Aesop's Fables 107, 213
affect heuristic 25–6, 66–7
age of mother 12
agenesis of mammary tissue 39
Akre, James 16
'all that matters is...' excuses 128
altercasting 223–4
anatomical excuses 118–21, 160, 213, 236 *see also* 'broken breasts' excuses for quitting
Angelou, Maya 212
anger, envy misinterpreted as 167, 175
antenatal period
    anticipatory excuses in 42, 43, 73–8, 214
    commitment to breastfeeding 39–44
    empowering mothers 68
    role of breastfeeding advocates in 234
    sabotage in 214
    tips for successful breastfeeding 238–41
anticipating visceral influences 61–2, 240–2
anticipation of criticism 114, 242
anticipatory excuses 42, 43, 73–8, 214
anticipatory grief 45
anxiety 26 *see also* depression
apologising for breastfeeding success 171
Aronson, Elliot 131, 157, 160, 184
*Art of Choosing, The* (Iyengar, 2010) 19, 21, 142
'artificial feeding' (non-use of term) 106–7
Asch, Solomon 53
assertiveness 210, 224
attachment
    mother's, to baby 103
    mother's, to breastfeeding 95
attentional resources 62, 84
Attitude 25–42, 195–6, 231

responsibility *see also* blame; personal
  responsibility
    cognitive dissonance 104–5
    and collectivist rhetoric 187
    and the contempt of the successful
      mother towards failures 182
    and the Culture of Truth 233–7
    and excuses 114–15
    false responsibility of the successful
      breastfeeder for others' envy 171
    and guilt triggering 94
    and the 'just world' hypothesis 182
    and justification for quitting
      129–31
    and mitigating excuses 121–3
    mothers trying to evade 70–87
    not needed when 'luck' is in charge
      165
    public responsibility of
      breastfeeding 190
    society as cause of breastfeeding
      failure 9–10, 13, 17, 49, 186, 189,
      202, 231
    and the 'worst possible
      interpretation of breastfeeding
      failure' 114–15
returning to work
  as excuse 126
  and successful breastfeeding 244–5
rewards
  contempt as reward 182
  guilt as reward 99
  from medical profession for
    quitting breastfeeding 75–6
  and 'secondary gain' 99
righteousness 180
rightousness 182
rights (of others), as excuse 126
risk
  and feelings of control 55
  hostility to the fact of formula risks
    200–2
  overweighing of tiny possibilities
    when overwhelmed 66
  perceptions of risk and mother's
    attitude 26
  remote risks 67
  risks of formula 58, 66–7, 102, 187,
    190, 196–7

seeking only information which
  confirms perceptions of 201–2
Rochefoucauld, François Due De La
  193
Rohn, Emanuel James 110
role-modelling of successful
  breastfeeding 167, 215
Roosevelt, Eleanor 82, 99
Rosen, Sidney 145
rose-tinted views 107
*Rough Guide to Babies and Toddlers*
  (Cooke, 2009) 47
routines, feeding 57, 58–9, 242

sabotage
  by others 175, 207–25, 232, 235
  self-sabotage 45, 72, 240
sadness 93, 97, 103, 219
scapegoating 74
*schadenfraude* 174, 208
Schlenker, Barry 155
Schulz, Kathryn 157, 182, 194, 231,
  233
scientific information
  denying credibility of 200–1
  outweighed by peer pressure 214
selective attention to information *see*
  confirmation bias
selective perception 130
self, three types of 88–9, 94–5, 98, 168
self-actualisation 88
self-deception 46–7, 155, 156
self-delusion 156–7
self-determination 67–8
self-efficacy, sense of 86
self-efficiency, low 43–7, 86, 217
self-esteem
  damaged by malicious envy 175
  damaged by the success of others
    208
  importance of acceptance of
    personal responsibility 158–62
  and internalisation of excuses
    155–6
  and mutual evaluation of mothers
    134
  and the need for feedback 169
  and positive deviants 83
  preserved by self-handicapping 78